Elastography - Applications in Clinical Medicine

Edited by Dana Stoian and Alina Popescu

Published in London, United Kingdom

Elastography – Applications in Clinical Medicine
http://dx.doi.org/10.5772/intechopen.98047
Edited by Dana Stoian and Alina Popescu

Contributors
Tomonori Kawai, Celik Halil Ibrahim, Karaduman Aynur Ayşe, Alina Popescu, Camelia Foncea, Monica Lupsor-Platon, Teodora Şerban, Alexandra Iulia Silion, Felix Bende, Tudor Moga, Natalia Kuzmina, Mikhail Pykov, Nikolay Rostovtsev, Cristina Mihaela Cepeha, Andreea Borlea, Corina Paul, Iulian Velea, Dana I Stoian, Ioan Sporea, Raluca Lupuşoru, Roxana Şirli, Iulia Raţiu, Byung Ihn Choi, Dong Ho Lee, Jae Young Lee, Ana-Maria Ghiuchici, Mirela Dănilă, Flaviu Bob, Laura Cotoi, Dana Amzar, Gheorghe Nicusor Pop, Calin Adela, Dominique Amy, Bogdan Silviu Ungureanu, Adrian Saftoiu

Notice
Statements and opinions expressed in the chapters are these of the individual contributors and not necessarily those of the editors or publisher. No responsibility is accepted for the accuracy of information contained in the published chapters. The publisher assumes no responsibility for any damage or injury to persons or property arising out of the use of any materials, instructions, methods or ideas contained in the book.

First published in London, United Kingdom, 2022 by IntechOpen
IntechOpen is the global imprint of INTECHOPEN LIMITED, registered in England and Wales, registration number: 11086078, 5 Princes Gate Court, London, SW7 2QJ, United Kingdom

British Library Cataloguing-in-Publication Data
A catalogue record for this book is available from the British Library

Additional hard and PDF copies can be obtained from orders@intechopen.com

Elastography – Applications in Clinical Medicine
Edited by Dana Stoian and Alina Popescu
p. cm.
Print ISBN 978-1-78984-637-9
Online ISBN 978-1-78985-354-4
eBook (PDF) ISBN 978-1-78985-603-3

We are IntechOpen,
the world's leading publisher of
Open Access books
Built by scientists, for scientists

6,000+
Open access books available

146,000+
International authors and editors

185M+
Downloads

156
Countries delivered to

Our authors are among the

Top 1%
most cited scientists

12.2%
Contributors from top 500 universities

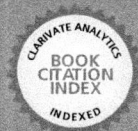

Interested in publishing with us?
Contact book.department@intechopen.com

Numbers displayed above are based on latest data collected.
For more information visit www.intechopen.com

Meet the editors

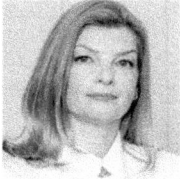

Dana Stoian, MD, Ph.D., DSc, FECSM, is a Professor of Endocrinology, Department of Endocrinology, "Victor Babeş" University of Medicine and Pharmacy, Romania. She is a senior attendant in endocrinology and an expert in endocrine ultrasonography. She is a member of the Endocrine Committee of the Romanian Ministry of Health and the National Committee of the Medical Proof and Degree Commission, National Council for Attestation of University Degrees, Diplomas and Certificates (CNATDCU). Since 2014, Dr. Stoian has been part of the World Federation of Ultrasound in Medicine and Biology Center of Education (WFUMB COE) in Timisoara, Romania. She has organized numerous postgraduate courses about the thyroid, parathyroid breast ultrasound, and elastography in daily practice. She has eight books, fourteen book chapters, and more than 100 journal papers to her credit. Dr. Stoian is the founder of Dr.D Medical Center, Timisoara.

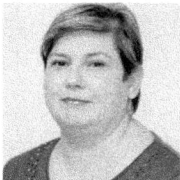

Alina Popescu, MD, Ph.D., is a Professor of Gastroenterology and Hepatology and head of the Department of Gastroenterology and Hepatology, "Victor Babeş" University of Medicine and Pharmacy Timişoara, Romania. She is also a senior attendant of gastroenterology and internal medicine and an expert in general ultrasonography. She was president of the Romanian Society of Ultrasound in Medicine and Biology (SRUMB) from 2020–2022. Dr. Popescu is a member of the Executive Bureau and the Education and Professional Standards Committee of the European Federation of Societies for Ultrasound in Medicine and Biology (EFSUMB) and of the World Federation of Ultrasound in Medicine and Biology (WFUMB) Student Education Committee. She is the secretary of the WFUMB Center of Education (COE) Timişoara, Romania. She has published more than 160 papers in medical journals.

Contents

Preface

Elastography is part of the daily practice of many medical specialists, including radiologists, gastroenterologists, rheumatologists, endocrinologists, gynecologists, urologists, nephrologists, and pediatricians. The role of elastography is emerging in adding quality information to the conventional ultrasound evaluation.

Ultrasound elastography comprises different techniques to measure tissue stiffness. There are either transversal or tangential forces that induce the deformation of the tissues, with deformation related to the degree of presented elasticity.

The value of elastography in chronic liver pathology is widely recognized. Shear wave techniques seem to be more appropriate for liver applications. They allow for the accurate screening, diagnosis, and follow-up of patients with alcohol-induced liver pathology. Metabolic-associated fatty liver disease is one of the most frequent chronic pathologies, affecting around one-quarter of the adult population. If the evaluation of steatosis is made by conventional ultrasound, quantification of steatosis, fibrosis, and inflammation, which are actually the predictors of the impact of the disease, is delivered by elastography. The ability of elastography, regardless of type, to rule out cirrhosis by assessing liver fibrosis has been described in chronic hepatitis C cases. The technique also brings valuable information regarding the severity and evolution of liver damage, even in children, in special situations of cystic fibrotic disease. In the case of progressive liver damage with the development of cirrhosis, regardless of background, elastography has a valuable predictive diagnostic capacity, identifying the presence and severity of portal hypertension, one of the most important complications of the disease.

The predictive value of elastography in the differential diagnosis of focal hepatic lesions is still to be evaluated since there is no consensus regarding the threshold values of the used elastographic parameters.

Extrapolation of the results obtained from chronic liver disease to chronic renal disease cannot be made. Future studies and the development of viscoelasticity evaluation should be done before recommending the use of elastography in renal pathology.

A particular aspect is the situation of pancreatic diseases, in which elastography is performed via an endoscopic approach. Both strain and shear wave is available for pancreatic pathology, with excellent discrimination of tumoral masses. Increased stiffness is associated with the vast majority of breast malignancies, elastography being currently used for risk upgrade or downgrade in breast nodular disease. and promising results in identifying the presence and the severity of the chronic disease.

The first application of elastography in cancer discrimination was for the breast. Increased stiffness is associated with the vast majority of breast malignancies, elastography being currently used for risk upgrade or downgrade in breast nodular disease. Moreover, the evolution of stiffness, measured by the shear wave technique, brings information about the response rate to cancer treatment. In thyroid nodular disease, elastography aids diagnostic prediction of thyroid cancer, as most thyroid cancers are stiff. The method is also important in the evaluation of diffuse thyroid pathology, with suggestive stiffness in autoimmune thyroid disease cases, both in adults and children. In hyperparathyroidism cases, elastography helps discriminate parathyroid versus thyroid tissue, showing promising results in identifying hyperplastic versus hypertrophic tissue.

Shear wave elastography demonstrates promising results in evaluating chronic muscle injuries, evaluating the degree of fibrosis, and the stage of healing after acute injuries. The same characteristics are described even in the pediatric population, monitoring the effectiveness of therapeutic interventions, altering the approach, or deciding the treatment duration.

I would like to thank my co-editor Professor Alina Popescu for the effort in gathering this team of experts with tremendous experience in the field of elastography. I would like to thank all the authors for their excellent work. All the authors are active both in the clinical field and in the academic milieu, and time is one of the most valuable assets that they have. I am grateful for the time they spent developing their excellent contributions. Finally, I would like to thank the team at IntechOpen for their constant support in developing this book.

Dana Stoian
Department of Internal Medicine,
Discipline of Endocrinology,
COE WFUMB,
"Victor Babes" University of Medicine and Pharmacy,
Timisoara, Romania

Alina Popescu
Department of Internal Medicine II,
Department of Gastroenterology and Hepatology,
Center for Advanced Research in Gastroenterology and Hepatology,
WFUMB Center of Education,
"Victor Babes" University of Medicine and Pharmacy,
Timisoara, Romania

Section 1

Abdominal Region Applications of Elastography

Chapter 1

Liver Elastography: Basic Principles, Evaluation Technique, and Confounding Factors

Felix Bende and Tudor Moga

Abstract

Ultrasound-based elastography techniques have received considerable attention in the last years for the noninvasive assessment of tissue mechanical properties. These techniques have the advantage of detecting tissue elasticity changes occurring in various pathological conditions and are able to provide qualitative and quantitative information that serves diagnostic and prognostic purposes. For liver applications and especially for the noninvasive assessment of liver fibrosis, ultrasound-based elastography has shown promising results. Several ultrasound elastography techniques using different excitation methods have been developed. In general, these techniques are classified into strain elastography, which is a semi-quantitative method that uses internal or external compression for tissue stimulation, and shear wave elastography, which measures the ultrasound-generated shear wave speed at different locations in the tissue. All liver elastography techniques have a standardized examination technique, with the patient in a supine position, while the measurements are performed through the right liver lobe. There are also some confounding factors that need to be taken into account when performing liver elastography such as a higher level of aminotransferases, infiltrative liver disease, liver congestion, cholestasis. This chapter briefly introduces the basic principles of liver elastography and discusses some important clinical aspects of elastography, such as the examination technique and the limitations.

Keywords: liver ultrasound elastography, shear wave elastography, transient elastography, acoustic radiation force impulse, strain elastography, liver fibrosis

1. Introduction

Chronic liver disease is a major health problem worldwide. This situation is generated by a wide range of chronic liver injuries such as chronic viral hepatitis, chronic alcohol abuse, non-alcoholic fatty liver disease, autoimmune hepatitis, primary biliary cirrhosis, and other less frequent causes. Regardless of the liver disease etiology, a common pathway of fibrosis is set up, which progresses and leads to liver cirrhosis that may be complicated by portal hypertension, liver failure, and hepatocellular carcinoma.

The evaluation of patients with chronic liver disease must be as simple as possible, cost efficient, and easily repeatable. While the liver biopsy is still considered the gold standard for liver fibrosis evaluation, due to its shortcomings (invasiveness, potential complications, inter-/intra-observer variability, sampling error) [1–3] scientific and practical interest has focused on the development of noninvasive techniques for the diagnosis of liver fibrosis.

Elastography can be used to assess liver fibrosis noninvasively. It measures the tissue behavior when mechanical stress is applied, either using ultrasound (ultrasound-based elastography) or magnetic resonance (magnetic resonance elastography).

Ultrasound elastography is perhaps the most important breakthrough in the evolution of ultrasound in the last 20 years. The basic idea behind liver elastography is that the elasticity of the tissue examined offers information on liver health. A stiffer liver tissue usually indicates the presence of chronic liver disease.

Mainly, most liver ultrasound elastography techniques are based on the principle of measuring the speed of the shear wave that propagates through the liver which is influenced by the stiffness of the tissue. The speed of the shear wave is proportional to the tissue stiffness. Basically, the stiffer the liver, the faster the shear wave will propagate through the liver.

The value of ultrasound-based elastography for staging chronic liver disease has been established by numerous studies [4–7]. Moreover, its value for evaluating and predicting chronic liver disease complications (portal hypertension, hepatocellular carcinoma) has been also proven in different studies [8–10].

The European Federation of Societies for Ultrasound in Medicine and Biology (EFSUMB) and the World Federation of Societies for Ultrasound in Medicine and Biology (WFUMB) have issued guidelines and recommendations on the clinical use of ultrasound-based elastography and describe in detail their basic principles [11–13].

This chapter focuses on the basic principles of elastography, which is an important aspect for every clinician or practitioner who is performing or learning liver elastography. Moreover, clinical features such as the examination techniques of different liver elastography methods and the factors that influence the liver elastography results are described and discussed.

2. Basic principles

Elastography assesses tissue elasticity, which is the tendency of tissue to resist deformation with an applied force or to resume its original form after removal of the force. Elastography can be considered a type of remote palpation that allows the measurement and display of the biomechanical properties in a tissue that acts against the shear deformation. Shear deformation is generated by applying a force either to a single location or broadly across the body surface. A force can be applied by vibrating the body surface that produces a natural internal physiological motion or using the ultrasound transducer to create focused acoustic radiation force at controlled depths [13, 14].

All ultrasound-based elastography methods use ultrasound to measure the tissue shear deformations resulting from an applied force. The type of force applied can be quasi-static or dynamic. Quasi-static forces do not allow the acquiring of images that are quantitative for tissue properties. Dynamic forces allow the quantification of the tissue properties. They include impulses that can be produced mechanically at the body surface or by acoustic radiation force impulse at controlled depths.

According to the EFSUMB guidelines [11], elastography techniques can be classified according to how the displacement data are shown. Three options are available as follows:

a. Display of displacement without further processing. This type of displacement is used in acoustic radiation force impulse (ARFI) imaging, which allows a quantitative measurement (units of μm), and the image displayed is scaled between bright (soft tissue) and dark (hard tissue). This technique is not used for liver elastography measurements.

b. Display of tissue strain or strain rate, which is calculated from the spatial gradient of displacement or velocity. This type of displacement works according to Hooke's law, which states that $E = \sigma/\varepsilon$, where stress is the applied force per unit area and strain is the change in length of the tissue divided by its original length. If the stress (not known in strain module) is assumed to be the same for all image locations, an image of strain can be thought of as an inverse relative to Young's modulus map. Strain is a quantitative measurement (%) and image brightness is typically scaled between bright (soft) and dark (hard).

c. Display of shear wave speed, which is calculated by measuring the arrival time of a shear wave at different locations in the tissue. This is possible only when the force is applied dynamically. Shear wave speed may be displayed in units of m/s. Alternatively, it may be converted to either Young's modulus E or shear modulus G, which are expressed in units of kilopascal (kPa). These elastography techniques are called shear wave elastography (SWE) and include transient elastography (TE), point shear wave elastography (pSWE), and multidimensional shear wave elastography (2D-SWE and 3D-SWE).

For liver applications, elastography methods that display the shear wave speed are the most commonly used in practice, followed by strain and displacement imaging (for liver lesions), which are less frequently used. The elastography methods integrated into clinical practice for the liver are described in **Table 1**.

2.1 Strain elastography

Strain elastography is the most widely implemented elastography method on commercial systems; however, it is the least used technique for liver applications. The force used in strain elastography is either produced with the ultrasound probe or due to the internal physiological motion. The axial displacement images are calculated using radiofrequency echo correlation tracking or Doppler processing, which converts the axial displacement images into strain images [14, 15]. Excitation with manual pressure measures elasticity in superficial tissues. A disadvantage of this excitation method is that manual stress is not efficiently transmitted to deeper tissues. Excitation from natural physiologic motion, such as cardiac pulsation and respiration, is another mechanism of generating tissue stress. Deep organs, such as the liver or the kidney, can be assessed with this method [14, 15].

Strain/displacement techniques	Strain elastography
Shear wave elastography techniques	Transient elastography
	Point shear wave elastography
	Multidimensional shear wave elastography (2D-SWE and 3D-SWE)

Table 1.
Elastography methods used for the liver.

Strain elastography is a semi-quantitative method for tissue elastic property analysis, which has not demonstrated high accuracy for liver applications.

2.2 Shear wave elastography (SWE)

2.2.1 Transient elastography (TE)

TE has been designed only for liver elasticity measurement. It uses an automated piston, which is also a disk-shaped ultrasound transducer, that applies a low-frequency (50 Hz) mechanical push to the body surface with controlled applied force [16]. A transient shear wave is created that propagates into the tissue. The shear wave propagation velocity is proportional to tissue stiffness, which increases with fibrosis [17]. TE measures tissue stiffness over a 1 cm diameter and 4 cm length region of tissue, which is 100 times larger than those evaluated with liver biopsy. The transient shear wave deformation is propagated at a constant speed, for 4 cm, and measured by a straight line automatically displayed in a displacement M-mode shown in the result (**Figure 1**) [11]. If the pulse is not transmitted and recorded successfully, the software does not provide a reading. Transient elastography is marketed under the trade name FibroScan®. Stiffness values are presented in kPa. Controlled attenuation parameter (CAP) is a technology that quantifies liver steatosis by measuring the energy loss as the sound wave passes through the medium. Total attenuation at 3.5 MHz is expressed in dB/m, and steatosis is estimated using the same radiofrequency data as elastography, in the same location that stiffness is measured [18]. A schematic representation of the basic principle of TE is presented in **Figure 2**.

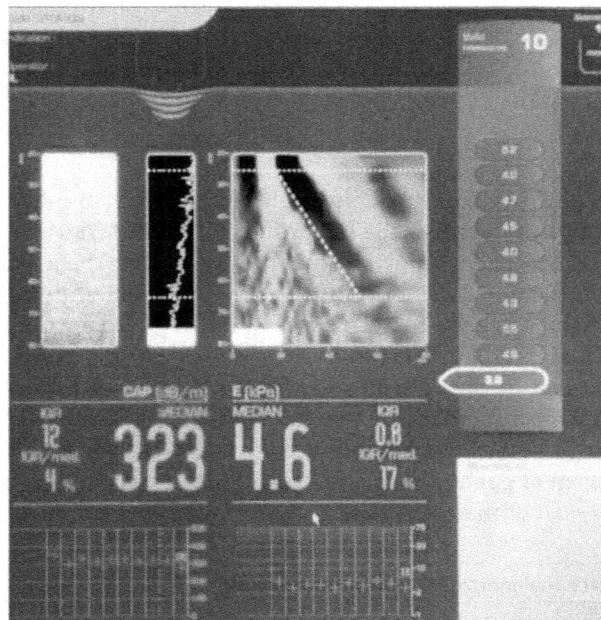

Figure 1.
Transient elastography (TE) and controlled attenuation parameter (CAP) with the Fibroscan® device. Sample display showing the echo M-scan on the left, single-line amplitude A-scan in the middle, and the displacement M-mode after a vibration-controlled impulse push on the surface on the right. Numeric values for CAP are displayed on the left side (db/m) and for TE on the right side (kPa).

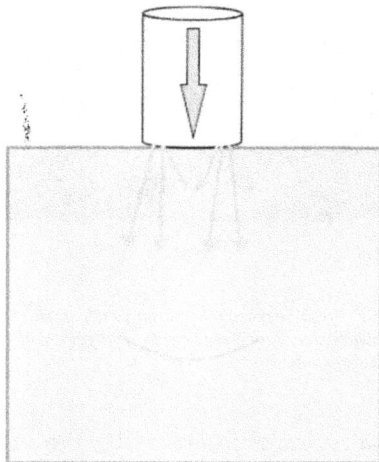

Figure 2.
Schematic representation of the principle of transient elastography. A mechanically induced impulse at the tissue surface with an A-mode transducer produces an axial shear wave pulse. The measured shear wave speed is proportional to the fibrosis.

2.2.2 Point shear wave elastography (pSWE)

Applying an ARFI at a controlled depth within a tissue generates a shear wave that propagates away from the pushing beam's axis and focal point (**Figure 3**). Its average speed of propagation from the focal point positioned on one lateral

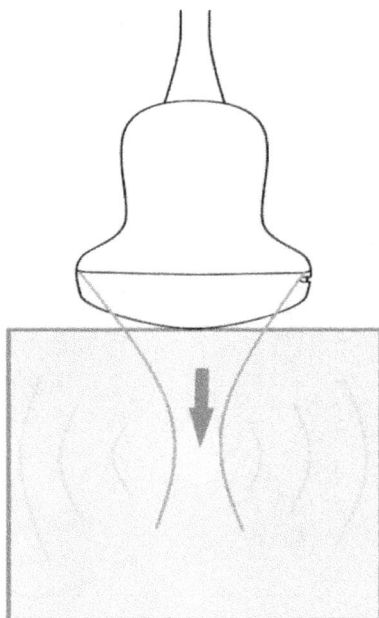

Figure 3.
Schematic representation of the principle of point shear wave elastography (pSWE). An ultrasound-induced focused radiation force impulse is produced at a controlled depth generating a lateral shear wave in a region of interest (ROI). The measured shear wave speed represents tissue stiffness.

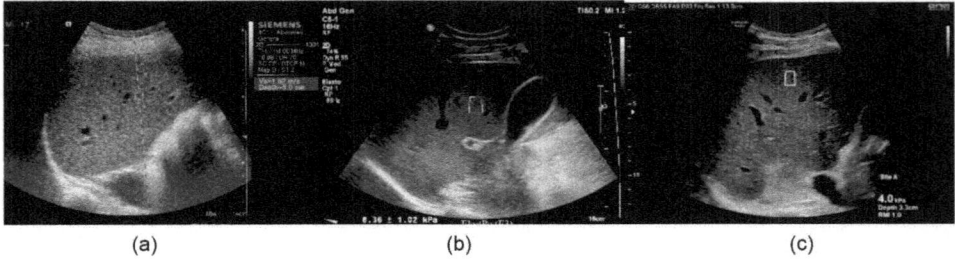

(a)   (b)   (c)

Figure 4.
Point shear wave elastography (pSWE) implemented on virtual touch quantification (VTQ) from Siemens (4a), ElastPQ from Philips (4b), and S-Shearwave from Samsung (4c). A region of interest (ROI) is placed 1–2 cm below the liver capsule for liver stiffness assessment.

boundary of a measurement region of interest (ROI) to another on the opposite lateral boundary of the ROI may be measured by detecting its time of arrival at that point, relative to that of the ARFI [14]. Ultrasound imaging is used to guide placement of the ROI; however, no elasticity images are produced (**Figure 4**). First introduced by Siemens, pSWE is available on different commercial systems from different vendors (e.g., Philips, Samsung, Hitachi, Esaote). The results can be expressed either in m/s or in kPa.

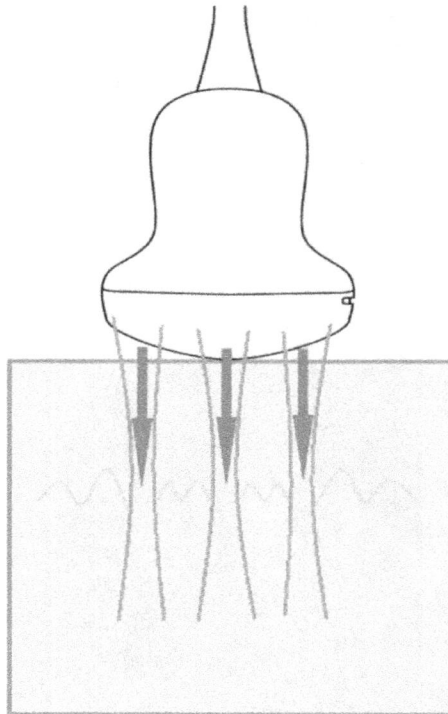

Figure 5.
Schematic representation of the principle of 2D shear wave elastography (2D-SWE). Multiple ultrasound-induced ARFI lines create transverse shear waves that produce quantitative images of their speed.

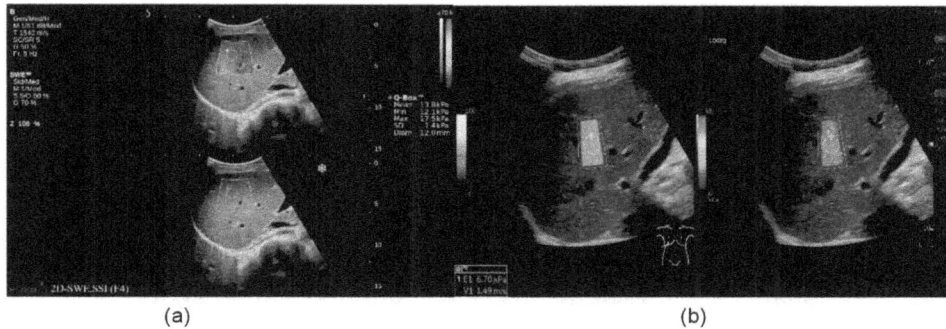

Figure 6.
2D shear wave elastography (2D-SWE) implemented by SuperSonic imagine (6a) and General Electric (6b). The elastogram, which is superimposed on the B-mode image, is placed 1–2 cm below the liver capsule. A circular ROI is placed inside the elastogram for tissue stiffness measurements. A color-coded scaled quality map (6b left image) can be available for guiding the measurement placement. The result is expressed in kPa and m/s.

2.2.3 Two-dimensional shear wave elastography (2D-SWE)

In this technique, acoustic radiation force impulse is used to create tissue displacement at multiple points (**Figure 5**). By placing the ARFI focus at multiple sequential locations and, at each, detecting the shear wave speed and arrival time, quantitative images of the shear wave speed can be produced [13, 14]. A large quantitative color-coded elasticity map (elastogram) is presented, which can be overlaid on the B-mode image or displayed separately, side by side (**Figure 6**). In addition to the visual impression of the elastogram against a color scale, a quantitative measurement can be obtained by placing smaller ROIs (measurement boxes) inside the elastogram. The result of one measurement is displayed usually as the mean and standard deviation either in m/s as shear wave propagation speed or in Young's modulus in kPa (**Figure 6**).

This technique is available on multiple ultrasound systems including SuperSonic Imagine, GE Healthcare, Canon, Philips, Siemens, Mindray.

3. Evaluation technique

All elastography methods follow an evaluation technique that enables a good approach toward the liver parenchyma. The patients will be positioned in a supine position with their right arm in maximal abduction in order to widen the intercostal spaces thus offering a better view of the right liver lobe. The measurements from the left liver lobe are not recommended due to higher values and significant variability. A minimum training is required that one may perform liver stiffness measurements, and the acquisition itself will take usually less than 5 minutes. Patients should be in fasting condition (for at least 3 hours) and rest for a minimum of 10 minutes prior to the evaluation. When scanning for the ultrasound section, large vessels and artifacts should be avoided in both A-mode (TE) and B-mode image (pSWE and 2D-SWE) as well as deep inspiratory movements [12, 19, 20]. A dedicated ultrasound gel is used as an interface between the probe and the patient's skin.

3.1 Transient elastography (TE)

For the TE technique, the transducer is placed between the 9th and 11th right intercostal spaces in order to penetrate at least 4 cm thickness of liver parenchyma. The device offers an A-mode image that will assist the examiner to choose the best section into the liver. TE probe will transmit a mechanical impulse to the liver through a special piston (cylinder-shaped) that will apply a controlled force and thus will generate an elastic share wave. The probe is able to detect the velocity of the shear wave propagation into the liver reflecting the liver stiffness. Measurements are expressed in kilopascals with a range between 1.5 and 75 kPa. If the system detects errors in the acquisition process, it will automatically discard the measurement. At the end of the examination, the median of 10 measurements is displayed as well with the quality parameters (IQR, SR) [12, 19, 20]. For more accurate evaluations, manufacturers provided M, XL, and S probes that are recommended in order to overcome the confounding factor of obesity and thoracic circumference variations [20]. Studies demonstrated that at least 100 measurements are needed for training for one to achieve reliable results and 500 for expert level [21, 22]. It is also a reproducible method with an excellent intra- and interobserver agreement [23].

3.2 Point shear wave elastography (pSWE)

pSWE is a different method integrated into an ultrasound machine that evaluates liver fibrosis by noninvasive means. The acoustic "push" of the probe will generate share waves that will be transferred to liver parenchyma. Being an ultrasound-assisted method, ultrasound experience plays an important role in performing reliably the technique; even so, the reproducibility of the method is excellent [20, 24]. Using this technique, ascites is not a barrier for liver stiffness measurement. The probe, as in TE, should be placed in the right intercostal spaces in order to depict full liver tissue, without large vessels or other structures. Following, ROI should be set at depths between 1 and 6 cm beneath the liver capsule, ideally at 1–2 cm or 2–3 cm [25]. Special attention should be given to breathing oscillations and to cardiac cycles, patients should hold their breath for a few seconds during the acquisition, and the operator should choose a fair distance from the heart when selecting the ultrasound section and the ROI. However, no elastogram is provided by pSWE. Ten valid measurements are recommended and the result (the median of the measurements) is shown in m/s or kPa. Quality parameters such as IQR/M and standard deviation (SD) are used to optimize the performance of the method [11, 26].

3.3 2D shear wave elastography (2D-SWE)

As in the other methods, 2D-SWE uses a section through the right live lobe free of large vessels and other structures that need a steady image in order to make the acquisition. Patients should hold their breath for 4 to 5 seconds or even longer so that the high frame rate should record the tissue displacement of the share wave propagation into the color-coded box. Tissue displacement by the share waves is displayed by a color-coded map; thus, the technique offers both quantitative and qualitative assessments of the tissue stiffness. The colored box should be positioned at least 1–2 cm below the liver capsule but not deeper than 7 cm into the liver parenchyma [27]. The ROI will express the results as the mean value and standard deviation in kPa or in m/s. The biggest advantage that this method is offering is the fact that it evaluates a larger area of the liver parenchyma (up to 10 cm^2). Usually, stiffer tissue will be depicted in red and softer tissue in blue. The operator should obtain as many elastogram loops to which in post-processing will select the ROI for LSM acquisition on the most homogeneous elastogram [26]. A minimum ultrasound training (>300) is necessary to be able to achieve good elastograms [28]. Recommended quality criteria are the IQR/M and measurement depth < 5.6 cm as quality technical [11, 29]. The median of at least three measurements should be used when performing LSM, but the examiner can choose between 3 and 15 measurements [30–32]. Even though it is a reproducible method [33], the inter- and intra-observer agreement in patients might be slightly inferior to pSWE [34, 35].

3.4 Real-time strain elastography (SE)

SE, offered by the Hitachi system (HI-RTE) [36], uses a regular ultrasound transducer that has embedded the SE module in it. It needs a good echoic window for the SE system to work properly; thus, a good ultrasound section is mandatory. The probe will generate echo signals under mild tissue compression and by this will produce a real-time elasticity image by overlapping a colored map on the B-mode image [37, 38]. It has all the advantages of the B-mode imaging and the examination approach will be as for the rest of the techniques with the patient in dorsal decubitus with the right arm in maximal abduction and a short breath hold when the acquisition is made, ascites and high BMI not being a contraindication for this method. However, the method is mainly used as a qualitative evaluation. Results will be displayed as blue for stiffer tissue and in red for soft tissue. Several methods have been developed in order to quantitatively assess tissue stiffness such as Elastic Ratio, Elastic Index, Elasticity Score, and Liver Fibrosis Index but without a proven consistency. The examiner must have ultrasound skills and special training is necessary for ROI setting and probe adjustment for homogeneous compression/relaxation index [20, 38]. Even though experience plays a role in SE, studies [39, 40] demonstrated that SE has a good and very good intra- and inter-observer variability and is a reproducible method.

4. Confounding factors

When measuring liver stiffness with ultrasound-based elastography, we have to acknowledge some factors that can influence the results. Some of the factors are related to a physiological state, and some are linked to pathology. Hepatic inflammation with a threshold of ASAT and/or ALAT >5 times the normal value, hepatic congestion, cholestasis, acute hepatitis, and infiltrative liver disease are known to increase liver stiffness [20]. It is also known that food intake and physical activity can falsely increase LSM; thus, a minimum of 2 hours fasting and resting for 10 minutes before the examination are recommended [20, 41, 42]. Confounding factors of the SWE according to their method are depicted in **Figure 7**.

For TE, BMI seemed to be the main factor influencing the results [43]; hence, a new dedicated XL probe (2.5 MHz) was produced for overweight and obese patients (BMI > 28 Kg/m2) with good clinical results [44, 45].

Besides BMI, TE results can be influenced by increased transaminase, cholestasis, hepatic congestion, infiltrative liver disease, food intake, and heavy alcohol consumption. Several limitations of TE that are worth mentioning are the contraindication of LSM in patients with ascites and the lack of B-mode imaging [26, 46].

Transient Elastography	pSWE	2D SWE	Strain elastograhpy
• BMI (partially surmounted with XL probe) [44] • Ascites [26]	• BMI [48] • Experience [28] • Moderate/Severe steatosis [51]	• BMI [52] • Experience [28]	• Experience & Operator dependency [12, 20, 38] • Inconsistent measurements [12, 20, 56]

Inflammation, infiltrative liver disease, cholestasis, congestion, bad cooperation are confounding factors that will influence all methods [12,20,26]

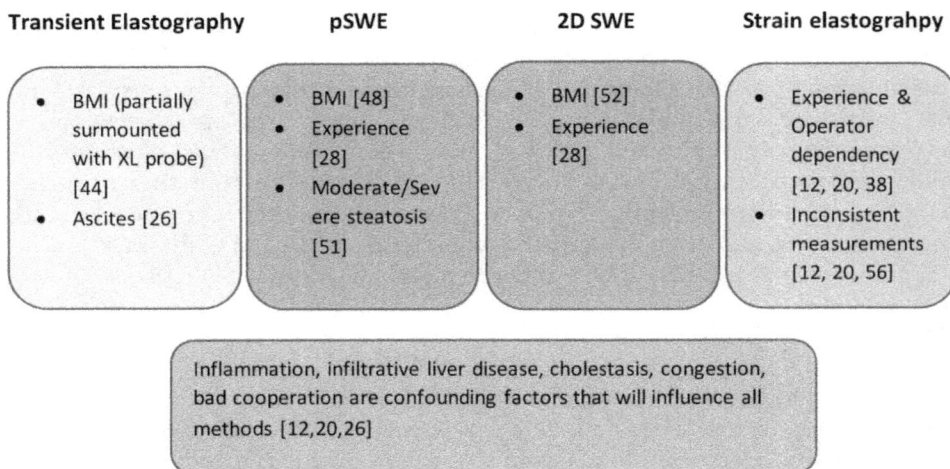

Figure 7.
Associated confounding factors in ultrasound-based liver elastography.

The pSWE technique uses a B-mode image to select a proper liver section where the acquisition will be made, therefore making it more dependent on ultrasound image selection ergo the operator [24]. Selection of ROI deepness and values obtained in the right vs. left lobe [47, 48] were the aspects that could influence the results. Increased BMI, moderate/severe steatosis, elevated transaminase, congestive liver, and cholestasis are influencing LSM as well as food intake. The examination should be done in fasting condition or at least after 3–4 hours from the last meal [49–51].

The 2D SWE technique is an operator-dependent method, with experience playing a role in obtaining reliable results [28]. Even though the method overcomes some of the previous limitations, it might have impaired results in patients with severe ascites, bad echoic window, obesity (BMI >30), inability to hold their breath, increased wall thickness (≥25 mm), steatosis, waist circumference (≥ 102 cm), and recent food intake [20, 52–55].

The real-time strain elastography method is an operator-dependent method, the clear echoic window being a prerequisite for a proper acquisition. Experience would be the front confounder. The method is not very common in daily practice due to its inconsistency [12, 20, 38, 56].

Ultrasound-based liver elastography confounding factors are described in **Figure 7**.

5. Conclusions

Ultrasound elastography comprises a set of techniques that noninvasively measure tissue stiffness. In this chapter, we have provided a brief introduction into the physical concepts of liver elastography and discussed several aspects important for clinical practice. In conclusion, elastography techniques that measure the shear wave speed are the most appropriate for liver applications. The liver elastography examination technique is standardized and co-founding factors need to be taken into consideration before performing liver stiffness measurements.

Author details

Felix Bende[1,2]* and Tudor Moga[1,2]

1 Department VII, Internal Medicine II, Center of Advanced Research in
Gastroenterology and Hepatology, "Victor Babes" University of Medicine and
Pharmacy Timisoara, Timisoara, Romania

2 Center for Advanced Hepatology Research of the Academy of Medical Sciences,
Timişoara, Romania

*Address all correspondence to: bende.felix@umft.ro

IntechOpen

References

[1] Papastergiou V, Tsochatzis E, Burroughs AK. Non- invasive assessment of liver fibrosis. Annals of Gastroenterology. 2012;**25**(3):218-231

[2] Seeff LB, Everson GT, Morgan TR, Curto TM, Lee WM, Ghany MG, et al. HALT–C trial group. Complication rate of percutaneous liver biopsies among persons with advanced chronic liver disease in the HALT-C trial. Clinical Gastroenterology and Hepatology. 2010;**8**(10):877-883

[3] Regev A, Berho M, Jeffers LJ, Milikowski C, Molina EG, Pyrsopoulos NT, et al. Sampling error and intraobserver variation in liver biopsy in patients with chronic HCV infection. The American Journal of Gastroenterology. 2002;**97**(10): 2614-2618

[4] Friedrich-Rust M, Ong MF, Martens S, Sarrazin C, Bojunga J, Zeuzem S, et al. Performance of transient elastography for the staging of liver fibrosis: A meta-analysis. Gastroenterology. 2008;**134**:960-974

[5] Tsochatzis EA, Gurusamy KS, Ntaoula S, Cholongitas E, Davidson BR, Burroughs AK. Elastography for the diagnosis of severity of fibrosis in chronic liver disease: A meta-analysis of diagnostic accuracy. Journal of Hepatology. 2011;**54**:650-659

[6] Herrmann E, de Lédinghen V, Cassinotto C, Chu WC, Leung VY, Ferraioli G, et al. Assessment of biopsy-proven liver fibrosis by two-dimensional shear wave elastography: An individual patient data-based meta-analysis. Hepatology. 2018;**67**(1):260-272. DOI: 10.1002/hep.29179. Epub 2017 Nov 15. PMID: 28370257; PMCID: PMC5765493

[7] Bende F, Sporea I, Șirli R, Nistorescu S, Fofiu R, Bâldea V, et al. The performance of a 2-dimensional shear-wave Elastography technique for predicting different stages of liver fibrosis using transient Elastography as the control method. Ultrasound Quarterly. 2020;**37**(2):97-104. DOI: 10.1097/RUQ.0000000000000527

[8] de Franchis R. Baveno VI Faculty. Expanding consensus in portal hypertension: Report of the Baveno VI consensus workshop: Stratifying risk and individualizing care for portal hypertension. Journal of Hepatology. 2015 Sep;**63**(3):743-752. DOI: 10.1016/j.jhep.2015.05.022. Epub 2015 Jun 3. PMID: 26047908

[9] Fofiu R, Bende F, Popescu A, Șirli R, Miuțescu B, Sporea I. Assessing Baveno VI criteria using liver stiffness measured with a 2D-shear wave Elastography technique. Diagnostics. 2021;**11**(5):737. DOI: 10.3390/diagnostics11050737. PMID: 33919033; PMCID: PMC8142982

[10] Wong GL, Chan HL, Wong CK, Leung C, Chan CY, Ho PP, et al. Liver stiffness-based optimization of hepatocellular carcinoma risk score in patients with chronic hepatitis B. Journal of Hepatology. 2014 Feb;**60**(2):339-345. DOI: 10.1016/j.jhep.2013.09.029 Epub 2013 Oct 12. PMID: 24128413

[11] Dietrich CF, Bamber J, Berzigotti A, Bota S, Cantisani V, Castera L, et al. EFSUMBguidelinesandrecommendations on the clinical use of liver ultrasound Elastography, update 2017 (long version). Ultraschall in der Medizin. 2017;**38**(4):e16-e47. DOI: 10.1055/s-0043-103952. Epub 2017 Apr 13. Erratum in: Ultraschall Med. 2017 Aug;38(4):e48. PMID: 28407655

[12] Ferraioli G, Filice C, Castera L, Choi BI, Sporea I, Wilson SR, et al. WFUMB guidelines and recommendations for clinical use of ultrasound elastography: Part 3: Liver. Ultrasound in Medicine & Biology. 2015;**41**(5):1161-1179. DOI: 10.1016/j. ultrasmedbio.2015.03.007 Epub 2015 Mar 20. PMID: 25800942

[13] Bamber J, Cosgrove D, Dietrich CF, Fromageau J, Bojunga J, Calliada F, et al. EFSUMB guidelines and recommendations on the clinical use of ultrasound elastography. Part 1: Basic principles and technology. Ultraschall in der Medizin. 2013;**34**(2):169-184. DOI: 10.1055/s-0033-1335205 Epub 2013 Apr 4. PMID: 23558397

[14] Shiina T, Nightingale KR, Palmeri ML, Hall TJ, Bamber JC, Barr RG, et al. WFUMB guidelines and recommendations for clinical use of ultrasound elastography: Part 1: Basic principles and terminology. Ultrasound in Medicine & Biology. 2015;**41**(5):1126-1147. DOI: 10.1016/j. ultrasmedbio.2015.03.009 Epub 2015 Mar 21. PMID: 25805059

[15] Sigrist RMS, Liau J, Kaffas AE, Chammas MC, Willmann JK. Ultrasound Elastography: Review of techniques and clinical applications. Theranostics. 2017;**7**(5):1303-1329. DOI: 10.7150/ thno.18650. PMID: 28435467; PMCID: PMC5399595

[16] Sandrin L, Tanter M, Gennisson JL, Catheline S, Fink M. Shear elasticity probe for soft tissues with 1-D transient elastography. IEEE Transactions on Ultrasonics, Ferroelectrics, and Frequency Control. 2002 Apr;**49**(4): 436-446. DOI: 10.1109/58.996561

[17] Srinivasa Babu A, Wells ML, Teytelboym OM, Mackey JE, Miller FH, Yeh BM, et al. Elastography in chronic liver disease: Modalities, techniques, limitations, and future directions. Radiographics. 2016;**36**(7):1987-2006. DOI: 10.1148/rg.2016160042

[18] Sasso M, Beaugrand M, de Ledinghen V, Douvin C, Marcellin P, Poupon R, et al. Controlled attenuation parameter (CAP): A novel VCTE™ guided ultrasonic attenuation measurement for the evaluation of hepatic steatosis: Preliminary study and validation in a cohort of patients with chronic liver disease from various causes. Ultrasound in Medicine & Biology. 2010 Nov;**36**(11):1825-1835. DOI: 10.1016/j. ultrasmedbio.2010.07.005

[19] Beaugrand M. Fibroscan: Instructions for use. Gastroentérologie Clinique et Biologique. 2006;**30**(4):513-514. DOI: 10.1016/S0399-8320(06)73219-5

[20] Cosgrove D, Piscaglia F, Bamber J, Bojunga J, Correas JM, Gilja OH, et al. EFSUMBguidelinesandrecommendations on the clinical use of ultrasound elastography. Part 2: Clinical applications. Ultraschall in der Medizin. 2013;**34**(3):238-253. DOI: 10.1055/s-0033-1335375

[21] Armstrong MJ, Corbett C, Hodson J, Marwah N, Parker R, Houlihan DD, et al. Operator training requirements and diagnostic accuracy of Fibroscan in routine clinical practice. Postgraduate Medical Journal. 2013;**89**(1058):685-692. DOI: 10.1136/postgradmedj-2012-131640

[22] Castéra L, Foucher J, Bernard PH, Carvalho F, Allaix D, Merrouche W, et al. Pitfalls of liver stiffness measurement: A 5-year prospective study of 13369 examinations. Hepatology. 2010;**51**: 828-835. DOI: 10.1002/hep.23425

[23] Afdhal NH, Bacon BR, Patel K, Lawitz EJ, Gordon SC, Nelson DR, et al. Accuracy of fibroscan, compared with

histology, in analysis of liver fibrosis in patients with hepatitis B or C: A United States multicenter study. Clinical Gastroenterology and Hepatology. 2015;**13**(4):772-779.e1-3. DOI: 10.1016/j. cgh.2014.12.014

[24] Bota S, Mare R, Sporea I. Point share wave Elastography (p-SWE). In: Sporea I, Şirli R, editors. Hepatic Elastography Using Ultrasound Waves. Revised Edition of Volume 1. Sharjah: Bentham Science E-Book; 2016. p. 44. DOI: 10.2174/9781608054633112010I

[25] Sporea I, Sirli RL, Deleanu A, Popescu A, Focsa M, Danila M, et al. Acoustic radiation force impulse elastography as compared to transient elastography and liver biopsy in patients with chronic hepatopathies. Ultraschall in der Medizin. 2011;**32**(Suppl. 1): S46-S52. DOI: 10.1055/s-0029-1245360

[26] Sporea I, Şirli R. Hepatic Elastography Using Ultrasound Waves. Bentham Science: E-Book2016. p. 178. DOI: 10.2174/9781608054633112010I

[27] Wang CZ, Zheng J, Huang ZP, Xiao Y, Song D, Zeng J, et al. Influence of measurement depth on the stiffness assessment of healthy liver with real-time shear wave elastography. Ultrasound in Medicine & Biology. 2014;**40**(3):461-469. DOI: 10.1016/j. ultrasmedbio.2013.10.021

[28] Grădinaru-Taşcău O, Sporea I, Bota S, Jurchiş A, Popescu A, Popescu M, et al. Does experience play a role in the ability to perform liver stiffness measurements by means of supersonic shear imaging (SSI)? Medical Ultrasonography. 2013;**15**:180-183. DOI: 10.11152/ mu.2013.2066.153.ogt1is2

[29] Colombo S, Buonocore M, Del Poggio A, Jamoletti C, Elia S, Mattiello M, et al. Head-to-head comparison of transient elastography (TE), real-time tissue elastography (RTE), and acoustic radiation force impulse (ARFI) imaging in the diagnosis of liver fibrosis. Journal of Gastroenterology. 2012;**47**(4):461-469. DOI: 10.1007/s00535-011-0509-4

[30] Ferraioli G, Tinelli C, Dal Bello B, Zicchetti M, Filice G, Filice C. Accuracy of real-time shear wave elastography for assessing liver fibrosis in chronic hepatitis C: A pilot study. Hepatology. 2012;**56**(6):2125-2133. DOI: 10.1002/ hep.25936

[31] Sporea I, Grădinaru-Taşcău O, Bota S, Popescu A, Şirli R, Jurchiş A, et al. How many measurements are needed for liver stiffness assessment by 2D-shear wave Elastography (2D-SWE) and which value should be used: The mean or median? Medical Ultrasonography. 2013;**15**(4):268-272. DOI: 10.11152/ mu.2013.2066.154.isp2

[32] Huang ZP, Zhang XL, Zeng J, Zheng J, Wang P, Zheng RQ. Study of detection times for liver stiffness evaluation by shear wave elastography. World Journal of Gastroenterology. 2014;**20**(28):9578-9584. DOI: 10.3748/wjg.v20.i28.9578

[33] Moga TV, Stepan AM, Pienar C, Bende F, Popescu A, Şirli R, et al. Intra- and inter-observer reproducibility of a 2-D shear wave Elastography technique and the impact of ultrasound experience in achieving reliable data. Ultrasound in Medicine & Biology. 2018;**44**(8):1627-1637. DOI: 10.1016/j. ultrasmedbio.2018.03.029

[34] Woo H, Lee JY, Yoon JH, Kim W, Cho B, Choi BI. Comparison of the reliability of acoustic radiation force impulse imaging and supersonic shear imaging in measurement of liver stiffness. Radiology. 2015;**277**:881-886. DOI: 10.1148/radiol.2015141975

[35] Popescu A, Bende F, Sporea I. 2D-share waves Elastography (2D-SWE). In: Sporea I, Șirli R, editors. Hepatic Elastography Using Ultrasound Waves. Revised Edition of Volume 1. Sharjah: Bentham Science E-Book; 2016. p. 88. DOI: 10.2174/97816080546331120101

[36] Friedrich-Rust M, Ong MF, Herrmann E, Dries V, Samaras P, Zeuzem S, et al. Real-time elastography for noninvasive assessment of liver fibrosis in chronic viral hepatitis. AJR. American Journal of Roentgenology. 2007;**188**(3):758-764. DOI: 10.2214/AJR.06.0322

[37] Frey H. Realtime elastography. A new ultrasound procedure for the reconstruction of tissue elasticity. Radiologe. 2003;**43**(10):850-855. DOI: 10.1007/s00117-003-0943-2

[38] Sandulescu R, Sporea I, Popescu A. Real-time strain Elastography (HI-RTE). In: Sporea I, Șirli R, editors. Hepatic Elastography Using Ultrasound Waves. Revised Edition of Volume 1. Sharjah: Bentham Science E-Book; 2016. p. 105. DOI: 10.2174/97816080546331120101

[39] Gheonea DI, Săftoiu A, Ciurea T, Gorunescu F, Iordache S, Popescu GL, et al. Real-time sono-elastography in the diagnosis of diffuse liver diseases. World Journal of Gastroenterology. 2010;**16**(14):1720-1726. DOI: 10.3748/wjg.v16.i14.1720

[40] Koizumi Y, Hirooka M, Kisaka Y, Konishi I, Abe M, Murakami H, et al. Liver fibrosis in patients with chronic hepatitis C: Noninvasive diagnosis by means of real-time tissue elastography establishment of the method for measurement. Radiology. 2011;**258**(2):610-617. DOI: 10.1148/radiol.10100319

[41] Arena U, Lupsor Platon M, Stasi C, Moscarella S, Assarat A, Bedogni G, et al. Liver stiffness is influenced by a standardized meal in patients with chronic hepatitis C virus at different stages of fibrotic evolution. Hepatology. 2013;**58**:65-72. DOI: 10.1002/hep.26343

[42] Gersak MM, Sorantin E, Windhaber J, Dudea SM, Riccabona M. The influence of acute physical effort on liver stiffness estimation using virtual touch quantification (VTQ). Preliminary results. Medical Ultrasonography. 2016;**18**:151-156. DOI: 10.11152/mu.2013.2066.182.vtq

[43] Gersak MM, Sorantin E, Windhaber J, Dudea SM, Riccabona M. Prevalence and factors associated with failure of liver stiffness measurement using FibroScan in a prospective study of 2114 examinations. European Journal of Gastroenterology & Hepatology. 2006;**18**(4):411-412. DOI: 10.1097/00042737-200604000-00015

[44] Myers RP, Pomier-Layrargues G, Kirsch R, Pollett A, Duarte-Rojo A, Wong D, et al. Feasibility and diagnostic performance of the fibroScan XL probe for liver stiffness measurement in overweight and obese patients. Hepatology. 2012;**55**(1):199-208. DOI: 10.1002/hep.24624

[45] Sporea I, Șirli R, Mare R, Popescu A, Ivașcu SC. Feasibility of transient elastography with M and XL probes in real life. Medical Ultrasonography. 2016;**18**(1):7-10. DOI: 10.1097/00042737-200604000-00015

[46] Castéra L, Foucher J, Bernard PH, Carvalho F, Allaix D, Merrouche W, et al. Pitfalls of liver stiffness measurement: A 5-year prospective study of 13,369 examinations. Hepatology. 2010;**51**(3):828-835. DOI: 10.1002/hep.23425

[47] DOnofrio M, Gallotti A, Mucelli RP. Tissue quantification with acoustic

radiation force impulse imaging: Measurement repeatability and normal values in the healthy liver. AJR. American Journal of Roentgenology. 2010;**195**(1):132-136. DOI: 10.2214/AJR.09.3923

[48] Liao LY, Kuo KL, Chiang HS, Lin CZ, Lin YP, Lin CL. Acoustic radiation force impulse elastography of the liver in healthy patients: Test location, reference range and influence of gender and body mass index. Ultrasound in Medicine & Biology. 2015;**41**(3):698-704. DOI: 10.1016/j.ultrasmedbio.2014.09.030

[49] Goertz RS, Egger C, Neurath MF, Strobel D. Impact of food intake, ultrasound transducer, breathing maneuvers and body position on acoustic radiation force impulse (ARFI) elastometry of the liver. Ultraschall in der Medizin. 2012;**33**(4):380-335. DOI: 10.1055/s-0032-1312816

[50] Bota S, Sporea I, Peck-Radosavljevic M, Sirli R, Tanaka H, I ijima H, et al. The influence of aminotransferase levels on liver stiffness assessed by acoustic radiation force impulse elastography: A retrospective multicentre study. Digestive and Liver Disease. 2013;**45**(9):762-768. DOI: 10.1016/j.dld.2013.02.008

[51] Bota S, Sporea I, Sirli R, Popescu A, Dănilă M, Sendroiu M. Factors that influence the correlation of acoustic radiation force impulse (ARFI), elastography with liver fibrosis. Medical Ultrasonography. 2011;**13**(2):135-140

[52] Yoon JH, Lee JM, Han JK, Choi BI. Shear wave elastography for liver stiffness measurement in clinical sonographic examinations: Evaluation of intraobserver reproducibility, technical failure, and unreliable stiffness measurements. Journal of Ultrasound in Medicine. 2014;**33**:437-447. DOI: 10.7863/ultra.33.3.437

[53] Staugaard B, Christensen PB, Mössner B, Hansen JF, Madsen BS, Søholm J, et al. Feasibility of transient elastography versus real-time two-dimensional shear wave elastography in difficult-to-scan patients. Scandinavian Journal of Gastroenterology. 2016;**51**:1354-1359. DOI: 10.1080/00365521.2016.1193217

[54] Cassinotto C, Lapuyade B, Mouries A, Hiriart JB, Vergniol J, Gaye D, et al. Noninvasive assessment of liver fibrosis with impulse elastography: Comparison of supersonic shear imaging with ARFI and Fibroscan. Journal of Hepatology. 2014;**61**:550-557. DOI: 10.1016/j.jhep.2014.04.044

[55] Vonghia L, Werlinden W, Pelckmans P, Michielsen P, Francque S. Liver stiffness by shear waves elastography is influenced by meal and meal-related haemodynamic modifications. Ultraschall Med. 2013;**34**:W_SL24_09. DOI: 10.1055/s-0033-1354961

[56] Morikawa H, Fukuda K, Kobayashi S, Fujii H, Iwai S, Enomoto M, et al. Real-time tissue elastography as a tool for the noninvasive assessment of liver stiffness in patients with chronic hepatitis C. Journal of Gastroenterology. 2011;**46**:350-358. DOI: 10.1007/s00535-010-0301-x

Chapter 2

Ultrasound Based Elastography Techniques for the Evaluation of Nonalcoholic Liver Disease

Ioan Sporea, Raluca Lupușoru and Roxana Șirli

Abstract

The number of NAFLD patients is increasing in the developed world and non-invasive modalities for their evaluation are needed. Ultrasound-based methods are very useful for this approach, starting with standard ultrasound used for steatosis detection, and continuing with new modalities for steatosis, fibrosis, and inflammation quantification. Modern ultrasound systems can quantify all these parameters in NAFLD patients, thus making ultrasound a real Multiparameter Ultrasound (MPUS). The performance of ultrasound-based methods is very well documented with liver stiffness assessment as a marker of fibrosis, and more recently, for quantification of steatosis and viscoelastic properties as a marker of inflammation.

Keywords: nonalcoholic fatty liver disease (NAFLD), fatty liver, ultrasound, liver elastography, fat quantification

1. Introduction

Currently, at least in the developed world, the focus of hepatology changed, from chronic viral hepatitis (B or C), which is now well controlled with efficient drugs, to the problem of fatty liver. This disease occurs in both non-alcoholic patients with metabolic conditions as well as in alcoholic patients [1]. Nonalcoholic fatty liver disease (NAFLD) become more and more present in clinical practice, since it currently affects more than a quarter of the world population [2] and the prevalence is increasing [3]. Overweight and obesity, type 2 diabetes, dyslipidemia, and sedentariness are increasing at a global level, at least in the developed world [4, 5]. For a long time, the fatty liver was considered to be a "benign" entity, but in the last years, the potential evolution of this disease to severe fibrosis and cirrhosis has been proven. Furthermore, in the last years, NAFLD became an important indication for liver transplantation [6–8].

Recently, new terminology for NAFLD was proposed, to better reflect its clinical spectrum: Metabolic Associated Fatty Liver Disease (MAFLD) [9, 10]. This new terminology is used more and more, having the advantage to underline the role of metabolic factors and to not exclude the use of alcohol. Thus, we must be focused to screen for fatty liver in the population at risk: patients with obesity, metabolic syndrome, and type 2 diabetes mellitus (DM).

Recent data showed that 650 million people around the world are obese and 1,9 billion are overweight (39% of the adult population)! Type 2 diabetes mellitus (type 2 DM) become a frequent cause of morbidity in the last decade (1 in 11 people of the developed countries have type 2 DM) [11]. Furthermore, many of type 2 DM patients are overweight and obese. Association of obesity and type 2 DM increases the risk for fatty liver infiltration. Features of metabolic syndrome are frequent in the adult population; thus, all these conditions explain the increased incidence of fatty liver in daily practice.

These huge cohorts of patients should be evaluated, especially in regard to fibrosis severity, the main driver of fibrosis. Simple non-invasive biologic tests to predict significant fibrosis in patients with NAFLD are available, such as Fibrosis-4 (FIB-4) or APRI (which uses only transaminases serum levels, platelet count and age), with acceptable accuracy [12]. Other biologic tests are more accurate [Enhanced Liver Fibrosis (ELF™) Test, FibroMax, others], but also more complex and more expensive.

In the last 15 years numerous ultrasound (US) based elastography techniques have been developed [Transient Elastography (TE), point Shear Wave Elastography (pSWE) or 2D-SWE], which have demonstrated their practical value in many studies. International Guidelines classify these US elastography techniques into: Strain Elastography (used mostly for breast, thyroid and prostate nodules) and Shear Waves Elastography (SWE - in which external impulses generate shear waves inside the liver, whose speed is measured by ultrasound) [13, 14]. The faster the shear-waves speed are, the stiffer the tissue and the fibrosis are more severe. Based on the generation of the external impulse and the technology used to measure the shear-waves speed, SWE elastography is subdivided into: Transient Elastography (with a mechanic external impulse), Point SWE (pSWE) [in which an Acoustic Radiation Force Impulse (ARFI) is used and the shear-waves speed is measured in a point], and real-time elastography which includes 2D-SWE and 3D-SWE (in which ARFI is used, shear-waves speed is measured in an area of interest and in the same time a color-coded elastogram is generated) [13, 14].

However, in patients with NAFLD, not only the evaluation of fibrosis is important, but also quantification of steatosis and inflammation is of practical value.

In this chapter, we aim to discuss the ultrasound-based methods for the evaluation of patients with NAFLD. In such patient's evaluation and quantification of steatosis, fibrosis and inflammation are important. In practice, these methods are frequently used and more and more data are collected regarding their value.

2. Steatosis evaluation

In patients with NAFLD, the presence of steatosis is a common fact and then the evaluation of its severity is necessary. *Ultrasonography* (US) is the simplest way to evaluate steatosis, and two signs are important: "bright" hyperechoic liver" with posterior attenuation (**Figure 1**) and increased hepato-renal index (**Figure 2**). Using these two signs, a semiquantitative assessment of steatosis severity can be performed. Many papers evaluated the performance of liver ultrasound for the assessment of the steatosis severity, some of them are quite old papers. Mathiesen et al. [15] compared the US with hepatic histology for steatosis assessment in a series of 165 patients. Steatosis was graded as none, mild, moderate or severe. In patients with increased echogenicity, 86.7% had at least moderate liver steatosis by histology. To detect steatosis, US had a sensitivity of 0.90, a specificity of 0.82, a positive predictive value of 0.87 and a negative predictive value of 0.87. In another study, Palmentieri et al. [16] compared the "bright liver" echo pattern to liver biopsy in 235 patients.

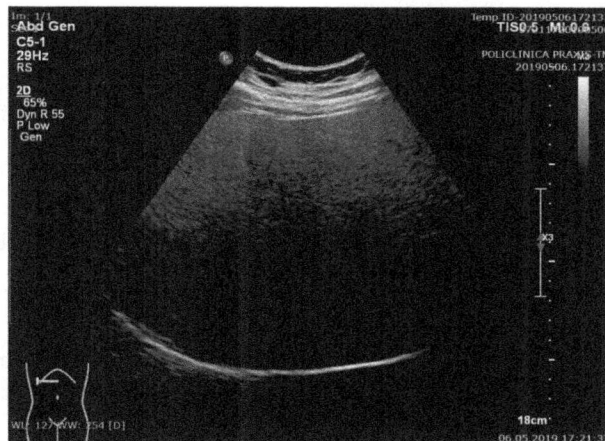

Figure 1.
"Bright liver" with posterior attenuation.

The study showed that the "bright liver" echo pattern was found in 67% of patients with steatosis of any degree and in 89% of patients with severe steatosis (≥30% of the hepatocytes involved). Among the subgroup of patients who had severe steatosis, the sensitivity and specificity of US were 91% and 93%, respectively.

Maybe the most important paper regarding the value of liver US for diagnosing fatty liver is a large meta-analysis [17], which included 49 studies and 4720 subjects. The sensitivity of US for moderate and severe steatosis was 84.8% (CI 95%: 79.5–88.9%), with a specificity of 93.6% (CI 95%: 87.2–97.0%).

Computer Assisted Diagnosis (CAD) was also evaluated as a tool to increase the accuracy of US for the detection and severity assessment of steatosis [18]. In a study including 120 patients [19], CAD was able to correctly classify the severity of steatosis with an accuracy of 82.2%. More recently, Artificial Intelligence (AI) has been used for the same purpose [20].

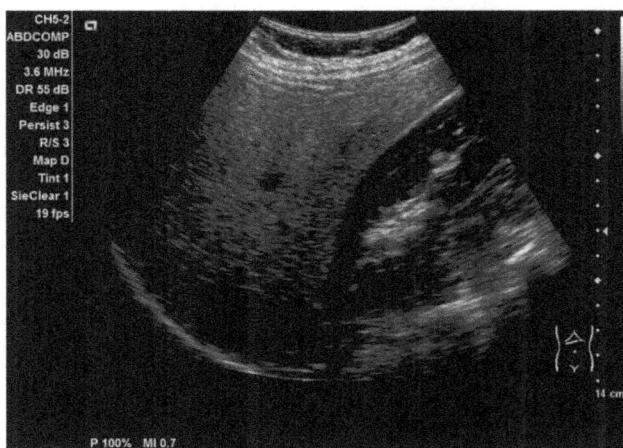

Figure 2.
Increased hepato-renal index.

All these papers are in favor to use liver ultrasound for the detection of steatosis in patients with risk factors. The latest update of the European Association for the Study of the Liver (EASL) Guidelines regarding the non-invasive evaluation in chronic liver disease [12] states that: "Conventional ultrasound should be used as a first-line tool for the diagnosis of steatosis in clinical practice, despite its well-known limitations". This method can be used for a semi-quantitative assessment of the severity of fatty infiltration.

For a quantitative evaluation of liver steatosis, the most used method in this moment is Controlled Attenuation Parameter (CAP). It is a module implemented on a FibroScan device (Echosens, Paris, France), which measures the attenuation of the ultrasound beams throughout the liver to assess steatosis severity. CAP was first used on the M probe and latter also on the XL probe (**Figure 3**).

Many papers have been published on the value of CAP for liver steatosis assessment, comparing it to liver biopsy. In the next table, we resumed the main published papers concerning the value of CAP (**Table 1**).

Having in mind that the CAP module is available both in M and XL probes, the next question is if the same cut-off values can be used in practice for both probes? Chan et al. evaluated a cohort of 180 patients by liver biopsy and CAP with both M and XL probes [36]. The group had a mean age of 53.7 ± 10.8 years and NAFLD was identified in 86.7% of them, the sensitivity, specificity, PPV, and NPV of CAP using the M/XL probe for the diagnosis of steatosis grade ≥ S1 was 93.9%/93.3%, 58.8%/58.8%, 95.6%/95.6%, and 50.0%/47.6%, respectively. Thus, the authors concluded that the same cut-off values for CAP may be used for the M and XL probes for the diagnosis of hepatic steatosis grade.

However, in another prospective study on 100 adults [37], which compared CAP with the M vs. the XL probe for quantification of hepatic fat content, using magnetic resonance imaging proton density fat fraction (MRI-PDFF) as the standard, the mean CAP values by M probe (310 ± 62 db/m) were significantly lower than by the XL probe (317 ± 63 db/m) ($P = 0.007$). The authors demonstrated that the M probe under-quantifies CAP values as compared with the XL probe and they proposed that the type of probe should be considered when interpreting CAP data from patients with fatty liver.

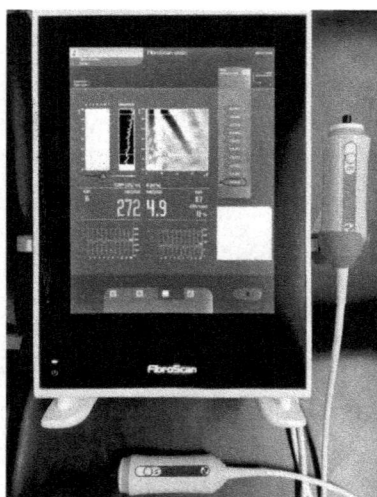

Figure 3.
FibroScan (Echosens, Paris, France) with M and XL probes (in light blue CAP values are shown, while in yellow the liver stiffness values).

Study	No. of patients	Cut-off values for each steatosis grade (dB/m)		
		$S \geq 1$	$S \geq 2$	$S \geq 3$
Chan 2014 [21]	105	263	281	283
De Ledinghen 2016 [22]	261	—	310	311
Imajo 2016 [23]	142	236	279	302
Park 2017 [24]	104	261	305	312
Naveau 2017 [25]	123	298	303	326
Sissiqui 2019 [26]	393	285	311	306
Shalimar 2020 [27]	219	285	331	348
Oeda 2019 [28]	137	—	264	289
Eddowes 2019 [29]	88	302	331	337
Petroff 2021 [30]	2346	294	310	331
Karlas 2017 [31]	2735	248	268	280
Kamali 2019 [32]	77	237	259	291
Zenovia 2021 [33]	204	245	273,5	333
Mikolasevic 2021 [34]	179	304	311	345
Park 2017 [24]	104	261	—	—
Gu 2021 [35]	1183/3295/2835	273.5	288.5	309

Table 1.
Value of CAP for liver steatosis assessment.

In the last years, *ultrasound modules for the quantification of liver steatosis* have been implemented in standard US machines, by several companies. The advantage of these systems is that when steatosis is seen by standard ultrasound, immediately a quantification can be performed. Several papers have been published in this area, with good results. In the following pages, we will present the most recent developments in this field.

Ultrasound Guided Attenuation Parameter (UGAP) from General Electric (**Figure 4**) was evaluated for the detection of hepatic steatosis as compared with CAP, using histopathology as the reference standard [38]. In a cohort of 163 chronic liver disease patients who underwent UGAP, CAP and liver biopsy on the same day, the AUROC's of UGAP for identifying >S1, >S2 and S3 were 0.900, 0.953 and 0.959, respectively, which were significantly better than the results obtained with CAP.

Attenuation imaging (ATI) from Canon (**Figure 5**) has shown promising results for fatty quantification in several published papers. In a study performed on 114 subjects potentially at risk of steatosis and 15 healthy controls, ATI results were compared to the ones obtained with CAP, using MRI-PDFF as the reference method [39]. ATI showed a better correlation with MRI-PDFF (r = 0.81) than CAP (r = 0.65). Similar good results have been obtained by the same group in a later paper [39]. In this study, the correlation between ATI and PDFF was better than with CAP (0.83 vs. 0.58).

In another study, in which liver histology was used as a reference in a series of 108 subjects, it has been reported that the degree of steatosis was the only significant determinant factor for the ATI results and that the AUROCs for different grades of steatosis ranged from 0.84 to 0.93 [40].

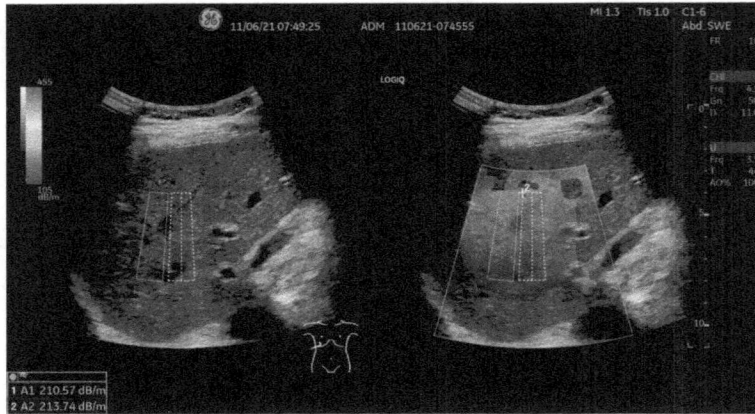

Figure 4.
UGAP (ultrasound-guided attenuation parameter).

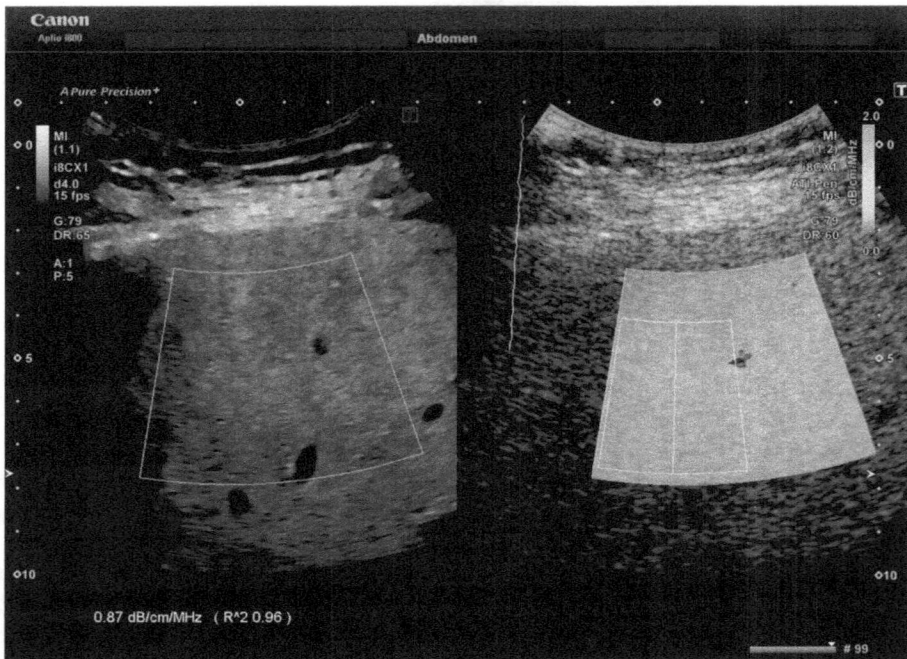

Figure 5.
Attenuation image from Canon.

In a study that used once again MRI-PDFF as reference [41], in a cohort of 87 patients, the AUROCs of ATI for detection of hepatic steatosis ≥5% and ≥ 10%, were 0.76 and 0.88, respectively (95% CI: 0.66–0.85 and 0.79–0.94) and the correlation of ATI with MRI-PDFF was moderate (p = 0.66).

The *Attenuation coefficient (ATT)* from Hitachi was used in a multicenter prospective study including patients who underwent liver biopsy and ATT measurements on the same day [42]. Correlations between ATT and steatosis grade were evaluated. In a total of 351 patients that were enrolled in this study, the median values of ATT for steatosis grades S0, S1, S2, and S3 were 0.55, 0.63, 0.69, and 0.85 dB/cm/MHz, respectively, and ATT increased with the increase in steatosis grade ($P < 0.001$). The AUROC's corresponding to $S \geq 1$, $S \geq 2$, and $S \geq 3$ were 0.79, 0.87, and 0.96, respectively.

Speed of sound estimation (SSE) (**Figure 6**) implemented in the Aixplorer US system - MACH 30 was compared with MRI-PDFF in a pilot study including 100 patients [43]. The technique's reproducibility was excellent, with an intraclass correlation coefficient (ICC) of 0.93. An SSE cutoff ≤1.537 mm/μs showed 80% sensitivity and 85.7% specificity in detecting any steatosis (S1–S3). In a multivariant regression analysis, only MRI-PDFF and BMI were associated with SSE values.

In another study in a cohort of 215 NAFLD patients using Aixplorer MACH 30 system [44] for the evaluation of steatosis, Sound Speed Plane-wave UltraSound (*SSp. PLUS*) and Attenuation Plane-wave UltraSound (*Att.PLUS*) were used in comparison with CAP. In this study, SSp.PLUS correlated better than Att.PLUS with CAP values: ($r = -0.74$ vs. $r = 0.45$) and the best SSp.PLUS cut-off value for predicting the presence significant steatosis by CAP was 1524 m/s.

Quantification of steatosis (AC-TAI and SC-TAI) using the Samsung ultrasound system (**Figures 7** and **8**) was evaluated in a cohort of 120 subjects suspected of having NAFLD [45]. The participants underwent US examination for radiofrequency (RF) data acquisition. Using RF data analysis, the attenuation coefficient (AC) based on tissue attenuation imaging (TAI) (AC-TAI) as well as a scatter-distribution coefficient (SC) based on tissue scatter-distribution imaging (TSI) (SC-TSI) were measured and compared with MRI-PDFF. In this study, AC-TAI and SC-TSI were significantly correlated with MRI-PDFF ($r = 0.659$ and 0.727, $p < 0.001$ for both). For detecting hepatic fat contents of ≥5% and ≥ 10%, the areas under the AUROCs of AC-TAI were 0.861 (95% CI: 0.786–0.918) and 0.835 (95% CI: 0.757–0.897), while those of SC-TSI were 0.964 (95% CI: 0.913–0.989) and 0.935 (95% CI: 0.875–0.972), respectively.

All these results concerning the quantification of liver steatosis using ultrasound are very promising and every day new papers are published in well-known medical journals considering the rapid development of this field.

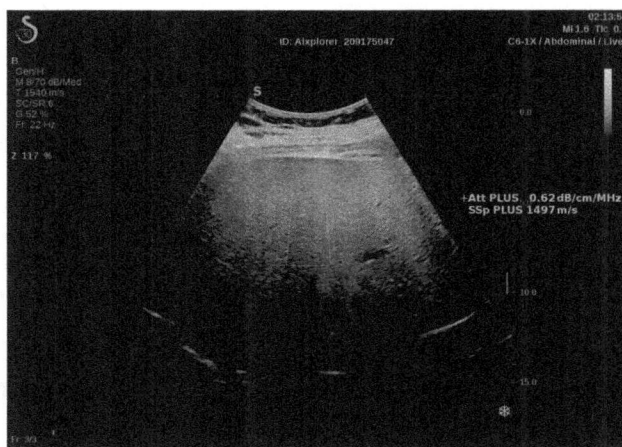

Figure 6.
Speed of sound estimation (SSE).

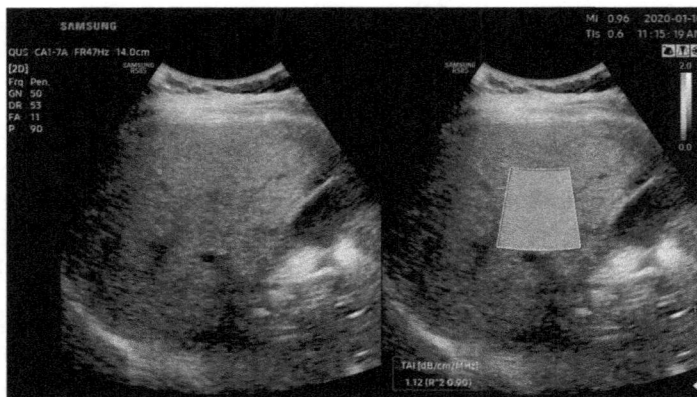

Figure 7.
AC-TAI- severe steatosis.

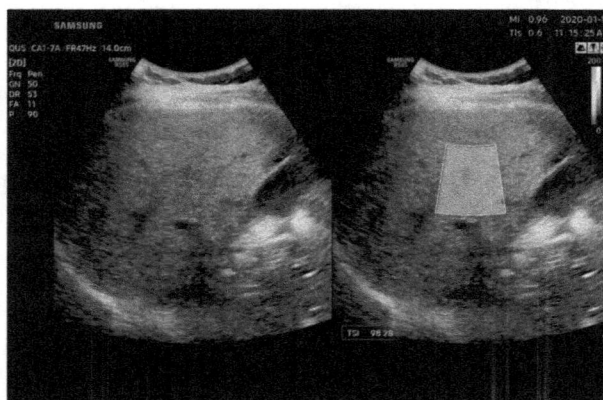

Figure 8.
AC-TSI severe steatosis.

3. Evaluation of fibrosis

In the early times of non-invasive assessment of patients with chronic liver disease, the main field of research was liver fibrosis. Replacing in many cases liver biopsy, this assessment is essential for the prognosis of patients [46, 47]. Early papers in this field evaluated Transient Elastography (TE) as a predictor of fibrosis in NAFLD [48]. Later, ARFI technologies (Acustic Radiation Force Impulse) with pSWE and 2D-SWE became fields of research [49]. In **Table 2** we presented the main papers evaluating TE and SWE methods for the assessment of liver fibrosis in NAFLD patients.

Considering the practical value of different systems, TE is the oldest system, a semi-blind method of evaluation, it can assess fibrosis severity as well as steatosis (with CAP) in the same machine, is not possible to be performed in patients with ascites and in some areas TE and CAP measurements are made by technicians. ARFI technologies (pSWE and 2D-SWE) are included in standard ultrasound systems and fibrosis assessment (and others parameters) can be performed immediately after B-mode examination and can evaluate to the patients with ascites. International

Study	No of patients	Elastography	Cut-off values for each fibrosis stage			
			F1	F2	F3	F4
Petta 2016 [50]	324	TE	—	>10.5 kPa	>12.5 kPa	—
Yoneda 2007 [51]	67	TE	>5.6 kPa	>6.65 kPa	>8 kPa	>17 kPa
Gaia 2011 [52]	72	TE	>5.5 kPa	>7 kPa	>8 kPa	>10.5 kPa
Kumar 2013 [53]	205	TE	>6.1 kPa	>7 kPa	>9 kPa	>11.8 kPa
Lupsor 2010 [54]	72	TE	—	>6.8 kPa	>10.4 kPa	—
Petta 2011 [55]	169	TE	—	>7.25 kPa	>8.75 kPa	—
Ratziu 2010 [56]	53	TE	>5.1 kPa	>9.1 kPa	>11.1 kPa	>14.5 kPa
Yoneda 2008 [57]	50	TE	—	>6.6 kPa	>9.8 kPa	>17.5 kPa
Nobili 2008 [58]	52	TE	—	>7.4 kPa	>10.2 kPa	—
Wong 2010 [48]	146	TE	—	>7 kPa	>8.7 kPa	>10.3 kPa
Wong 2012 [59]	193	TE	—	>6.2 kPa	>7.2 kPa	>7.9 kPa
Musso 2011 [60]	60	TE	—	>7 kPa	>8.7 kPa	—
Yoneda 2010 [61]	54	TE	—	—	>9.9 kPa	>16 kPa
Mahadeva 2013 [62]	131	TE	—	>6.65 kPa	>7.1 kPa	>10.6 kPa
Imajo 2016 [23]	152	TE	—	>11 kPa	>11.4 kPa	>14 kPa
Pathik 2015 [63]	89	TE	—	>9.1 kPa	>12 kPa	>20 kPa
Kumar 2013 [53]	207	TE	—	>7 kPa	>9 kPa	>11.8 kPa
Cassinotto 2016 [49]	291	TE	—	>6.2 kPa	>8.2 kPa	>9.5 kPa
Kamali 2019 [32]	77	TE	—	>8 kPa	>11 kPa	>16 kPa
Eddowes 2019 [29]	88	TE	—	>8.2 kPa	>9.7 kPa	>13.6 kPa
Park 2017 [24]	104	TE	—	>6.10 kPa	—	—
Seki 2017 [64]	171	TE	>7.2 kPa	—	>10.0 kPa	—
Lee 2017 [65]	94	TE	—	>7.4 kPa	> 8 kPa	>10.8 kPa
Hsu 2018 [66]	230	TE	>6.2 kPa	>7.6 kPa	>8.8 kPa	>11.8 kPa
Attia 2016 [67]	61	TE	—	>7.0 kPa	>11.8 kPa	>15.0 kPa
Myers 2010 [68]	50	TE	—	—	>10.3 kPa	>11.1 kPa
Myers 2012 [69]	276	TE	—	—	—	>16 kPa
Furlan 2020 [70]	59	TE	—	>8.8 kPa	>6.7 kPa	—
Leong 2020 [71]	100	TE	>7.68 kPa	>9.13 kPa	>9.28 kPa	>13.4 kPa
Imajo 2020 [72]	221	TE	>6.95 kPa	>8.14 kPa	>13.8 kPa	>19.5 kPa
Yoneda 2010 [61]	54	pSWE	—	—	>1.77 m/s	>1.9 m/s
Fierbinteanu 2013 [73]	64	pSWE	—	—	>1.48 m/s	>1.63 m/s
Cassinotto 2013 [74]	165	pSWE	—	>1.3 m/s	>1.51 m/s	>1.61 m/s
Friedrich-Rust 2012 [75]	50	pSWE	—	>1.37 m/s	—	—

Study	No of patients	Elastography	Cut-off values for each fibrosis stage			
			F1	F2	F3	F4
Osaki 2010 [76]	101	pSWE	>1.34 m/s	>1.79 m/s	>2.2 m/s	>2.9 m/s
Lee 2017 [65]	94	pSWE	—	>1.35 m/s	>1.43 m/s	>1.50 m/s
Attia 2016 [66]	61	pSWE	—	>1.18 m.s	>1.45 m/s	>1.95 m/s
Palmeri 2011 [77]	172	pSWE	—	—	>1.49 m/s	—
Cui 2016 [78]	114	pSWE	—	>1.29 m/s	>1.34 m/s	>2.48 m/s
Li 2016 [79]	136	pSWE	—	>1.30 m/s	>1.36 m/s	>1.41 m/s
Leong 2020 [72]	100	pSWE	>6.83 kPa	>6.98 kPa	>7.02 kPa	>11.5 kPa
Sharpton 2021 [80]	114	pSWE	>7.8 kPa	>6.8 kPa	>8.7 kPa	>10.6 kPa
Cassinotto 2016 [49]	291	2D-SWE	—	>6.3 kPa	>8.3 kPa	>10.5 kPa
Herrmann 2017 [81]	156	2D-SWE	—	>7.1 kPa	>9.2 kPa	>13 kPa
Takeuchi 2018 [82]	71	2D-SWE	>6.6 kPa	>11.6 kPa	>13.1 kPa	>15.7 kPa
Jamialahmadi 2019 [83]	90	2D-SWE	>5.6 kPa	>6.6 kPa	>6.8 kPa	>6.8 kPa
Lee 2017 [65]	94	2D-SWE	—	>8.3 kPa	>10.7 kPa	>15.1 kPa
Furlan 2020 [70]	57	2D-SWE	—	>5.7 kPa	>8.1 kPa	—
Sharpton 2021 [80]	114	2D-SWE	>7.5 kPa	>7.7 kPa	>7.7 kPa	>9.3 kPa
Imajo 2020 [72]	221	2D-SWE	>6.65 kPa	>8.04 kPa	>10.6 kPa	>12.37 kPa

Table 2.
Value of TE, pSWE and 2D-SWE for liver fibrosis assessment in NAFLD patients.

published guidelines regarding the practical values of all these techniques have been published [13, 14]. Barr et al. [84] showed the advantages and disadvantages of each method. The most recent guideline (from 2021) is the EASL Guideline for the use of the main non-invasive tests, with the important recommendations in this field [12].

4. Evaluation of inflammation

In patients with NAFLD, it is of crucial importance to differentiate between simple steatosis and steatohepatitis (NASH: non-alcoholic steatohepatitis). The best method for this is liver biopsy. However, having in mind the huge number of subjects with NAFLD (1/4 of the population in the developed countries), this invasive technique is not feasible in practice for all the patients. It has been demonstrated that using only biologic tests (such as aminotransferases or Cytokeratin 18) is not enough, thus new methods that accurately assess inflammation are necessary [85].

The newest high-end US machines include modules that evaluate the viscoelastic properties of the liver. This parameter is considered to be an expression of inflammation in the fatty liver, useful for the diagnosis of steatohepatitis (NASH).

Such a paper was published recently. Detection of steatosis, fibrosis and inflammation in 102 patients with NAFLD in comparison with liver biopsy was performed using a high-end US machine [86]. *Attenuation coefficient* (dB/cm/MHz) from attenuation imaging, *liver stiffness* measurements, and *shear wave dispersion slope* (SWDS, [m/s]/kHz) from 2D-SWE were evaluated. The AUROC values for steatosis grades S1, S2 or S3, were 0.93, 0.88, and 0.83, respectively, while for lobular inflammatory activity (SWDS) the system detected inflammation grades 1, 2 and 3 with an AUROCs of 0.89, 0.85, and 0.78, respectively.

In a prospective study performed in a cohort of 120 consecutive adults who underwent liver biopsy for suspected NAFLD, Multiparametric US was used for liver assessment [87]. Three US parameters: *dispersion slope* [(m/s)/kHz], *attenuation coefficient* [dB/cm/MHz], and *shear-wave speed* (m/s), were evaluated with a 2D-SWE system, immediately before biopsy. This study has shown that dispersion slope identified lobular inflammation with an AUC of 0.95 (95% CI: 0.91, 0.10) for an inflammation grade $\geq$ A1 (mild), of 0.81 (95% CI: 0.72, 0.89) for an inflammation grade $\geq$ A2 (moderate), and of 0.85 (95% CI: 0.74, 0.97) for an inflammation grade A3 (marked). Considering the attenuation coefficient, it identified steatosis with an AUC of 0.88 (95% CI: 0.80, 0.97) for S $\geq$ 1 (mild), 0.86 (95% CI: 0.79, 0.93) for $\geq$S2 (moderate), and 0.79 (95% CI: 0.68, 0.89) for S3 (severe). Shear-wave speed identified fibrosis with an AUC of 0.79 (95% CI: 0.69, 0.88) for fibrosis stage F $\geq$ 1, of 0.88 (95% CI: 0.82, 0.94) for F $\geq$ 2, of 0.90 (95% CI: 0.84, 0.96) for F $\geq$ 3 and of 0.95 (95% CI: 0.91, 0.99) for F4 (cirrhosis). Probably the most important fact is that this combination of dispersion slope, attenuation coefficient, and shear-wave speed showed an AUC of 0.81 (95% CI: 0.71, 0.91) for the diagnosis of NASH.

Although, there are still many steps to go to reach an accurate software for the detection of inflammation using US waves, these early papers are encouraging for the noninvasive assessment of patients with NAFLD. All necessary information can be obtained using the Multiparametric Ultrasound (MPUS), and this is an ideal technique for NAFLD patients (quantification of fibrosis, steatosis and inflammation in less than 5 minutes) (**Figure 9**).

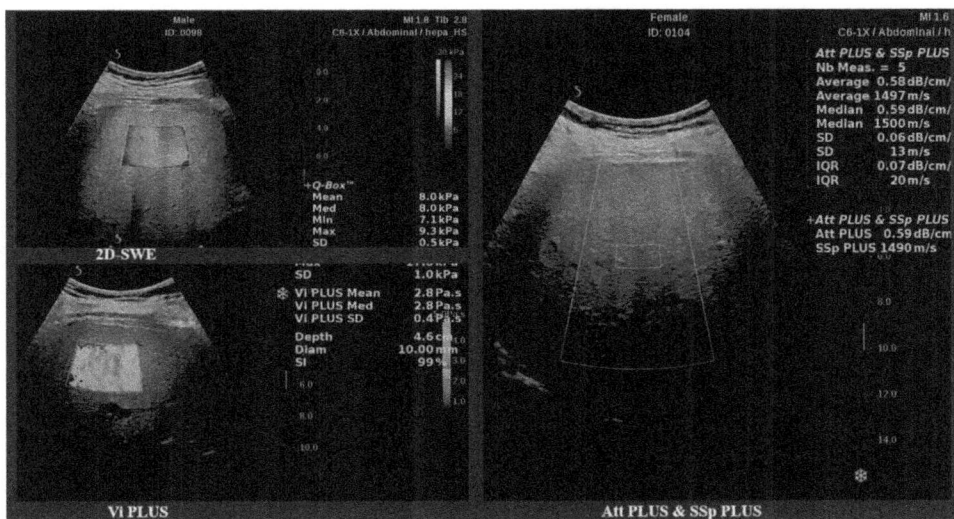

Figure 9.
Multiparameter ultrasound: 2D-SWE, Vi PLUS (viscosity index) and AttPLUS and SSpPLUS quantification.

In this moment, the main challenge in this field is to start the screening of the population at risk (MAFLD patients) for all the parameters of NAFLD [88]. Using simple biological tests [89] or maybe more sophisticated systems, such as ultrasound based or maybe MRI-based elastography, we can identify patients with advanced disease. Then intensive measures for such patients must be implemented.

5. Conclusion

Ultrasound methods are very useful for the evaluation of NAFLD patients. Identification of steatosis can be performed with standard ultrasound. Quantification of steatosis, fibrosis and inflammation can be assessed quickly with new high-tech ultrasound machines. Screening of patients at risk for the fatty liver with these modern tools is a challenge for the near future.

Author details

Ioan Sporea[1*], Raluca Lupuşoru[1,2] and Roxana Şirli[1,3]

1 Regional Center of Research in Advanced Hepatology, Academy of Medical Sciences, Timişoara, Romania

2 Center of Modelling Biomedical Systems and Data Analysis, Department of Functional Sciences, "Victor Babeş" University of Medicine and Pharmacy Timişoara, Romania

3 Department of Internal Medicine II, Division of Gastroenterology and Hepatology, Center for Advanced Research in Gastroenterology and Hepatology, "Victor Babeş" University of Medicine and Pharmacy Timişoara, Romania

*Address all correspondence to: isporea@umft.ro

IntechOpen

References

[1] Mitra S, De A, Chowdhury A. Epidemiology of non-alcoholic and alcoholic fatty liver diseases. Translational Gastroenterology and Hepatology. 2020;**5**:16. DOI: 10.21037/tgh.2019.09.08

[2] Younossi ZM, Koenig AB, Abdelatif D, Fazel Y, Henry L, Wymer M. Global epidemiology of nonalcoholic fatty liver disease-meta-analytic assessment of prevalence, incidence, and outcomes. Hepatology. 2016;**64**(1):73-84. DOI: 10.1002/hep.28431

[3] Estes C, Razavi H, Loomba R, Younossi Z, Sanyal AJ. Modeling the epidemic of nonalcoholic fatty liver disease demonstrates an exponential increase in burden of disease. Hepatology. 2018;**67**(1):123-133. DOI: 10.1002/hep.29466

[4] Perumpail BJ, Khan MA, Yoo ER, Cholankeril G, Kim D, Ahmed A. Clinical epidemiology and disease burden of nonalcoholic fatty liver disease. World Journal of Gastroenterology. 2017;**23**(47):8263-8276. DOI: 10.3748/wjg.v23.i47.8263

[5] Björkström K, Franzén S, Eliasson B, Miftaraj M, Gudbjörnsdottir S, Trolle-Lagerros Y, et al. Risk factors for severe liver disease in patients with type 2 diabetes. Clinical Gastroenterology and Hepatology. 2019;**17**(13):2769-2775.e4. DOI: 10.1016/j.cgh.2019.04.038

[6] Wong RJ, Aguilar M, Cheung R, Perumpail RB, Harrison SA, Younossi ZM, et al. Nonalcoholic steatohepatitis is the second leading etiology of liver disease among adults awaiting liver transplantation in the United States. Gastroenterology. 2015;**148**(3):547-555. DOI: 10.1053/j.gastro.2014.11.039

[7] Noureddin M, Vipani A, Bresee C, Todo T, Kim IK, Alkhouri N, et al. NASH leading cause of liver transplant in women: Updated analysis of indications for liver transplant and ethnic and gender variances. The American Journal of Gastroenterology. 2018;**113**(11):1649-1659. DOI: 10.1038/s41395-018-0088-6

[8] Younossi ZM, Stepanova M, Ong J, Trimble G, AlQahtani S, Younossi I, et al. Nonalcoholic steatohepatitis is the Most rapidly increasing indication for liver transplantation in the United States. Clinical Gastroenterology and Hepatology. 2021;**19**(3):580-589.e5. DOI: 10.1016/j.cgh.2020.05.064

[9] Eslam M, Sanyal AJ, George J. International consensus panel. MAFLD: A consensus-driven proposed nomenclature for metabolic associated fatty liver disease. Gastroenterology. 2020;**158**(7):1999-2014.e1. DOI: 10.1053/j.gastro.2019.11.312

[10] Lin S, Huang J, Wang M, Kumar R, Liu Y, Liu S, et al. Comparison of MAFLD and NAFLD diagnostic criteria in real world. Liver International. 2020;**40**(9):2082-2089. DOI: 10.1111/liv.14548

[11] Sporea I, Popescu A, Dumitraşcu D, Brisc C, Nedelcu L, Trifan A, et al. Nonalcoholic fatty liver disease: Status quo. Journal of Gastrointestinal and Liver Diseases. 2018;**27**(4):439-448. DOI: 10.15403/jgld.2014.1121.274.quo

[12] European Association for the Study of the Liver. Clinical Practice Guideline Panel; Chair: EASL Governing Board representative: Panel members. EASL clinical practice guidelines on non-invasive tests for evaluation of liver disease severity and prognosis - 2021

update. Journal of Hepatology. 2021;**75**(3):659-689. DOI: 10.1016/j.jhep.2021.05.025

[13] Dietrich CF, Bamber J, Berzigotti A, Bota S, Cantisani V, et al. EFSUMB guidelines and recommendations on the clinical use of liver ultrasound Elastography, update 2017 (long version). Ultraschall in der Medizin-European Journal of Ultrasound. 2017;**38**(4):e16-e47. English. DOI: 10.1055/s-0043-103952 Erratum in: Ultraschall Med. 2017 Aug;38(4):e48.

[14] Ferraioli G, Wong VW, Castera L, Berzigotti A, Sporea I, Dietrich CF, et al. Liver ultrasound Elastography: An update to the world Federation for Ultrasound in medicine and biology guidelines and recommendations. Ultrasound in Medicine & Biology. 2018;**44**(12):2419-2440. DOI: 10.1016/j.ultrasmedbio.2018.07.008

[15] Mathiesen UL, Franzén LE, Aselius H, Resjö M, Jacobsson L, Foberg U, et al. Increased liver echogenicity at ultrasound examination reflects degree of steatosis but not of fibrosis in asymptomatic patients with mild/moderate abnormalities of liver transaminases. Digestive and Liver Disease. 2002;**34**(7):516-522. DOI: 10.1016/s1590-8658(02)80111-6

[16] Palmentieri B, de Sio I, La Mura V, Masarone M, Vecchione R, Bruno S, et al. The role of bright liver echo pattern on ultrasound B-mode examination in the diagnosis of liver steatosis. Digestive and Liver Disease. 2006;**38**(7):485-489. DOI: 10.1016/j.dld.2006.03.021

[17] Hernaez R, Lazo M, Bonekamp S, Kamel I, Brancati FL, Guallar E, et al. Diagnostic accuracy and reliability of ultrasonography for the detection of fatty liver: A meta-analysis. Hepatology.

2011;**54**(3):1082-1090. DOI: 10.1002/hep.24452

[18] Gaitini D, Baruch Y, Ghersin E, Veitsman E, Kerner H, Shalem B, et al. Feasibility study of ultrasonic fatty liver biopsy: Texture vs. attenuation and backscatter. Ultrasound in Medicine & Biology. 2004;**30**(10):1321-1327. DOI: 10.1016/j.ultrasmedbio.2004.08.001

[19] Mihăilescu DM, Gui V, Toma CI, Popescu A, Sporea I. Computer aided diagnosis method for steatosis rating in ultrasound images using random forests. Medical Ultrasonography. 2013;**15**(3):184-190. DOI: 10.11152/mu.2013.2066.153.dmm1vg2

[20] Byra M, Styczynski G, Szmigielski C, Kalinowski P, Michałowski Ł, Paluszkiewicz R, et al. Transfer learning with deep convolutional neural network for liver steatosis assessment in ultrasound images. International Journal of Computer Assisted Radiology and Surgery. 2018;**13**(12):1895-1903. DOI: 10.1007/s11548-018-1843-2

[21] Chan WK, Nik Mustapha NR, Mahadeva S. Controlled attenuation parameter for the detection and quantification of hepatic steatosis in nonalcoholic fatty liver disease. Journal of Gastroenterology and Hepatology. 2014;**29**(7):1470-1476. DOI: 10.1111/jgh.12557

[22] de Lédinghen V, Wong GL, Vergniol J, Chan HL, Hiriart JB, Chan AW, et al. Controlled attenuation parameter for the diagnosis of steatosis in non-alcoholic fatty liver disease. Journal of Gastroenterology and Hepatology. 2016;**31**(4):848-855. DOI: 10.1111/jgh.13219

[23] Imajo K, Kessoku T, Honda Y, Tomeno W, Ogawa Y, Mawatari H, et al.

Magnetic resonance imaging more accurately classifies steatosis and fibrosis in patients with nonalcoholic fatty liver disease than transient Elastography. Gastroenterology. 2016;**150**(3):626-637.e7. DOI: 10.1053/j.gastro.2015.11.048

[24] Park CC, Nguyen P, Hernandez C, Bettencourt R, Ramirez K, Fortney L, et al. Magnetic resonance Elastography vs transient Elastography in detection of fibrosis and noninvasive measurement of steatosis in patients with biopsy-proven nonalcoholic fatty liver disease. Gastroenterology. 2017;**152**(3):598-607.e2. DOI: 10.1053/j.gastro.2016.10.026

[25] Naveau S, Voican CS, Lebrun A, Gaillard M, Lamouri K, Njiké-Nakseu M, et al. Controlled attenuation parameter for diagnosing steatosis in bariatric surgery candidates with suspected nonalcoholic fatty liver disease. European Journal of Gastroenterology & Hepatology. 2017;**29**(9):1022-1030. DOI: 10.1097/MEG.0000000000000919

[26] Siddiqui MS, Vuppalanchi R, Van Natta ML, Hallinan E, Kowdley KV, Abdelmalek M, et al. NASH clinical research network. Vibration-controlled transient Elastography to assess fibrosis and steatosis in patients with nonalcoholic fatty liver disease. Clinical Gastroenterology and Hepatology. 2019;**17**(1):156-163.e2. DOI: 10.1016/j.cgh.2018.04.043

[27] Shalimar KR, Rout G, Kumar R, Yadav R, Das P, Aggarwal S, et al. Body mass index-based controlled attenuation parameter cut-offs for assessment of hepatic steatosis in non-alcoholic fatty liver disease. Indian Journal of Gastroenterology. 2020;**39**(1):32-41. DOI: 10.1007/s12664-019-00991-2

[28] Oeda S, Takahashi H, Imajo K, Seko Y, Ogawa Y, Moriguchi M, et al. Accuracy of liver stiffness measurement and controlled attenuation parameter using FibroScan® M/XL probes to diagnose liver fibrosis and steatosis in patients with nonalcoholic fatty liver disease: A multicenter prospective study. Journal of Gastroenterology. 2020;**55**(4):428-440. DOI: 10.1007/s00535-019-01635-0

[29] Eddowes PJ, Sasso M, Allison M, Tsochatzis E, Anstee QM, Sheridan D, et al. Accuracy of FibroScan controlled attenuation parameter and liver stiffness measurement in assessing steatosis and fibrosis in patients with nonalcoholic fatty liver disease. Gastroenterology. 2019;**156**(6):1717-1730. DOI: 10.1053/j.gastro.2019.01.042

[30] Petroff D, Blank V, Newsome PN, Shalimar VCS, Thiele M, et al. Assessment of hepatic steatosis by controlled attenuation parameter using the M and XL probes: An individual patient data meta-analysis. The Lancet Gastroenterology & Hepatology. 2021;**6**(3):185-198. DOI: 10.1016/S2468-1253(20)30357-5

[31] Karlas T, Petroff D, Sasso M, Fan JG, Mi YQ, de Lédinghen V, et al. Individual patient data meta-analysis of controlled attenuation parameter (CAP) technology for assessing steatosis. Journal of Hepatology. 2017;**66**(5):1022-1030. DOI: 10.1016/j.jhep.2016.12.022

[32] Kamali L, Adibi A, Ebrahimian S, Jafari F, Sharifi M. Diagnostic performance of ultrasonography in detecting fatty liver disease in comparison with Fibroscan in people suspected of fatty liver. Advanced Biomedical Research. 2019;**8**:69. DOI: 10.4103/abr.abr_114_19

[33] Zenovia S, Stanciu C, Sfarti C, Singeap AM, Cojocariu C, Girleanu I, et al. Vibration-controlled transient Elastography and controlled attenuation parameter for the diagnosis of liver steatosis and fibrosis in patients

with nonalcoholic fatty liver disease. Diagnostics (Basel). 2021;**11**(5):787. DOI: 10.3390/diagnostics11050787

[34] Mikolasevic I, Domislovic V, Klapan M, Juric T, Lukic A, Krznaric-Zrnic I, et al. Accuracy of controlled attenuation parameter and liver stiffness measurement in patients with non-alcoholic fatty liver disease. Ultrasound in Medicine & Biology. 2021;**47**(3):428-437. DOI: 10.1016/j.ultrasmedbio.2020.11.015

[35] Gu Q, Cen L, Lai J, Zhang Z, Pan J, Zhao F, et al. A meta-analysis on the diagnostic performance of magnetic resonance imaging and transient elastography in nonalcoholic fatty liver disease. European Journal of Clinical Investigation. 2021;**51**(2):e13446. DOI: 10.1111/eci.13446

[36] Chan WK, Nik Mustapha NR, Mahadeva S, Wong VW, Cheng JY, Wong GL. Can the same controlled attenuation parameter cut-offs be used for M and XL probes for diagnosing hepatic steatosis? Journal of Gastroenterology and Hepatology. 2018;**33**(10):1787-1794. DOI: 10.1111/jgh.14150

[37] Caussy C, Brissot J, Singh S, Bassirian S, Hernandez C, Bettencourt R, et al. Prospective, same-day, direct comparison of controlled attenuation parameter with the M vs the XL probe in patients with nonalcoholic fatty liver disease, using magnetic resonance imaging-proton density fat fraction as the standard. Clinical Gastroenterology and Hepatology. 2020;**18**(8):1842-1850. e6. DOI: 10.1016/j.cgh.2019.11.060

[38] Fujiwara Y, Kuroda H, Abe T, Ishida K, Oguri T, Noguchi S, et al. The B-mode image-guided ultrasound attenuation parameter accurately detects hepatic steatosis in chronic liver disease. Ultrasound in Medicine & Biology. 2018;**44**(11):2223-2232. DOI: 10.1016/j. ultrasmedbio.2018.06.017

[39] Ferraioli G, Maiocchi L, Savietto G, Tinelli C, Nichetti M, Rondanelli M, et al. Performance of the attenuation imaging Technology in the Detection of liver steatosis. Journal of Ultrasound in Medicine. 2021;**40**(7):1325-1332. DOI: 10.1002/jum.15512

[40] Bae JS, Lee DH, Lee JY, Kim H, Yu SJ, Lee JH, et al. Assessment of hepatic steatosis by using attenuation imaging: A quantitative, easy-to-perform ultrasound technique. European Radiology. 2019;**29**(12):6499-6507. DOI: 10.1007/ s00330-019-06272-y

[41] Jeon SK, Lee JM, Joo I, Yoon JH, Lee DH, Lee JY, et al. Prospective evaluation of hepatic steatosis using ultrasound attenuation imaging in patients with chronic liver disease with magnetic resonance imaging proton density fat fraction as the reference standard. Ultrasound in Medicine & Biology. 2019;**45**(6):1407-1416. DOI: 10.1016/j.ultrasmedbio.2019.02.008

[42] Tamaki N, Koizumi Y, Hirooka M, Yada N, Takada H, Nakashima O, et al. Novel quantitative assessment system of liver steatosis using a newly developed attenuation measurement method. Hepatology Research. 2018;**48**(10):821-828. DOI: 10.1111/hepr.13179

[43] Dioguardi Burgio M, Imbault M, Ronot M, Faccinetto A, Van Beers BE, Rautou PE, et al. Ultrasonic adaptive sound speed estimation for the diagnosis and quantification of hepatic steatosis: A pilot study. Ultraschall in der Medizin-European Journal of Ultrasound. 2019;**40**(6):722-733. English. DOI: 10.1055/a-0660-9465

[44] Popa A, Bende F, Șirli R, Popescu A, Bâldea V, Lupușoru R, et al. Quantification of liver fibrosis, steatosis, and viscosity using multiparametric ultrasound in patients with non-alcoholic

liver disease: A "real-life" cohort study. Diagnostics (Basel). 2021;**11**(5):783. DOI: 10.3390/diagnostics11050783

[45] Jeon SK, Lee JM, Joo I, Park SJ. Quantitative ultrasound radiofrequency data analysis for the assessment of hepatic steatosis in nonalcoholic fatty liver disease using magnetic resonance imaging proton density fat fraction as the reference standard. Korean Journal of Radiology. 2021;**22**(7):1077-1086. DOI: 10.3348/kjr.2020.1262

[46] Ekstedt M, Hagström H, Nasr P, Fredrikson M, Stål P, Kechagias S, et al. Fibrosis stage is the strongest predictor for disease-specific mortality in NAFLD after up to 33 years of follow-up. Hepatology. 2015;**61**(5):1547-1554. DOI: 10.1002/hep.27368

[47] Hagström H, Nasr P, Ekstedt M, Hammar U, Stål P, Hultcrantz R, et al. Fibrosis stage but not NASH predicts mortality and time to development of severe liver disease in biopsy-proven NAFLD. Journal of Hepatology. 2017;**67**(6):1265-1273. DOI: 10.1016/j. jhep.2017.07.027

[48] Wong VW, Vergniol J, Wong GL, Foucher J, Chan HL, Le Bail B, et al. Diagnosis of fibrosis and cirrhosis using liver stiffness measurement in nonalcoholic fatty liver disease. Hepatology. 2010;**51**(2):454-462. DOI: 10.1002/hep.23312

[49] Cassinotto C, Boursier J, de Lédinghen V, Lebigot J, Lapuyade B, et al. Liver stiffness in nonalcoholic fatty liver disease: A comparison of supersonic shear imaging, FibroScan, and ARFI with liver biopsy. Hepatology. 2016;**63**(6):1817-1827. DOI: 10.1002/hep.28394

[50] Petta S, Wong VW, Cammà C, Hiriart JB, Wong GL, Marra F, et al. Improved noninvasive prediction of liver fibrosis by liver stiffness measurement in patients with nonalcoholic fatty liver disease accounting for controlled attenuation parameter values. Hepatology. 2017;**65**(4):1145-1155. DOI: 10.1002/hep.28843

[51] Yoneda M et al. Transient elastography in patients with non-alcoholic fatty liver disease (NAFLD). Gut. 2007;**56**:1330-1331. DOI: 10.1136/gut.2007.126417

[52] Gaia S, Carenzi S, Barilli AL, Bugianesi E, Smedile A, Brunello F, et al. Reliability of transient elastography for the detection of fibrosis in non-alcoholic fatty liver disease and chronic viral hepatitis. Journal of Hepatology. 2011;**54**(1):64-71. DOI: 10.1016/j. jhep.2010.06.022

[53] Kumar R, Rastogi A, Sharma MK, Bhatia V, Tyagi P, Sharma P, et al. Liver stiffness measurements in patients with different stages of nonalcoholic fatty liver disease: Diagnostic performance and clinicopathological correlation. Digestive Diseases and Sciences. 2013;**58**(1):265-274. DOI: 10.1007/s10620-012-2306-1

[54] Lupsor M, Badea R, Stefanescu H, Grigorescu M, Serban A, Radu C, et al. Performance of unidimensional transient elastography in staging non-alcoholic steatohepatitis. Journal of Gastrointestinal and Liver Diseases. 2010;**19**(1):53-60

[55] Petta S, Di Marco V, Cammà C, Butera G, Cabibi D, Craxì A. Reliability of liver stiffness measurement in non-alcoholic fatty liver disease: The effects of body mass index. Alimentary Pharmacology & Therapeutics. 2011;**33**(12):1350-1360. DOI: 10.1111/j.1365-2036.2011.04668.x

[56] Ratziu V, Bugianesi E, Dixon J, Fassio E, Ekstedt M, Charlotte F, et al. Histological progression of non-alcoholic fatty liver disease: A critical reassessment

based on liver sampling variability. Alimentary Pharmacology & Therapeutics. 2007;**26**(6):821-830. DOI: 10.1111/j.1365-2036.2007.03425.x

[57] Yoneda M, Yoneda M, Mawatari H, Fujita K, Endo H, et al. Noninvasive assessment of liver fibrosis by measurement of stiffness in patients with nonalcoholic fatty liver disease (NAFLD). Digestive and Liver Disease. 2008;**40**(5):371-378. DOI: 10.1016/j.dld.2007.10.019

[58] Nobili V, Vizzutti F, Arena U, Abraldes JG, Marra F, Pietrobattista A, et al. Accuracy and reproducibility of transient elastography for the diagnosis of fibrosis in pediatric nonalcoholic steatohepatitis. Hepatology. 2008;**48**(2):442-448. DOI: 10.1002/hep.22376

[59] Wong VW, Vergniol J, Wong GL, Foucher J, Chan AW, Chermak F, et al. Liver stiffness measurement using XL probe in patients with nonalcoholic fatty liver disease. The American Journal of Gastroenterology. 2012;**107**:1862-1871. DOI: 10.1038/ajg.2012.331

[60] Musso G, Gambino R, Cassader M, Pagano G. Meta-analysis: Natural history of non-alcoholic fatty liver disease (NAFLD) and diagnostic accuracy of non-invasive tests for liver disease severity. Annals of Medicine. 2011;**43**(8):617-649. DOI: 10.3109/07853890.2010.518623

[61] Yoneda M, Suzuki K, Kato S, Fujita K, Nozaki Y, Hosono K, et al. Nonalcoholic fatty liver disease: US-based acoustic radiation force impulse elastography. Radiology. 2010;**256**(2):640-647. DOI: 10.1148/radiol.10091662

[62] Mahadeva S, Mahfudz AS, Vijayanathan A, Goh KL, Kulenthran A, Cheah PL. Performance of transient elastography (TE) and factors associated with discordance in non-alcoholic fatty liver disease. Journal of Digestive Diseases. 2013;**14**(11):604-610. DOI: 10.1111/1751-2980.12088

[63] Pathik P, Ravindra S, Ajay C, Prasad B, Jatin P, Prabha S. Fibroscan versus simple noninvasive screening tools in predicting fibrosis in high-risk nonalcoholic fatty liver disease patients from Western India. Annals of Gastroenterology. 2015;**28**(2):281-286

[64] Seki K, Shima T, Oya H, Mitsumoto Y, Mizuno M, Okanoue T. Assessment of transient elastography in Japanese patients with non-alcoholic fatty liver disease. Hepatology Research. 2017;**47**(9):882-889. DOI: 10.1111/hepr.12829

[65] Lee MS, Bae JM, Joo SK, Woo H, Lee DH, Jung YJ, et al. Prospective comparison among transient elastography, supersonic shear imaging, and ARFI imaging for predicting fibrosis in nonalcoholic fatty liver disease. PLoS One. 2017;**12**(11):e0188321. DOI: 10.1371/journal.pone.0188321 Erratum in: PLoS One. 2018 Jun 26;13(6):e0200055.

[66] Hsu C, Caussy C, Imajo K, Chen J, Singh S, Kaulback K, et al. Magnetic resonance vs transient Elastography analysis of patients with nonalcoholic fatty liver disease: A systematic review and pooled analysis of individual participants. Clinical Gastroenterology and Hepatology. 2019;**17**(4):630-637.e8. DOI: 10.1016/j.cgh.2018.05.059

[67] Attia D, Bantel H, Lenzen H, Manns MP, Gebel MJ, Potthoff A. Liver stiffness measurement using acoustic radiation force impulse elastography in overweight and obese patients. Alimentary Pharmacology & Therapeutics. 2016;**44**(4):366-379. DOI: 10.1111/apt.13710

[68] Myers RP, Pomier-Layrargues G, Kirsch R, Pollett A, Duarte-Rojo A, Wong D, et al. Feasibility and diagnostic performance of the FibroScan XL probe for liver stiffness measurement in overweight and obese patients. Hepatology. 2012;**55**(1):199-208. DOI: 10.1002/hep.24624

[69] Myers RP, Elkashab M, Ma M, Crotty P, Pomier-Layrargues G. Transient elastography for the noninvasive assessment of liver fibrosis: A multicentre Canadian study. Canadian Journal of Gastroenterology. 2010;**24**(11):661-670. DOI: 10.1155/2010/153986

[70] Furlan A, Tublin ME, Yu L, Chopra KB, Lippello A, Behari J. Comparison of 2D shear wave Elastography, transient Elastography, and MR Elastography for the diagnosis of fibrosis in patients with nonalcoholic fatty liver disease. AJR. American Journal of Roentgenology. 2020 Jan;**214**(1):W20-W26. DOI: 10.2214/AJR.19.21267

[71] Leong WL, Lai LL, Nik Mustapha NR, Vijayananthan A, Rahmat K, Mahadeva S, et al. Comparing point shear wave elastography (ElastPQ) and transient elastography for diagnosis of fibrosis stage in non-alcoholic fatty liver disease. Journal of Gastroenterology and Hepatology. 2020;**35**(1):135-141. DOI: 10.1111/jgh.14782

[72] Imajo K, Honda Y, Kobayashi T, Nagai K, Ozaki A, Iwaki M, et al. Direct comparison of US and MR Elastography for staging liver fibrosis in patients with nonalcoholic fatty liver disease. Clinical Gastroenterology and Hepatology. 2020;**S1542-3565**(20):31673-31676. DOI: 10.1016/j.cgh.2020.12.016

[73] Fierbinteanu Braticevici C, Sporea I, Panaitescu E, Tribus L. Value of acoustic radiation force impulse imaging elastography for non-invasive evaluation of patients with nonalcoholic fatty liver disease. Ultrasound in Medicine & Biology. 2013;**39**(11):1942-1950. DOI: 10.1016/j.ultrasmedbio.2013.04.019

[74] Cassinotto C, Lapuyade B, Aït-Ali A, Vergniol J, Gaye D, Foucher J, et al. Liver fibrosis: Noninvasive assessment with acoustic radiation force impulse elastography--comparison with FibroScan M and XL probes and FibroTest in patients with chronic liver disease. Radiology. 2013;**269**(1):283-292. DOI: 10.1148/radiol.13122208

[75] Friedrich-Rust M, Romen D, Vermehren J, Kriener S, Sadet D, Herrmann E, et al. Acoustic radiation force impulse-imaging and transient elastography for non-invasive assessment of liver fibrosis and steatosis in NAFLD. European Journal of Radiology. 2012;**81**(3):e325-ee31. DOI: 10.1016/j.ejrad.2011.10.029

[76] Osaki A, Kubota T, Suda T, Igarashi M, Nagasaki K, Tsuchiya A, et al. Shear wave velocity is a useful marker for managing nonalcoholic steatohepatitis. World Journal of Gastroenterology: WJG. 2010;**16**(23):2918

[77] Palmeri ML, Wang MH, Rouze NC, Abdelmalek MF, Guy CD, Moser B, et al. Noninvasive evaluation of hepatic fibrosis using acoustic radiation force-based shear stiffness in patients with nonalcoholic fatty liver disease. Journal of Hepatology. 2011;**55**(3):666-672. DOI: 10.1016/j.jhep.2010.12.019

[78] Cui J, Heba E, Hernandez C, Haufe W, Hooker J, Andre MP, et al. Magnetic resonance elastography is superior to acoustic radiation force impulse for the diagnosis of fibrosis in patients with biopsy-proven nonalcoholic fatty liver disease: A prospective study. Hepatology.

2016;**63**(2):453-461. DOI: 10.1002/hep.28337

[79] Li Y, Dong C. Diagnostic value of acoustic radiation force impluse imaging and APRI ratio index for quantitative for evaluating the degree of liver fibrosis in non-alcoholic fatty liver disease patients. Chinese Journal of Ultrasound in Medicine. 2017;(12):544-548

[80] Sharpton SR, Tamaki N, Bettencourt R, Madamba E, Jung J, Liu A, et al. Diagnostic accuracy of two-dimensional shear wave elastography and transient elastography in non-alcoholic fatty liver disease. Therapeutic Advances in Gastroenterology. 2021;**14**:17562848211050436. DOI: 10.1177/17562848211050436. PMID: 34646360; PMCID: PMC8504217

[81] Herrmann E, de Lédinghen V, Cassinotto C, Chu WC, Leung VY, Ferraioli G, et al. Assessment of biopsy-proven liver fibrosis by two-dimensional shear wave elastography: An individual patient data-based meta-analysis. Hepatology. 2018;**67**(1):260-272. DOI: 10.1002/hep.29179

[82] Takeuchi H, Sugimoto K, Oshiro H, Iwatsuka K, Kono S, Yoshimasu Y, et al. Liver fibrosis: Noninvasive assessment using supersonic shear imaging and FIB4 index in patients with non-alcoholic fatty liver disease. Journal of Medical Ultrasonics (2001). 2018;**45**(2):243-249. DOI: 10.1007/s10396-017-0840-3

[83] Jamialahmadi T, Nematy M, Jangjoo A, Goshayeshi L, Rezvani R, Ghaffarzadegan K, et al. Measurement of liver stiffness with 2D-shear wave Elastography (2D-SWE) in bariatric surgery candidates reveals acceptable diagnostic yield compared to liver biopsy. Obesity Surgery. 2019;**29**(8):2585-2592. DOI: 10.1007/s11695-019-03889-2

[84] Barr RG, Wilson SR, Rubens D, Garcia-Tsao G, Ferraioli G. Update to the Society of Radiologists in ultrasound liver Elastography consensus statement. Radiology. 2020;**296**(2):263-274. DOI: 10.1148/radiol.2020192437

[85] Castera L, Friedrich-Rust M, Loomba R. Noninvasive assessment of liver disease in patients with nonalcoholic fatty liver disease. Gastroenterology. 2019;**156**(5):1264-1281.e4. DOI: 10.1053/j.gastro.2018.12.036

[86] Lee DH, Cho EJ, Bae JS, Lee JY, Yu SJ, Kim H, et al. Accuracy of two-dimensional shear wave Elastography and attenuation imaging for evaluation of patients with nonalcoholic steatohepatitis. Clinical Gastroenterology and Hepatology. 2021;**19**(4):797-805.e7. DOI: 10.1016/j.cgh.2020.05.034

[87] Sugimoto K, Moriyasu F, Oshiro H, Takeuchi H, Abe M, Yoshimasu Y, et al. The role of multiparametric US of the liver for the evaluation of nonalcoholic steatohepatitis. Radiology. 2020;**296**(3):532-540. DOI: 10.1148/radiol.2020192665

[88] Sporea I. To screen or not to screen for NAFLD? Medical Ultrasonography. 2021;**23**(2):133-134. DOI: 10.11152/mu-3251

[89] Pandyarajan V, Gish RG, Alkhouri N, Noureddin M. Screening for nonalcoholic fatty liver disease in the primary care clinic. Gastroenterology & Hepatology (NY). 2019;**15**(7):357-365

Chapter 3

The Place of Liver Elastography in Diagnosis of Alcohol-Related Liver Disease

Alina Popescu and Camelia Foncea

Abstract

Harmful use of alcohol is associated with more than 200 diseases and types of injuries, the liver being one of the most important targets. Alcoholic liver disease (ALD) is the most frequent cause of severe chronic liver disease in Europe and worldwide. ALD can progress from alcoholic fatty liver to alcoholic steatohepatitis and alcoholic liver cirrhosis, the grade of fibrosis being the key prognostic factor for the severity of the diseases. This chapter will present the place of liver elastography in the noninvasive assessment of ALD. It will describe the data available in the literature regarding the different elastography techniques for liver stiffness assessment and also the potential of these techniques for screening ALD.

Keywords: liver elastography, alcoholic liver disease, alcoholic steatohepatitis, alcoholic liver cirrhosis, liver fibrosis

1. Introduction

Alcohol-related liver disease (ALD) is one of the major causes of liver injury worldwide, according to WHO [1]. More than 40% of the liver deaths are attributed to alcohol [2] and the indication for liver transplant in patients with ALD has significantly increased, being the top health burden. ALD is rarely detected at early stages, most of the patients being diagnosticated at the decompensation stage, when liver cirrhosis and its complications occur [3].

Diagnosis of ALD is suspected when alcohol consumption is >20 g/d in females and > 30 g/d in males and clinical and/or biological modifications suggestive of liver injury or extrahepatic manifestations of alcohol use disorder (AUD) occur [4]. Because a high proportion of patients with AUD do not express clinical symptoms or laboratory abnormalities, asymptomatic patients with harmful use of alcohol should undergo appropriate screening investigations [5].

ALD follows the typical progression of chronic liver diseases including alcoholic liver steatosis, steatohepatitis, fibrosis, and liver cirrhosis. Approximately 90% of heavy drinkers will develop liver steatosis and 5–10% liver cirrhosis in 5 years [6]. Liver cirrhosis is the main predictor of survival [7], so early recognition of fibrosis is the most important objective in this category of patients. On the other hand, another argument for early detection and diagnosis of patients with harmful use of alcohol is that the risk of developing liver disease decreases with abstinence [4]. ALD remains underestimated due to bad reporting of real alcohol consumption and a lack of specific investigations.

The main points to address in front of a patient with ALD from the hepatological point of view would be the evaluation of liver steatosis, inflammation, and fibrosis.

Liver biopsy remains the "gold standard" of diagnosis and staging for diffuse liver changes [4] since it is able to evaluate all points presented above; however, it is an invasive method, less likely accepted by patients, with a 7% rate of complications and sampling errors [8]. Noninvasive methods for evaluating steatosis and fibrosis in ALD gained a lot of interest lately, with many studies supporting their usefulness [9], but we still lack reliable noninvasive methods for grading liver inflammation. The main advantages of these noninvasive methods are the easy acceptability by patients, repeatability, and low costs. They consist of serum markers and elastography methods [9].

Noninvasive liver fibrosis evaluation in ALD by serum markers/biological scores can be performed by patented or non-patented serum biomarkers. Enhanced Liver Fibrosis (ELF™) and FibroTest (FT) are most commonly used as patented biomarkers. In a meta-analysis performed on nine studies, the ELF test showed good performance for the prediction of histological fibrosis stage [10]. A prospective study found that ELF and FT also had comparable diagnostic accuracy for ALD when it comes to AUROC, 0.92 for ELF and 0.9 for FT, and can rule out advanced fibrosis for ALD based on an ELF <10.5 or an FT value below 0.58 [11].

Nonpatented serum markers have been assessed in ALD for the diagnosis of liver fibrosis—age-platelet index, the aspartate transaminase (AST)-platelet-ratio index APRI [12], fibrosis-4 index-FIB-4 [13], and AST/alanine aminotransferase (ALT) ratio-AST/ALT [14]. A comparison of the performance of the different biological scores suggests that ELF and FT are better in the diagnosis of LF in ALD (**Table 1**) [9, 16].

From an economical point of view, patented scores for ALD have higher costs than nonpatented but provide the best diagnostic performance of advanced liver fibrosis. Lifetime health costs in ALD are very high in decompensated stages, so noninvasive methods were proven to be cost-effective [17].

For liver steatosis assessment several methods can be used as noninvasive techniques such as ultrasound-based methods or magnetic resonance imaging (MRI)-based methods. In the following part of this chapter, ultrasound-based methods will be

Test	AUC	Se (%)	Sp (%)
APRI cut off 0.5 [15]	0.79	84	41
APRI ≥ 1 [11]	0.80	38	90
FIB-4 ≥ 3.25 [11]	0.85	58	91
AST/ALT ratio ≥ 1 [11]	0.76	85	46
Age-platelet index ≥ 6.0 [11]	0.81	65	85
ELF ≥ 10.5 [11]	0.92	79	91
FT ≥ 0.58 [11]	0.90	67	87

APRI – aspartate transaminase-platelet ratio index; FIB-4 – fibrosis 4 index; ELF-Enhanced Liver Fibrosis; FT – Fibrotest; AUC – area under the curve; Se – sensitivity; and Sp – specificity.

Table 1.
Comparison and performance of biological tests for the diagnosis of advanced fibrosis (F3) in studies with biopsy-proven ALD.

introduced. MRI methods use MRI-PDFF (proton density fat fraction) and a routinely used MRI scanner to identify liver steatosis. MRI sensitivity and specificity are 76.7–90.0% and 80.2–87.0%, respectively. It is not affected by the etiology of liver disease or other abnormalities such as inflammation, most seen in ALD or iron overload. It has several advantages such as the highest accuracy following liver biopsy for liver steatosis diagnosis, but the major disadvantages include the high cost, long time of examination, and the inability to be used in claustrophobic or overweight patients [18, 19].

Liver elastography by means of transient elastography compared to serum markers is superior when it comes to liver stiffness assessment [20], and in the following sections, the place of noninvasive ultrasound-based steatosis quantification methods and ultrasound-based elastography techniques in ALD are presented in detail.

In patients with suspected ALD (presence of alcohol use disorder-AUD, abnormal liver test or extrahepatic manifestations of AUD, and no other causes of chronic liver disease), noninvasive tests can be transferred into clinical practice for the detection of advanced fibrosis. Physical and biological approaches are complementary and both methods should be used starting from primary care to facilitate the early detection of ALD. First of all, patients should be routinely screened for AUD using AUDIT questionnaire [4]. Further, patients can be easily assessed by primary care using patented or nonpatented biological scores and in case of liver fibrosis presence, redirected to second-line assessment made by a liver specialist, to validate the results by elastography methods. All patients with AUD need to be referred to a specialized withdrawal center. Follow-up can be performed by primary care or in case of advanced liver fibrosis by liver clinic units for specific investigations [7, 16].

2. Alcoholic liver steatosis assessment by ultrasound-based methods

Hepatic steatosis is characterized by accumulation of fat-lipids, especially triglycerides in hepatocytes, and when is over 5%, it is considered pathological. It is usually asymptomatic and is mainly caused by alcohol use and metabolic factors. In patients with AUD, liver steatosis can be reversible with abstinence. Steatosis severity is associated with lobular inflammation and fibrosis [21]. Approximately 90% of patients with AUD will develop liver steatosis [6].

Liver biopsy remains the gold standard of steatosis assessment, but has many drawbacks, like potential complications, sampling error, invasive, and is difficult for patients to accept this method as a follow-up method [8]. Noninvasive methods were developed to easily assess patients at risk of developing liver steatosis.

Because fat accumulation alters liver imagistic appearance, B-mode ultrasound (US) is the first-line technique used for screening and assessment of fatty liver [9]. It is a safe method, available, accessible, repeatable, and cost-efficient, with a sensitivity between 60 and 94% and specificity between 88 and 95% in detecting steatosis [22]. However, it has a better performance in detecting severe liver steatosis as compared to mild steatosis, is operator-dependent, and cannot give information related to fibrosis presence [23]. Magnetic resonance imaging (MRI)-proton density fat fraction (PDFF) is considered the most specific and sensitive technique for liver steatosis assessment [24], but it is not appropriate as a point of care technique because it requires complex evaluation by specialized radiologists, has high costs, and is not available in all centers. Also, it is not possible in the case of obese, claustrophobic patients and with metallic devices implanted [24].

A novel noninvasive ultrasound-based elastographic parameter called CAP-controlled attenuation parameter has been developed for life's steatosis assessment. It is based on vibration controlled transient elastography (VTCE) and is incorporated in FibroScan (Echosens, Paris, France) device and allows, in the same session, the evaluation of steatosis and fibrosis [25]. It is based on ultrasound attenuation, a physical characteristic of the propagation medium, which means the loss of energy when ultrasound spreads through this medium, and fat is known to be an attenuating medium [26]. CAP has been first developed on the M probe with a center frequency of 3.5 MHz [26], but when applied to overweight and obese patients the performance was impaired because of the thick subcutaneous fat layer. XL probe was then developed on 2.5 MHz and it measures to a depth of 7.5 cm [27]. The results are given in decibels per meter (dB/m) with a range from 100 to 400 dB/m. CAP is displayed only when liver stiffness measurements (LSMs) are valid, and it is recommended as a point-of-care technique for the detection of liver steatosis by the World Federation for Ultrasound in Medicine and Biology (WFUMB) [28].

CAP proved to have good accuracy for diagnosing steatosis in studies and meta-analysis including mixed cohorts [25] and especially in NAFLD [29]. In ALD, only one study is available from Thiele M. et al. [30], including 562 patients with ALD who underwent CAP, B-mode ultrasound, and liver biopsy. CAP proved to be superior to steatosis liver pattern by standard ultrasound. A CAP value over 290 dB/m ruled in any steatosis with 88% specificity, while CAP below 220 dB/m ruled out liver steatosis with 90% sensitivity. Moreover, CAP showed AUROCs of 0.77, 0.78, and 0.82 for mild, moderate, and severe steatosis, respectively. CAP had higher values for patients with ALD and metabolic syndrome (MetS) over imposed, with an average difference of 40 dB/m (302 ± 64 in patients with MetS vs. 262 ± 55 in patients without MetS; $P < 0.001$). The same was observed in patients with a BMI ≥ 30 kg/m^2 with a difference of 49 dB/m (311 ± 48 in obese patients versus 261 ± 57 in patients with BMI < 30; $P < 0.001$). In the same multicentric study, 293 patients were admitted for detoxification and CAP showed a decrease by 32 ± 47 dB/m, decreasing equally in patients with ALD with or without MetS, but did not significantly decrease in obese patients after detoxification. There was no evidence that CAP influences liver stiffness measurements by TE or vice-versa. Diagnostic accuracy of CAP seems to be lower in mild steatosis compared to other etiologies and optimal cut-offs, which varies in the different studies performed; variation is possibly explained by the pattern of alcohol consumption in the moment of investigations; hence, evaluation of CAP in ALD remains a challenge.

Several other ultrasound equipment developers designed new ultrasound-based steatosis quantification software embedded in ultrasound machines, based mainly also on the evaluation of the ultrasound beam attenuation. Such examples are Ultrasound-Guided Attenuation Parameter (UGAP) from General Electric Healthcare, Attenuation imaging (ATI) developed by Canon, Attenuation (ATT) from Hitachi, SSp.PLUS (Sound Speed Plane-wave UltraSound) and Att.PLUS (Attenuation Plane-wave UltraSound) from Supersonic Imagine, and TAI™ (Tissue Attenuation Image) & TSI™ (Tissue Scatter-distribution Image) from Samsung; all emerging techniques are under evaluation but with no data yet related to ALD.

3. Alcoholic-induced liver fibrosis evaluation by ultrasound-based elastography

Because the presence of liver fibrosis and liver cirrhosis is the main predictor of survival in patients with ALD, liver stiffness (LS) assessment is very important in high-risk patients [7]. Liver fibrosis assessment can be performed by biological

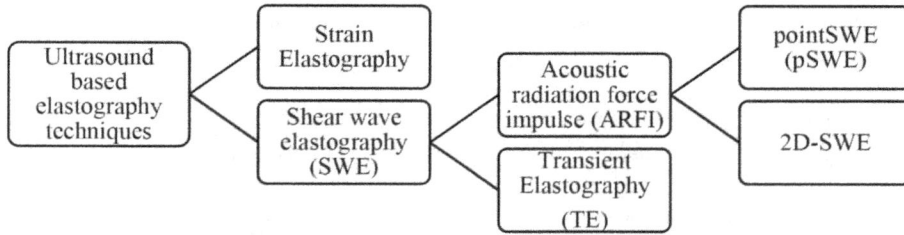

Figure 1.
Classification of ultrasound-based elastography methods.

and elastography methods in the detriment of liver biopsy. Direct comparison with serum markers showed a better performance of TE in patients with ALD [20] with an AUROCs >0.9 for F4 cirrhosis diagnosis. In this chapter, we will discuss only the ultrasound-based elastography methods.

Liver elastography methods became more and more reliable in the liver stiffness measurement (LSM), being supported by recently published guidelines [28, 31]. The methods are classified into shear wave elastography (SWE) and strain elastography (SE) (**Figure 1**). Both guidelines support that SWE is the best for clinical use in LSM.

4. Ultrasound-based elastography techniques

Transient elastography (TE) (FibroScan, EchoSens, Paris, and France), the first elastography technique developed, is the most widely used method, and it is noninvasive, rapid, and reproducible, with lower sampling errors [9]. The most important published studies in ALD are listed in the table below, majority of them biopsy-proven (**Table 2**). These studies showed good performance in the diagnosis of liver cirrhosis with AUROCs from 0.87 [41] to 0.97 [40], but the cut-off values differ quite a bit, most likely due to the presence of inflammation in these patients, given by recent alcohol consumption and assessed by AST levels. Several studies performed by Mueller et al. [40, 45, 46] show that absolute alcohol withdrawal leads to a 13% reduction of LS after one week and even a reduction of 40% in alcohol consumption can lead to a 17% reduction of LS [24]. In another study, LS improved in almost 80% of patients admitted for alcohol detoxification due to the coexistence of inflammation seen by AST >100 U/ml [25]. Preliminary observational data on long-term abstinence, observed over a period of more than 5 years, show LS decreases by 50% and also LS again increases by 22% if alcohol consumption continues [46]. **Table 3** resumes the data on alcohol abstinence/ relapse and LS improvement.

TE is followed by other ultrasound-based methods, such as point Share Wave Elastography (pSWE), Two-Dimensional Share Wave Elastography (2D-SWE), or Time-Harmonic Elastography embedded in ultrasound systems [47–53]. There are few studies that show data on the performance of pSWE or 2D-SWE in ALD (**Table 4**), with a small number of included patients, and in some studies, data show a wide range of values.

An important aspect of liver elastography in alcohol-induced liver fibrosis, compared to the rest of liver fibrosis etiologies is the presence of inflammation given by the levels of AST. In alcoholic liver disease, AST levels are typically higher as compared to ALT [58]. Although in cirrhotic stages, liver transaminases normalize, if alcohol consumption is continued, AST may be continuously increased.

Reference	Number of patients (n)	Elastography method	Cut-off values for different fibrosis stage		
			F2	F3	F4
Anastasiou 2010 [32]	14 patients	TE	>7.15 kPa		>12.5 kPa
Bardou-Jacquet 2013 [33]	8 patients	TE	>7.15 kPa		>17 kPa
Boursier 2009 [34]	106 patients	TE	>7.15 kPa	>9.5 kPa	>17.3 kPa
de Ledinghen 2012 [35]	34 patients	TE	>7.15 kPa	>9.5 kPa	>12.5 kPa
Fernandez 2012 [36]	139 patients	TE	>7.15 kPa	>10.5 kPa	>18 kPa
Janssens 2010 [37]	49 patients	TE	>7.15 kPa		>21.1 kPa
Lannerstedt 2013 [38]	16 patients	TE	>7.15 kPa	>9.5 kPa	>12.5 kPa
Lemoine 2008 [39]	48 patients	TE	>7.15 kPa		>34.9 kPa
Mueller 2010 [40]	101 patients	TE	>7.15 kPa	>8 kPa	>11.5 kPa
Nahon 2008 [41]	147 patients	TE	>7.15 kPa		>22.6 kPa
Nguyen-Khac 2008 [20]	103 patients	TE	>7.15 kPa	>11 kPa	>19.5 kPa
Muller 2015 [42]	364 patients	TE	>6 kPa	>8 kPa	>12.5 kPa
Voican 2017 [43]	188 patients	TE	—	>13 kPa	>20.8 kPa
Kim 2009 [44]	45 patients	TE	>7.15 kPa	>9.5 kPa	>25.8 kPa

Table 2.
Elastography in ALD patients performed by TE.

Reference	Patients (n)	Time	Mean LS Before/after	LS improvement
Mueller 2020 [45]	45- reduction of alcohol consumption and treatment with Nalmefene	12 weeks	10.5 kPa–8.7 kPa	−13%
Mueller 2010 [40]	50- detoxification	5 days	20.1 kPa–16.5 kPa	−17%
Mueller 2020 [46]	23- abstinence 23-relapse	5.7 years 5.3 years	20.5–10.5 kPa 14.8 kPa–18.1 kPa	−48% +22%

Table 3.
Alcohol abstinence/relapse and liver stiffness improvement.

The presence of steatohepatitis with AST >100 U/ml will increase liver stiffness in patients with ALD, so it was proposed to assess the presence of advanced fibrosis when AST decreases below <100 U/ml [40]. For that, an algorithm was developed for inflammation-adapted cut-off values in ALD [42], based on a multicentric study that included over 2000 patients with biopsy-proven HCV and ALD. In the absence of inflammation given by elevated transaminases, cut-off values for ALD and HCV were similar. The cut-off values increased exponentially in relation to median AST. After the formula was applied there was an improved agreement of the AST cut-off values with the histological stage for both HCV and ALD, so using inflammation-adapted cut-off values avoid repetitive assessment of LS in ALD.

In a recent meta-analysis [43], it was proved that in addition to AST, bilirubin can have a significant effect on LS assessment in ALD. Bilirubin was independently

Reference	Number of patients (n)	Elastography technique	Cut-off values for different fibrosis stage		
			F2	F3	F4
Thiele 2016 [54]	199 patients	2D-SWE	>10.2 kPa	—	>16.4 kPa
Kiani 2016 [55]	69 patients	pSWE	>1.63 m/s	>1.84 m/s	>1.94 m/s
Zhang 2015 [56]	112 patients	pSWE	>1.27 m/s	>1.40 m/s	>1.65 m/s
Cho Y 2020 [57]	251 patients	pSWE	>1.46 m/s	>1.47 m/s	>1.66 m/s

Table 4.
Elastography in ALD patients performed by 2D-SWE and pSWE.

associated with the presence of asymptomatic and non-severe steatohepatitis on histological features.

From an economical perspective, lifetime health care costs associated with ALD in advanced stages are very high, so noninvasive elastography methods for the diagnosis of advanced alcohol liver fibrosis were proven to be cost-effective [17] and may be used also for screening.

5. Conclusion

Because alcohol-related liver diseases are increasing, there is an unmet need for the identification and evaluation of patients at risk. Noninvasive elastography methods allow screening, diagnosis, and follow-up of liver steatosis and liver fibrosis in patients with ALD, with good accuracy and performance.

Conflict of interest

Alina Popescu has received speaker fees from Philips, General Electric Healthcare. Camelia Foncea has nothing to declare.

Author details

Alina Popescu[1,2]* and Camelia Foncea[1,2]

1 Division of Gastroenterology and Hepatology, Department of Internal Medicine II, Center for Advanced Research in Gastroenterology and Hepatology "Victor Babes" University of Medicine and Pharmacy Timisoara, Romania

2 Center for Advanced Hepatology Research of the Academy of Medical Sciences Timişoara, Romania

*Address all correspondence to: alinamircea.popescu@gmail.com

IntechOpen

References

[1] Kim D, Li AA, Gadiparthi C, Khan MA, Cholankeril G, Glenn JS, et al. Chronic liver disease, from 2007 through 2016. Gastroenterology. 2018;**155**:1154-1163.e3. DOI: 10.1053/j. gastro.2018.07.008.Changing

[2] Sepanlou SG, Safiri S, Bisignano C, Ikuta KS, Merat S, Saberifiroozi M, et al. The global, regional, and national burden of cirrhosis by cause in 195 countries and territories, 1990-2017: A systematic analysis for the Global Burden of Disease Study 2017. The Lancet Gastroenterology & Hepatology. 2020;**5**:245-266. DOI: 10.1016/S2468-1253(19)30349-8

[3] Sweatt SK, Gower BA, Chieh AY, Liu Y, Li L. 乳鼠心肌提取 HHS public access. Physiology & Behavior. 2016;**176**:139-148. DOI: 10.1016/j. cgh.2019.01.026.Alcohol-related

[4] Thursz M, Gual A, Lackner C, Mathurin P, Moreno C, Spahr L, et al. EASL clinical practice guidelines: Management of alcohol-related liver disease. Journal of Hepatology. 2018;**69**:154-181. DOI: 10.1016/j. jhep.2018.03.018

[5] Askgaard G, Leon DA, Kjær MS, Deleuran T, Gerds TA, Tolstrup JS. Risk for alcoholic liver cirrhosis after an initial hospital contact with alcohol problems: A nationwide prospective cohort study. Hepatology. 2017;**65**:929-937. DOI: 10.1002/hep.28943

[6] Gao B, Bataller R. Alcoholic liver disease: Pathogenesis and new therapeutic targets. Gastroenterology. 2011;**141**:1572-1585. DOI: 10.1053/j. gastro.2011.09.002

[7] Seitz HK, Bataller R, Cortez-Pinto H, Gao B, Gual A, Lackner C, et al. Alcoholic liver disease. Nature Reviews. Disease Primers. 28 Aug 2018;**4**(1):18

[8] Filingeri V, Francioso S, Sforza D, Santopaolo F, Oddi FM, Tisone G. A retrospective analysis of 1.011 percutaneous liver biopsies performed in patients with liver transplantation or liver disease: Ultrasonography can reduce complications? European Review for Medical and Pharmacological Sciences. 2016;**20**:3609-3617

[9] Moreno C, Mueller S, Szabo G. Non-invasive diagnosis and biomarkers in alcohol-related liver disease. Journal of Hepatology. 2019;**70**:273-283. DOI: 10.1016/j.jhep.2018.11.025

[10] Xie Q, Zhou X, Huang P, Wei J, Wang W, Zheng S. The performance of enhanced liver fibrosis (ELF) test for the staging of liver fibrosis: A meta-analysis. PLoS ONE. 2014;**9**(4):e92772. DOI: 10.1371/journal.pone.0092772

[11] Thiele M, Madsen BS, Hansen JF, Detlefsen S, Antonsen S, Krag A. Accuracy of the enhanced liver fibrosis test vs fibrotest, elastography, and indirect markers in detection of advanced fibrosis in patients with alcoholic liver disease. Gastroenterology. 2018;**154**:1369-1379. DOI: 10.1053/j. gastro.2018.01.005

[12] Wai CT, Greenson JK, Fontana RJ, Kalbfleisch JD, Marrero JA, Conjeevaram HS, et al. A simple noninvasive index can predict both significant fibrosis and cirrhosis in patients with chronic hepatitis C. Hepatology. 2003;**38**:518-526. DOI: 10.1053/jhep.2003.50346

[13] Sterling RK, Lissen E, Clumeck N, Sola R, Correa MC, Montaner J, et al.

Development of a simple noninvasive index to predict significant fibrosis in patients with HIV/HCV coinfection. Hepatology. 2006;**43**:1317-1325. DOI: 10.1002/hep.21178

[14] Williams ALB, Hoofnagle JH. Ratio of serum aspartate to alanine aminotransferase in chronic hepatitis relationship to cirrhosis. Gastroenterology. 1988;**95**:734-739. DOI: 10.1016/S0016-5085(88)80022-2

[15] Jin W, Lin Z, Xin Y, Jiang X, Dong Q, Xuan S. Diagnostic accuracy of the aspartate aminotransferase-to-platelet ratio index for the prediction of hepatitis B-related fibrosis: A leading meta-analysis. BMC Gastroenterology. 2012;**12**:14. DOI: 10.1186/1471-230X-12-14

[16] Hadefi A, Degré D, Trépo E, Moreno C. Noninvasive diagnosis in alcohol-related liver disease. Health Scientific Reports. 2020;**3**(1):e146. DOI: 10.1002/hsr2.146

[17] Asphaug L, Thiele M, Krag A, Melberg HO. Cost-effectiveness of noninvasive screening for alcohol-related liver fibrosis. Hepatology. 2020;**71**:2093-2104. DOI: 10.1002/hep.30979

[18] Noureddin M, Lam J, Peterson MR, Middleton M, Hamilton G, Le TA, et al. Utility of magnetic resonance imaging versus histology for quantifying changes in liver fat in nonalcoholic fatty liver disease trials. Hepatology. 2013;**58**:1930-1940. DOI: 10.1002/hep.26455

[19] Lee SS, Park SH. Radiologic evaluation of nonalcoholic fatty liver disease. World Journal of Gastroenterology. 2014;**20**:7392-7402. DOI: 10.3748/wjg.v20.i23.7392

[20] Nguyen-Khac E, Chatelain D, Tramier B, Decrombecque C, Robert B, Joly JP, et al. Assessment of asymptomatic liver fibrosis in alcoholic patients using fibroscan: Prospective comparison with seven non-invasive laboratory tests. Alimentary Pharmacology & Therapeutics. 2008;**28**:1188-1198. DOI: 10.1111/j.1365-2036.2008.03831.x

[21] Chalasani N, Wilson L, Kleiner DE, Cummings OW, Brunt EM, Ünalp A. Relationship of steatosis grade and zonal location to histological features of steatohepatitis in adult patients with non-alcoholic fatty liver disease. Journal of Hepatology. 2008;**48**:829-834. DOI: 10.1016/j.jhep.2008.01.016

[22] Lupşor-Platon M, Stefănescu H, Mureşcan D, Florea M, Erzsébet Szász M, Maniu A, et al. Noninvasive assessment of liver steatosis using ultrasound methods. Medical Ultrasonography. 2014;**16**:236-245. DOI: 10.11152/mu.2013.2066.163.1mlp

[23] Schwenzer NF, Springer F, Schraml C, Stefan N, Machann J, Schick F. Non-invasive assessment and quantification of liver steatosis by ultrasound, computed tomography and magnetic resonance. Journal of Hepatology. 2009;**51**:433-445. DOI: 10.1016/j.jhep.2009.05.023

[24] Zhang Y, Fowler KJ, Hamilton G, Cui JY, Sy EZ, Balanay M, et al. Liver fat imaging-a clinical overview of ultrasound, CT, and M R imaging. The British Journal of Radiology. Sep 2018;**91**(1089):20170959. DOI:10.1259/bjr.20170959

[25] Karlas T, Petroff D, Sasso M, Fan JG, Mi YQ, de Lédinghen V, et al. Individual patient data meta-analysis of controlled attenuation parameter (CAP) technology for assessing steatosis. Journal of Hepatology. 2017;**66**:1022-1030. DOI: 10.1016/j.jhep.2016.12.022

[26] Sasso M, Beaugrand M, de Ledinghen V, Douvin C, Marcellin P,

Poupon R, et al. Controlled attenuation parameter (CAP): A novel VCTE™ guided ultrasonic attenuation measurement for the evaluation of hepatic steatosis: Preliminary study and validation in a cohort of patients with chronic liver disease from various causes. Ultrasound in Medicine & Biology. 2010;**36**:1825-1835. DOI: 10.1016/j.ultrasmedbio.2010.07.005

[27] Sasso M, Audière S, Kemgang A, Gaouar F, Corpechot C, Chazouillères O, et al. Liver Steatosis Assessed by Controlled Attenuation Parameter (CAP) measured with the XL Probe of the FibroScan: A Pilot Study Assessing Diagnostic Accuracy. Ultrasound in Medicine & Biology. 2016;**42**:92-103. DOI: 10.1016/j.ultrasmedbio.2015.08.008

[28] Ferraioli G, Wong VWS, Castera L, Berzigotti A, Sporea I, Dietrich CF, et al. Liver ultrasound elastography: An update to the world federation for ultrasound in medicine and biology guidelines and recommendations. Ultrasound in Medicine & Biology. 2018;**44**:2419-2440. DOI: 10.1016/j.ultrasmedbio.2018.07.008

[29] Eddowes PJ, Sasso M, Allison M, Tsochatzis E, Anstee QM, Sheridan D, et al. Accuracy of FibroScan controlled attenuation parameter and liver stiffness measurement in assessing steatosis and fibrosis in patients with nonalcoholic fatty liver disease. Gastroenterology. 2019;**156**:1717-1730. DOI: 10.1053/j.gastro.2019.01.042

[30] Thiele M, Rausch V, Fluhr G, Kjærgaard M, Piecha F, Mueller J, et al. Controlled attenuation parameter and alcoholic hepatic steatosis: Diagnostic accuracy and role of alcohol detoxification. Journal of Hepatology. 2018;**68**:1025-1032. DOI: 10.1016/j.jhep.2017.12.029

[31] Dietrich CF, Bamber J, Berzigotti A, Bota S, Cantisani V, Castera L, et al. EFSUMB guidelines and

recommendations on the clinical use of liver ultrasound elastography. Ultraschall in der Medizin - European Journal of Ultrasound. Aug 2017;**38**(4):e16-e47. DOI: 10.1055/s-0043-103952

[32] Anastasiou J, Alisa A, Virtue S, Portmann B, Murray-Lyon I, Williams R. Noninvasive markers of fibrosis and inflammation in clinical practice: Prospective comparison with liver biopsy. European Journal of Gastroenterology & Hepatology. 2010;**22**:474-480. DOI: 10.1097/MEG.0b013e328332dd0a

[33] Bardou-Jacquet E, Legros L, Soro D, Latournerie M, Guillygomarc A, Le Lan C, et al. Effect of alcohol consumption on liver stiffness measured by transient elastography. World Journal of Gastroenterology. 2013;**19**:516-522. DOI: 10.3748/wjg.v19.i4.516

[34] Boursier J, Vergniol J, Sawadogo A, Dakka T, Michalak S, Gallois Y, et al. The combination of a blood test and Fibroscan improves the non-invasive diagnosis of liver fibrosis. Liver International. 2009;**29**:1507-1515. DOI: 10.1111/j.1478-3231.2009.02101.x

[35] De Lédinghen V, Wong VWS, Vergniol J, Wong GLH, Foucher J, Chu SHT, et al. Diagnosis of liver fibrosis and cirrhosis using liver stiffness measurement: Comparison between M and XL probe of FibroScan®. Journal of Hepatology. 2012;**56**:833-839. DOI: 10.1016/j.jhep.2011.10.017

[36] Fernandez M, Trépo E, Degré D, Gustot T, Verset L, Demetter P, et al. Transient elastography using Fibroscan is the most reliable noninvasive method for the diagnosis of advanced fibrosis and cirrhosis in alcoholic liver disease. European Journal of Gastroenterology & Hepatology. 2015;**27**:1074-1079. DOI: 10.1097/MEG.0000000000000392

[37] Janssens F, De Suray N, Piessevaux H, Horsmans Y, De Timary P,

Stärkel P. Can transient elastography replace liver histology for determination of advanced fibrosis in alcoholic patients: A real-life study. Journal of Clinical Gastroenterology. 2010;**44**:575-582. DOI: 10.1097/MCG.0b013e3181cb4216

[38] Lannerstedt H, Konopski Z, Sandvik L, Haaland T, Loberg EM, Haukeland JW. Combining transient elastography with FIB4 enhances sensitivity in detecting advanced fibrosis of the liver. Scandinavian Journal of Gastroenterology. 2013;**48**:93-100. DOI: 10.3109/00365521.2012.746389

[39] Lemoine M, Katsahian S, Ziol M, Nahon P, Ganne-Carrie N, Kazemi F, et al. Liver stiffness measurement as a predictive tool of clinically significant portal hypertension in patients with compensated hepatitis C virus or alcohol-related cirrhosis. Alimentary Pharmacology & Therapeutics. 2008;**28**:1102-1110. DOI: 10.1111/j.1365-2036.2008.03825.x

[40] Mueller S, Millonig G, Sarovska L, Friedrich S, Reimann FM, Pritsch M, et al. Increased liver stiffness in alcoholic liver disease: Differentiating fibrosis from steatohepatitis. World Journal of Gastroenterology. 2010;**16**:966-972. DOI: 10.3748/wjg.v16.i8.966

[41] Nahon P, Kettaneh A, Tengher-Barna I, Ziol M, de Lédinghen V, Douvin C, et al. Assessment of liver fibrosis using transient elastography in patients with alcoholic liver disease. Journal of Hepatology. 2008;**49**:1062-1068. DOI: 10.1016/j.jhep.2008.08.011

[42] Mueller S, Englert S, Seitz HK, Badea RI, Erhardt A, Bozaari B, et al. Inflammation-adapted liver stiffness values for improved fibrosis staging in patients with hepatitis C virus and alcoholic liver disease. Liver

International. 2015;**35**:2514-2521. DOI: 10.1111/liv.12904

[43] Nguyen-Khac E, Thiele M, Voican C, Nahon P, Moreno C, Boursier J, et al. Non-invasive diagnosis of liver fibrosis in patients with alcohol-related liver disease by transient elastography: An individual patient data meta-analysis. The Lancet Gastroenterology & Hepatology. 2018;**3**:614-625. DOI: 10.1016/S2468-1253(18)30124-9

[44] Kim SG, Kim YS, Jung SW, Kim HK, Jang JY, Moon JH, et al. The usefulness of transient elastography to diagnose cirrhosis in patients with alcoholic liver disease. The Korean Journal of Hepatology. Korean. Mar 2009;**15**(1):42-51. DOI: 10.3350/kjhep.2009.15.1.42

[45] Mueller S, Luderer M, Zhang D, Meulien D, Brach BS, Schou MB. Open-label study with nalmefene as needed use in alcohol-dependent patients with evidence of elevated liver stiffness and/or hepatic steatosis. Alcohol and Alcoholism. 2020;**55**:63-70. DOI: 10.1093/alcalc/agz078

[46] Mueller S. Liver Elastography: Clinical Use and Interpretation. Springer. 2020

[47] Popa A, Șirli R, Popescu A, Bâldea V, Lupușoru R, Bende F, et al. Ultrasound-based quantification of fibrosis and steatosis with a new software considering transient elastography as reference in patients with chronic liver diseases. Ultrasound in Medicine and Biology. 2021;**47**(7):1692. DOI: 10.1016/j.ultrasmedbio.2021.02.029

[48] Voicu Moga T, Sporea I, Lupus R, Popescu A, Popa A, Bota S, et al. Performance of a noninvasive time-harmonic elastography technique for liver fibrosis evaluation using vibration controlled transient

elastography as reference method. Diagnostics. 2020;**10**:653. DOI: 10.3390/diagnostics10090653

[49] Popa A, Bende F, Şirli R, Popescu A, Bâldea V, Lupuşoru R, et al. Quantification of liver fibrosis, steatosis, and viscosity using multiparametric ultrasound in patients with non-alcoholic liver disease: A "Real-Life" Cohort Study. Diagnostics. 2021;**11**:783. DOI: 10.3390/diagnostics11050783

[50] Ferraioli G, Maiocchi L, Lissandrin R, Tinelli C, De Silvestri A, Filice C. Accuracy of the ElastPQ technique for the assessment of liver fibrosis in patients with chronic Hepatitis C: A "Real Life" Single Center Study. Journal of Gastrointestinal and Liver Diseases. 2016;**25**:331-335. DOI: 10.15403/jgld.2014.1121.253.epq

[51] Herrmann E, de Lédinghen V, Cassinotto C, Chu WCW, Leung VYF, Ferraioli G, et al. Assessment of biopsy-proven liver fibrosis by two-dimensional shear wave elastography: An individual patient data-based meta-analysis. Hepatology. 2018;**67**:260-272. DOI: 10.1002/hep.29179

[52] Bende F, Sporea I, Şirli R, Nistorescu S, Fofiu R, Bâldea V, et al. The performance of a 2-dimensional shear-wave elastography technique for predicting different stages of liver fibrosis using transient elastography as the control method. Ultrasound Quarterly. 2020;**37**(2):97-104. DOI: 10.1097/ruq.00000000000000527

[53] Foncea C, Popescu A, Lupuşoru R, Fofiu R, Şirli R, Danilă M, et al. Comparative study between pSWE and 2D-SWE techniques integrated in the same ultrasound machine, with Transient Elastography as the reference method. Medical Ultrasonography. 2020;**22**:13-19. DOI: 10.11152/mu-2179

[54] Thiele M, Detlefsen S, Sevelsted Møller L, Madsen BS, Fuglsang Hansen J, Fialla AD, et al. Transient and 2-dimensional shear-wave elastography provide comparable assessment of alcoholic liver fibrosis and cirrhosis. Gastroenterology. 2016;**150**:123-133. DOI: 10.1053/j.gastro.2015.09.040

[55] Kiani A, Brun V, Lainé F, Turlin B, Morcet J, Michalak S, et al. Acoustic radiation force impulse imaging for assessing liver fibrosis in alcoholic liver disease. World Journal of Gastroenterology. 2016;**22**:4926-4935. DOI: 10.3748/wjg.v22.i20.4926

[56] Zhang D, Li P, Chen M, Liu L, Liu Y, Zhao Y, et al. Non-invasive assessment of liver fibrosis in patients with alcoholic liver disease using acoustic radiation force impulse elastography. Abdominal Imaging. 2014;**40**:723-729. DOI: 10.1007/s00261-014-0154-5

[57] Cho Y, Choi YI, Oh S, Han J, Joo SK, Lee DH, et al. Point shear wave elastography predicts fibrosis severity and steatohepatitis in alcohol-related liver disease. Hepatology International. 2020;**14**:270-280. DOI: 10.1007/s12072-019-10009-w

[58] Mukai M, Ozasa K, Hayashi K, Kawai K. Various S-GOT/S-GPT ratios in nonviral liver disorders and related physical conditions and life-style. Digestive Diseases and Sciences. 2002;**47**:549-555. DOI: 10.1023/A:1017959801493

Chapter 4

Evaluation of Liver Fibrosis Using Shear Wave Elastography: An Overview

Dong Ho Lee, Jae Young Lee and Byung Ihn Choi

Abstract

All kinds of chronic liver disease can progress into liver fibrosis, and the stage of liver fibrosis is an important prognostic factor. Therefore, assessment of liver fibrosis is of importance for the management of the chronic liver disease. Although liver biopsy is considered the standard method, its invasive nature limits clinical use. In this regard, shear wave-based ultrasound elastography has been emerged as a noninvasive method to evaluate liver fibrosis. Among various techniques, transient elastography (TE) has been the most extensively used and validated method. TE provides good diagnostic performance in staging liver fibrosis. In addition to TE, point shear wave elastography (pSWE) and two-dimensional SWE (2D-SWE) have been developed as another noninvasive method, and also reported good diagnostic performance in staging liver fibrosis. Although TE, pSWE, and 2D-SWE show good performance in assessing liver fibrosis, concurrent inflammatory activity and/or hepatic congestion are important limitations in the current elastography technique.

Keywords: liver fibrosis, liver cirrhosis, shear wave elastography

1. Introduction

Chronic liver disease is a major healthcare problem worldwide, and various etiologies including viral hepatitis caused by hepatitis B virus (HBV) or hepatitis C virus (HCV), alcohol abuse, and non-alcoholic fatty liver disease (NAFLD) can induce chronic liver disease [1]. Moreover, chronic liver disease is an evolving and dynamic process, progressing into liver fibrosis [2–4]. When appropriate management is not given, liver injury and fibrosis can continuously progress, eventually leading to the development of liver cirrhosis, portal hypertension, hepatic insufficiency as well as hepatocellular carinoma (HCC) which can increase morbidity and mortality [5, 6]. In addition, the stage of liver fibrosis is associated with the risk of HCC development and liver-related mortality. Therefore, information regarding the stage of liver fibrosis is important for both surveillance and personalized treatment [7–9]. Owing to the dynamic and evolving nature, liver fibrosis would be reversible under the adequate management, especially in early stage of the disease. In contrast, liver cirrhosis is generally considered as an irreversible process [10–13]. Therefore, evaluation, as well as detection of liver fibrosis in the early stage, is of importance for the management of the chronic liver disease.

IntechOpen

For the assessment of liver fibrosis, liver biopsy with histopathologic examination has been used as the reference standard method [14]. In addition, histopathologic examination enables the evaluation of concurrent inflammatory activity in the liver, in addition to the assessment of liver fibrosis. However, liver biopsy has several important drawbacks limiting its clinical use. First, liver biopsy is an invasive procedure that can cause potentially lethal complications, such as bleeding. Due to the invasive nature, repeated biopsy for the monitoring of liver fibrosis during the disease course in the same patient can hardly be performed in clinical practice [15]. The small sample volume of liver biopsy, generally 1/50000th of total liver parenchyma, is another important limitation. When the distribution of liver fibrosis is heterogeneous, a small volume with sampling variability of liver biopsy can lead to either overestimation or under-estimation of liver fibrosis [16, 17]. Another important limitation of liver biopsy is considerable inter-reader variability, and the reported kappa value among the different pathologists varies from 0.5 to 0.9 [18, 19]. Therefore, there has been a continuous need for a reliable and noninvasive methods for the evaluation of liver fibrosis in clinical practice, and tremendous effort has been made to develop non-invasive diagnostic methods for the assessment of liver fibrosis [13]. In this regard, shear wave based ultrasound elastography has been developed and introduced as an accurate noninvasive diagnostic method for the evaluation of liver fibrosis. After the introduction of transient elastography (TE) which was the first commercially available liver elastography technique, various ultrasound-based shear wave elastography methods including point shear wave elastography (pSWE) and two-dimensional shear wave elastography (2D-SWE) have been introduced in clinical practice and reported a good diagnostic performance in assessing liver fibrosis [20, 21].

2. Principle of shear wave elastography

Elastography is an imaging technique measuring a tissue mechanical characteristic such as elasticity, that was firstly described by Ophir et al. [22]. Tissue elasticity is defined as the resistance to the deformation of a certain tissue against applied stress [15], and stiff tissue is more resistant to the deformation than soft tissue in given applied stress. For the superficial organs such as the breast and thyroid, tissue elasticity can be measured by using strain elastography. In strain elastography, stress to tissue is directly applied by manual compression of an ultrasound transducer, and then the degree of tissue deformation after compression is measured by ultrasound imaging [22]. Manual compression works fairly well for superficial organs, and therefore, strain elastography is a useful technique for the evaluation of breast or thyroid lesion, providing information regarding tissue stiffness [23]. However, it is very challenging to induce stress to deeper located organs by manual compression such as the liver, limiting the application of strain elastography to the liver [24]. For deeper located organs such as the liver, the stress can be employed by acoustic radiation force impulse (ARFI) or mechanical push pulse to generate a shear wave within the target tissue [15]. Since shear wave propagation velocity is related to tissue elasticity and the shear wave velocity is faster in stiff tissue than in soft tissue, measurement of shear wave velocity generated by either ARFI or mechanical push pulse leads to the quantitative assessment of tissue elasticity [23]. Given that, the type of ultrasound-based shear wave elastography for the liver can be determined by following two factors: 1) how to generate shear wave within the liver tissue?; and 2) how to measure the velocity of generated shear wave within the liver tissue?. Based on these two factors, currently, there are three available ultrasound-based shear wave elastography techniques for the liver: 1) one-dimensional transient elastography (TE); 2) point shear wave elastography (pSWE), and 3) two-dimensional shear wave elastography (2D-SWE) [23]. The characteristics of these three elastography techniques are summarized in **Table 1** and **Figure 1**.

2.1 Transient elastography

The FibroScan system (Echosens, Paris, France), which is TE system, was the first commercially available ultrasound-based shear wave elastography system for the liver [25]. The FibroScan probe contains both a mechanical vibrating device and an ultrasound transducer [23]. When the mechanical vibrating device part of FibroScan probe employs a 50 Hz mechanical impulse to the skin surface, the shear wave is generated and propagated within the liver tissue [15]. The generated shear wave within the liver tissue by mechanical push pulse applied to the skin surface is traced by an ultrasound transducer for the measurement of shear wave velocity. Then, liver stiffness can be calculated by measured shear wave velocity. The frequency of generated shear wave within liver tissue by mechanical push pulse in TE is 50 Hz. Although TE is an ultrasound-based technique, it is impossible to provide B-mode images of the liver in TE system, and therefore, TE is performed without direct B-mode image guidance [23]. The size of the measurement area of TE is approximately 1 cm width × 4 cm length, which is >100 times larger than the tissue volume assessed by a liver biopsy [26, 27]. There are several available probes for TE, and M probe with an operating center frequency of 3.5 MHz is used for the standard examination [15]. Since TE applies a mechanical push pulse to the skin surface for the generation of shear wave within the liver tissue, the presence of ascites and obesity limiting the

	Excitation method	Frequency of generated shear wave	Shear wave velocity measurement direction	Measurement area	Placement of region of interest	Reported parameter
TE	Mechanical push pulse	50 Hz	Parallel to excitation	Small	Restricted, no guidance	Young modulus (kPa)
pSWE	ARFI, single focal location	Wideband (100–500 Hz)	Perpendicular to ARFI application	Small	Flexible under B-mode guidance	Young modulus (kPa) or shear wave velocity (m/s)
2D-SWE	ARFI, multiple focal zones	Wideband (100–500 Hz)	Perpendicular to ARFI application	Medium	Flexible under B-mode guidance	Young modulus (kPa) or shear wave velocity (m/s)

Note: TE, transient elastography; pSWE, point shear wave elastography; 2D-SWE, two-dimensional shear wave elastography; ARFI, acoustic radiation force impulse; kPa, kilopascal.

Table 1.
Characteristics of currently available ultrasound based shear wave elastography techniques for the liver.

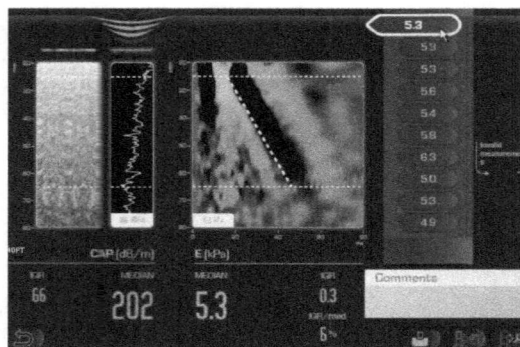

(a)

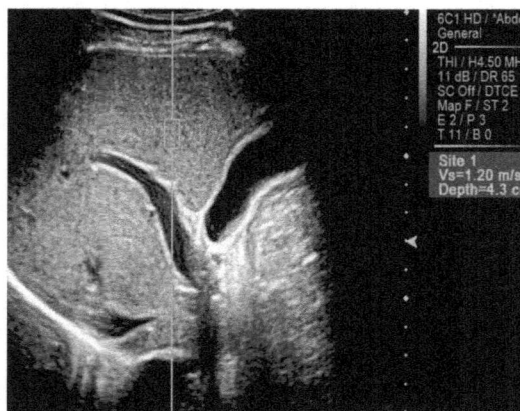

(b)

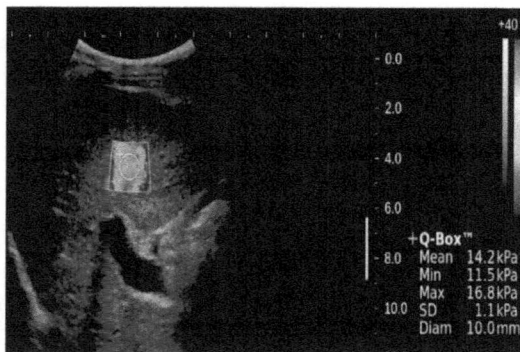

(c)

Figure 1.
*Currently available ultrasound-based shear wave elastography methods for the liver. (a) Transient elastography
(TE). In TE, B-mode images of the liver are not provided, and thus the measurement area cannot be selected.
Ten valid measurements were performed for this patient, and the IQR/M value was 6%, indicating reliable
measurement result. (b) Point shear wave elastography (pSWE) (Virtual touch quantification, Siemens Acouson
S2000). The measurement box is placed within liver parenchyma 2.5 cm apart from liver capsule. Since pSWE
provides B-mode images of the liver simultaneously, the placement of measurement box is undertaken under the
B-mode image guidance, avoiding large hepatic vessels or areas showing artifact. (c) Two-dimensional shear wave
elastography (2D-SWE) (Aixplorer, Supersonic Imagine). The size of measurement box of 2D-SWE is larger
than that of pSWE, and placed within liver parenchyma under the B-mode image guidance. 2D-SWE can also
provide color-coded elastogram, superimposed on B-mode image of the liver.*

shear wave generation by mechanical push pulse would be a drawback. In addition, M probe would have a limited ultrasound penetration for obese patients, hampering the accurate measurement of shear wave velocity. To overcome this limitation of M probe, XL probe with a lower operating frequency (2.5 MHz for XL probe vs. 3.5 MHz for M probe) enabling measurement at a greater depth (35–75 mm for XL probe vs. 25–65 mm for M probe) is introduced. Using XL probe, accurate and reliable measurement can be possible for obese patients.

2.2 Point shear wave elastography (pSWE)

In contrast to TE which uses a mechanical push pulse to generate a shear wave within the liver tissue, pSWE uses ARFI technique to induce stress and to generate a shear wave within the liver tissue. When ARFI is delivered in the liver tissue, the longitudinal waves along with the plane of applied ARFI are generated. At the same time, a portion of longitudinal waves is converted to shear waves within the liver tissue, and propagate perpendicular to the plane of longitudinal waves [28]. The frequency of generated shear wave by applied ARFI is wideband, ranging from 100 to 500 Hz. In pSWE, the velocity of the shear wave generated by ARFI is measured, which is either directly reported in meters per second or changed to Young's modulus E in kilopascal for the estimation of tissue elasticity [27]. Under the assumption of incompressibility, shear wave velocity can be converted to Young's modulus E by the following equation: E (kilopascal) = $3\rho c^2$, where c is the measured shear wave velocity in meter per second and ρ is the tissue density, assumed to be 1 of water [15]. Unlike TE, pSWE can be performed using a conventional ultrasound probe equipped with standard diagnostic ultrasound machine [27]. Therefore, pSWE can provide B-mode images of the liver simultaneously during the examination, enabling the selection of a uniform area of liver parenchyma without any large vessels, focal lesions, or artifacts where the shear wave velocity will be measured [23]. Given that, the accuracy and measurement reliability of pSWE are expected to be higher than those of TE. In addition, since the shear wave is generated by ARFI which is introduced inside the liver parenchyma, pSWE would be less affected by the presence of ascites and obesity than TE [9, 29, 30].

2.3 Two-dimensional shear wave elastography (2D-SWE)

2D-SWE is the newest ultrasound-based shear wave elastography technique, which also utilizes ARFI. In contrast to the pSWE which introduces ARFI in a single focal location, 2D-SWE uses multiple focused ultrasound push pulses to create multiple focal zones interrogated in rapid succession, faster than shear wave speed [23]. Those multiple push pulses in 2D-SWE generate a near cylindrical shear wave cone, allowing the real-time tracing of shear waves in 2D to measure the velocity of induced shear wave or Young's modulus E [23, 31]. The same as the pSWE, the frequency of generated shear wave by multiple push pulses in 2D-SWE is wideband, ranging from 100 to 500 Hz. Since 2D-SWE utilizes the conventional ultrasound probe for standard diagnostic imaging, it can also provide B-mode images of the liver simultaneously, and real-time visualization of a color-coded quantitative elastogram can be superimposed on a B-mide image. This merit of 2D-SWE allows the operator to obtain both anatomical and tissue stiffness information [20]. Currently, most of the major ultrasound vendors provide their own shear wave elastography technique for the liver, either form of pSWE or 2D-SWE.

3. Measurement protocol and reliability criteria

Regarding patient preparation, ultrasound-based shear wave elastography techniques including TE, pSWE, and 2D-SWE share the same recommended protocols [6, 32, 33]. Since the amount of portal flow can affect the result of liver stiffness measurement obtained by shear wave elastography, fasting for at least 4 hours before the examination is recommended for patients who undergo shear wave elastography examination to minimize the effect of portal flow. The liver stiffness measurement using shear wave elastography is usually performed in either supine or slightly left lateral decubitus position (not more than 30 degrees) with the right arm extended above the head to obtain the optimal sonic window via the stretching of the intercostal muscles [6, 34]. It has been known that both deep inspiration and deep expiration can have an influence on the result of liver stiffness measurement using shear wave elastography, and therefore, the neutral breath-hold is recommended for shear wave elastography examination to minimize the effect of breath-hold status. In addition to the aforementioned protocols for patient preparation, current guidelines for both pSWE and 2D-SWE have several recommendations for imaging acquisitions since pSWE as well as 2D-SWE provide B-mode images of the liver simultaneously, and the measurement area of pSWE and 2D-SWE can be selected under the real-time B-mode imaging guidance [6, 32, 33]. The transducer should be placed perpendicular to the liver capsule to ensure proper generation and propagation of the shear wave. The measurement box for both pSWE and 2D-SWE is placed parallel to the liver capsule, and the upper edge of the measurement box should be placed 1.5 to 2.0 cm apart from the liver capsule to minimize the effect of reverberation artifact which is generally seen in the area adjacent to the liver capsule. In most currently available ultrasound systems, the ARFI pulse reaches the maximum intensity at 4.0 to 4.5 cm apart from the transducer and is attenuated by 6.0–7.0 cm [6]. Given that, the area located at 4.0 to 4.5 cm apart from the transducer would be the optimal location for liver stiffness measurement. Since B-mode image is utilized to trace the shear wave in both pSWE and 2D-SWE, high-quality B-mode images without artifacts should be acquired for accurate and reliable

	Recommendation	Aim
Patient preparation	Fasting for at least 4 hours before examination	To minimize effect of portal flow
	Position: supine or slight left lateral decubitus (not more than 30°) with right arm extended above the head	To obtain optimal sonic window via stretching of the intercostal muscles
	Neutral breath hold, neither deep inspiration nor expiration	To minimize effect of breath-hold status
Imaging acquisition for pSWE and 2D-SWE	Transducer placed perpendicular to the liver capsule	To ensure proper shear wave generation
	Upper portion of measurement box placed at least 1.5–2.0 cm apart from liver capsule	To minimize effect of reverberation artifact
	Ideal location of measurement box: 4–4.5 cm apart from the transducer	To maximize intensity of ARFI pulse

Note: pSWE, point shear wave elastography; 2D-SWE, two-dimensional shear wave elastography; ARFI, acoustic radiation force impulse.

Table 2.
Recommendation for patient preparation and imaging acquisition.

liver stiffness measurement. The recommended protocols for both patient preparation and imaging acquisition are summarized in **Table 2**.

Regarding the acquisition number of liver stiffness measurements using TE, ten valid measurements are recommended. In addition, the interquartile range (IQR)-to-median ratio of ten valid measurements (subsequently referred to as IQR/M) is usually used as the quality criteria: IQR/M equal to or less than 30% indicates reliable measurement results [6, 32, 33]. According to the result of a study including 13,369 TE examinations using M probe [35], the failure rate of obtaining valid liver stiffness measurement and unreliable measurements rates was 3.1% of cases and 15.8% of cases, respectively. Regarding the contributory factors for failed and/or unreliable measurements of TE was body mass index [15, 35], and high body mass index was significantly associated with the failed and/or unreliable measurements. With the introduction of XL probe for TE examination, the reliability of liver stiffness measurements using TE has been improved, especially for NAFLD patients [36–40]. Regarding the measurement reproducibility of TE, excellent inter-reader agreement with the intraclass coefficient (ICC) of 0.98 was reported in a cohort of 188 patients having chronic HCV infection [41].

The recommended acquisition number of liver stiffness measurements using pSWE is also ten valid measurements. The same as the TE, the result with IQR/M equal to or less than 30% for measurement given in kilopascals is considered a reliable result. Regarding the 2D-SWE, the area for liver stiffness measurement is larger than pSWE, and thus, each liver stiffness measurement value is actually an average value of several measurements [6]. In addition, several manufacturers provide quality assessment methods for their 2D-SWE systems such as propagation map, stability index, and reliable measurement index [6]. Given that, the current guideline recommends five measurements for 2D-SWE when a quality assessment method is provided by the manufacturer. However, when a quality assessment method is not available, ten measurements for 2D-SWE are recommended, the same as the TE or pSWE [6]. IQR/M for measurement given in kilopascals is also used as the quality criteria for 2D-SWE, the same as the TE or pSWE. Result with IQR/M equal to or less than 30% of five or ten measurements given in kilopascals indicates reliable measurement results. It has been reported that when IQR/M for measurement given in kilopascals was higher than 30%, the accuracy of liver stiffness value obtained from shear wave elastography was reduced [33, 42, 43]. According to the result of a study comparing pSWE and 2D-SWE in 79 patients at the same day [44], the failure rate was 1.3% for pSWE and 5.1% for 2D-SWE, respectively. The overall intra-reader agreement was higher for pSWE than 2D-SWE (ICC of 0.915 for pSWE vs. ICC of 0.829 for 2D-SWE, P < 0.001). In addition, intra-reader reproducibility between liver stiffness measurements by using 2D-SWE performed in the same participant on different days was higher for the experienced operator than novice operator (ICC of 0.84 for experienced reader vs. 0.65 for novice reader) [45], indicating that reader experience has an influence on the measurement reliability. Ferraioli et al. also reported that the liver stiffness measurement by using pSWE was affected by operator experience [46]. Given that, operators doing pSWE and/or 2D-SWE examinations need to be properly trained and to follow the recommendations for patient preparation and imaging acquisition [15].

4. Diagnostic performance for staging liver fibrosis

Liver fibrosis is the result of chronic liver injury and is defined as an abnormal and excessive deposition of collagen and other extracellular matrix components in the liver [9, 47]. Essentially, any kind of chronic liver disease caused by HBV or HCV infection, alcohol abuse, and NAFLD lead to steatosis, inflammation with necrosis in response to an injury [9]. Without appropriate management, these liver cell injury continuously progresses, eventually developing liver cirrhosis. Information regarding the liver fibrosis stage is beneficial for the prediction of prognosis, personalized follow-up, and treatment decisions. For example, antiviral therapy for HBV or HCV infection might be guided by the information regarding the liver fibrosis stage [48, 49]. Therefore, an accurate assessment of the liver fibrosis stage is an important step for chronic liver disease management. For this purpose, liver biopsy with histopathologic examinations using various staging systems including Ishak, METAVIR, and Batts-Ludwig systems has been traditionally used as the standard reference method [18, 50]. However, liver biopsy is limited for widespread application in clinical practice, mainly due to its invasive nature. To overcome the limitation of liver biopsy, ultrasound-based shear wave elastography techniques including TE, pSWE, and 2D-SWE have been emerged as noninvasive methods for the evaluation of liver fibrosis and reported a good diagnostic performance.

4.1 *Transient elastography*

Since TE was the first approved and commercially available ultrasound-based elastography technique for the liver, there have been a lot of studies including meta-analyses reporting the diagnostic performance of TE in assessing liver fibrosis stage for chronic liver disease patients with various etiologies. Currently, TE is the most widely used and extensively validated elastography technique for liver stiffness measurement. Regarding the detection of advanced fibrosis and liver cirrhosis originated from HBV or HCV infection by using TE, early studies reported an excellent diagnostic performance with areas under the receiver operating characteristic curve (AUROCs) of 0.88–0.99 [51–57]. Several meta-analyses also reported the excellent diagnostic capability of TE to detect liver cirrhosis with AUROCs of 0.93–0.96, better than those for diagnosing moderate fibrosis (F2-F4) with AUROCs ranging from 0.83 to 0.88 [58–62]. The reported cut-off liver stiffness value was 7.0–7.9 kPa for the detection of moderate fibrosis (F2-F4) and 11.3–15.6 kPa for the diagnosis of cirrhosis (F4) [58–60, 63]. In addition to the HBV and HCV infection, TE also showed a good diagnostic performance in assessing liver fibrosis for NAFLD patients. However, the application of TE for NAFLD patients is challenging, mainly due to the high failure rate and poor measurement reliability in obese patients, especially when standard M probe is used. The reported rate of unreliable and/or failed measurement of TE for NAFLD patients ranged from 3.8% to 50.0% [38, 64, 65]. According to the result of a meta-analysis including 854 NAFLD patients with individual data, the reported pooled sensitivity and specificity of TE using the standard M probe was 79% and 75% to detect F2-F4, 85% and 82% to detect F3–4, and 92% and 92% to detect F4, respectively [66]. The AUROCs of TE ranged from 0.79–0.87 for detection of F2-F4, 0.76–0.98 for detection of F3-F4, and 0.91–0.99 for the diagnosis of F4, respectively, in NAFLD patients [15]. The introduction of XL probe for obese patients has improved the measurement reliability of TE [67].

4.2 Point shear wave elastography (pSWE) and two-dimensional shear wave elastography (2D-SWE)

Since both pSWE and 2D-SWE have become commercially available more lately than TE, the number of studies and the amount of data are less than those of TE.

Thus, the level of evidence for the diagnostic performance of pSWE or 2D-SWE in assessing the liver fibrosis stage is usually lower than that for TE.

Regarding the pSWE, several early studies reported a high accuracy for liver fibrosis staging in both HBV patients [68–71] and HCV patients [72–75]. For example, a study using pSWE done by Sporea et al. reported an AUROCs of 0.91 for detecting F3-F4 stage fibrosis and 0.94 for detecting cirrhosis (F4), respectively, in 274 patients having chronic HCV infection [72]. A meta-analysis including 21 studies containing 2691 individual data with chronic HBV or HCV infections showed an AUROCs of 0.88 for the detection of F2-F4, and 0.91 for the diagnosis of cirrhosis, respectively [76]. pSWE also provides a good diagnostic performance in diagnosing liver fibrosis stage for NAFLD patients, and the reported AUROCs of pSWE to detect liver cirrhosis (F4) was greater than 0.97 [77–80]. When pSWE was compared to TE for NAFLD patients in assessing liver fibrosis stage, there was no significant difference in diagnostic capability between the two elastography methods, although pSWE provided a significantly higher rate of reliable measurement [81].

In addition to pSWE, 2D-SWE also provides excellent diagnostic performance in assessing the liver fibrosis stage for patients having chronic HBV or HCV infection [20, 82–84]. However, since 2D-SWE is the newest elastography method, it has been less validated than TE or pSWE. A meta-analysis including seven studies using 2D-SWE in assessing liver fibrosis stage showed an AUROCs of 0.91 for detection of F2-F4 stage fibrosis and 0.95 for the diagnosis of liver cirrhosis (F4) [85]. In addition, recent studies reported that 2D-SWE showed a significant better diagnostic capability in detecting both F3-F4 stage fibrosis and cirrhosis (F4) than TE [86, 87]. The same as the chronic HBV or HCV patients, 2D-SWE is less well-validated for NAFLD patients than TE or pSWE. Several prospective studies showed a good diagnostic performance of 2D-SWE in detecting liver cirrhosis for NAFLD patients with AUROCs ranging from 0.88 to 0.95 [88–90].

5. Limitation of ultrasound-based shear wave elastography for the liver

Although currently available ultrasound-based shear wave elastography systems including TE, pSWE, and 2D-SWE provide an excellent diagnostic capability in assessing liver fibrosis stage and are widely used in clinical practice, ultrasound-based shear wave elastography systems have some limitations. Operators should be aware of the limitations of current ultrasound-based shear wave elastography techniques for accurate measurement of liver stiffness value as well as for the appropriate interpretation of the results. After the introduction of pSWE and 2D-SWE that can be incorporated into commercial ultrasound systems for routine B-mode imaging, many of manufacturers provide their own SWE systems for liver stiffness measurement. Therefore, inter-platform variability among the different SWE systems from the various vendors may be an issue [15]. In the view of physics, the liver stiffness measurement values obtained by different SWE systems from different vendors can not be interchangeable. Thus, vendor-specific cut-off values for the assessment of the liver fibrosis stage are needed since the frequencies of shear wave generated within the liver tissue are different among the various SWE systems from different vendors: 50 Hz for TE and wideband ranging from 100 to 500 Hz for pSWE and 2D-SWE [31, 91, 92]. However, the application of vendor-specific cut-off might be infeasible in clinical practice and it is hardly possible to follow up patients with the same SWE system during the disease course. According to the result of the study evaluating inter-observer variability of liver stiffness measurements among seven different SWE systems including TE, four pSWE methods, and two 2D-SWE methods, the overall agreement among the liver stiffness measurements performed with different SWE systems was good to excellent having ICCs ranging from 0.74 to 0.97 [93]. There would be an approximately 10% variability of the liver stiffness measurements among the different vendor SWE systems [93]. Therefore, these inter-platform variabilities should be taken into account in the application of various SWE systems from different vendors for the assessment of liver fibrosis staging.

To calculate the liver stiffness value from the measured shear wave propagation velocity, the current SWE systems assume that the tissue in that a stress is applied is purely elastic, and neglect the tissue viscosity. However, in some clinical situations, the assumption of pure tissue elasticity does not work well, leading to errors in the liver stiffness measurements. These conditions include acute hepatitis, liver inflammation with necrosis, obstructive cholangitis, hepatic congestion, and infiltrative disease such as amyloidosis or lymphoma [15], and have been known to increase tissue viscosity. When the tissue viscosity is increased by various causes, the liver stiffness values measured by SWE systems are usually higher than without those conditions, leading to the over-estimation of the liver fibrosis stage [94]. Therefore, current guidelines for liver elastography examination do not recommend the liver stiffness measurement for the assessment of liver fibrosis stage when the serum level of aspartate amino-transaminase (AST) and/or alanine aminotransaminase (ALT) is elevated greater than five times upper normal limits [15]. The assessment of the liver fibrosis stage by using liver SWE can be performed after the normalization of AST and/or ALT level to minimize the effect of liver inflammation on the results of liver stiffness measurement. In addition, tissue viscosity introduces a dependency of shear wave propagation velocity on excitation frequencies [23, 95]. Given that, more complex modeling taking tissue viscoelasticity into account is warranted to overcome the current limitation of ultrasound-based shear wave elastography for the liver.

6. Conclusion

Many studies reported an excellent diagnostic performance of ultrasound-based shear wave elastography in the evaluation of liver fibrosis and detection of liver cirrhosis. Among the various shear wave elastography techniques, TE has been the most widely used and extensively validated method for the assessment of liver fibrosis, subsequently having a higher level of evidence compared to the other elastography methods. In addition to TE, pSWE, and 2D-SWE have emerged as another noninvasive methods for the assessment of liver fibrosis. Since both pSWE and 2D-SWE utilize the conventional ultrasound probe for routine B-mode imaging equipped in standard diagnostic ultrasound machines, pSWE, and 2D-SWE can provide B-mode images of the liver simultaneously during the examination, enabling the liver stiffness measurement under the real-time B-mode image guidance. Although current ultrasound-based shear wave elastography techniques including TE, pSWE, and 2D-SWE provide an excellent diagnostic capability in assessing liver fibrosis stage, interchangeability of liver stiffness measurement results among the different SWE systems from different vendors may be an issue. In addition, the presence of concurrent liver inflammation with/without necrosis, hepatic congestion, obstructive cholestasis, and diffuse infiltrative disease in the liver, which can increase the tissue viscosity, is another limitation of the current liver elastography technique for the diagnosis of liver fibrosis and cirrhosis, leading to over-estimation of liver fibrosis stage. Therefore, operators should be aware of the limitations of current SWE systems for proper use of SWE technique in assessing liver fibrosis stage as well as for the accurate interpretation of the liver stiffness measurement results.

Author details

Dong Ho Lee[1,2,3]*, Jae Young Lee[1,2,3] and Byung Ihn Choi[4]

1 Department of Radiology, Seoul National University Hospital, South Korea

2 Institute of Radiation Medicine, Seoul National University Medical Research Center, South Korea

3 Department of Radiology, Seoul National University, College of Medicine, South Korea

4 Department of Radiology, Chung-Ang University Hospital, South Korea

*Address all correspondence to: dhlee.rad@gmail.com

IntechOpen

References

[1] Tsochatzis EA, Bosch J, Burroughs AK. Liver cirrhosis. Lancet. 2014;**383**(9930): 1749-1761. DOI: 10.1016/S0140-6736(14) 60121-5

[2] Friedman SL, Maher JJ, Bissell DM. Mechanisms and therapy of hepatic fibrosis: Report of the AASLD single topic basic research conference. Hepatology. 2000;**32**(6):1403-1408. DOI: 10.1053/jhep.2000.20243

[3] Friedman SL. Liver fibrosis -- from bench to bedside. Journal of Hepatology. 2003;**38**(Suppl. 1):S38-S53. DOI: 10.1016/ s0168-8278(02)00429-4

[4] Sebastiani G, Gkouvatsos K, Pantopoulos K. Chronic hepatitis C and liver fibrosis. World Journal of Gastroenterology. 2014;**20**(32):11033-11053. DOI: 10.3748/wjg.v20.i32.11033

[5] Deffieux T, Gennisson JL, Bousquet L, Corouge M, Cosconea S, Amroun D, et al. Investigating liver stiffness and viscosity for fibrosis, steatosis and activity staging using shear wave elastography. Journal of Hepatology. 2015;**62**(2):317-324. DOI: 10.1016/j.jhep.2014.09.020

[6] Barr RG, Wilson SR, Rubens D, Garcia-Tsao G, Ferraioli G. Update to the Society of Radiologists in ultrasound liver elastography consensus statement. Radiology. 2020;**296**(2):263-274. DOI: 10.1148/radiol.2020192437

[7] Ellis EL, Mann DA. Clinical evidence for the regression of liver fibrosis. Journal of Hepatology. 2012;**56**(5):1171-1180. DOI: 10.1016/j.jhep.2011.09.024

[8] Marcellin P, Gane E, Buti M, Afdhal N, Sievert W, Jacobson IM, et al. Regression of cirrhosis during treatment with tenofovir disoproxil fumarate for chronic hepatitis B: A 5-year open-label follow-up study. Lancet. 2013;**381**(9865):468-475. DOI: 10.1016/ S0140-6736(12)61425-1

[9] Barr RG, Ferraioli G, Palmeri ML, Goodman ZD, Garcia-Tsao G, Rubin J, et al. Elastography assessment of liver fibrosis: Society of Radiologists in ultrasound consensus conference statement. Radiology. 2015;**276**(3):845-861. DOI: 10.1148/radiol.2015150619

[10] Rockey DC. Antifibrotic therapy in chronic liver disease. Clinical Gastroenterology and Hepatology: The Official Clinical Practice Journal of the American Gastroenterological Association. 2005;**3**(2):95-107. DOI: 10.1016/s1542-3565(04)00445-8

[11] Rockey DC, Bissell DM. Noninvasive measures of liver fibrosis. Hepatology. 2006;**43**(2 Suppl. 1):S113-S120. DOI: 10.1002/hep.21046

[12] Lee DH, Lee JM, Han JK, Choi BI. MR elastography of healthy liver parenchyma: Normal value and reliability of the liver stiffness value measurement. Journal of Magnetic Resonance Imaging: JMRI. 2013;**38**(5):1215-1223. DOI: 10.1002/jmri.23958

[13] Lee DH, Lee ES, Lee JY, Bae JS, Kim H, Lee KB, et al. Two-dimensional-shear wave elastography with a propagation map: Prospective evaluation of liver fibrosis using histopathology as the reference standard. Korean Journal of Radiology. 2020;**21**(12):1317-1325. DOI: 10.3348/kjr.2019.0978

[14] Bravo AA, Sheth SG, Chopra S. Liver biopsy. The New England Journal of Medicine. 2001;**344**(7):495-500. DOI: 10.1056/NEJM200102153440706

[15] Kennedy P, Wagner M, Castera L, Hong CW, Johnson CL, Sirlin CB, et al. Quantitative elastography methods in liver disease: Current evidence and future directions. Radiology. 2018;**286**(3):738-763. DOI: 10.1148/radiol.2018170601

[16] Regev A, Berho M, Jeffers LJ, Milikowski C, Molina EG, Pyrsopoulos NT, et al. Sampling error and intraobserver variation in liver biopsy in patients with chronic HCV infection. The American Journal of Gastroenterology. 2002;**97**(10):2614-2618. DOI: 10.1111/j.1572-0241.2002.06038.x

[17] Rousselet MC, Michalak S, Dupre F, Croue A, Bedossa P, Saint-Andre JP, et al. Sources of variability in histological scoring of chronic viral hepatitis. Hepatology. 2005;**41**(2):257-264. DOI: 10.1002/hep.20535

[18] Goodman ZD. Grading and staging systems for inflammation and fibrosis in chronic liver diseases. Journal of Hepatology. 2007;**47**(4):598-607. DOI: 10.1016/j.jhep.2007.07.006

[19] Pavlides M, Birks J, Fryer E, Delaney D, Sarania N, Banerjee R, et al. Interobserver variability in histologic evaluation of liver fibrosis using categorical and quantitative scores. American Journal of Clinical Pathology. 2017;**147**(4):364-369. DOI: 10.1093/ajcp/aqx011

[20] Ferraioli G, Tinelli C, Dal Bello B, Zicchetti M, Filice G, Filice C. Liver fibrosis study G. accuracy of real-time shear wave elastography for assessing liver fibrosis in chronic hepatitis C: A pilot study. Hepatology. 2012;**56**(6):2125-2133. DOI: 10.1002/hep.25936

[21] Park SH, Kim SY, Suh CH, Lee SS, Kim KW, Lee SJ, et al. What we need to know when performing and interpreting US elastography. Clinical and Molecular Hepatology. 2016;**22**(3):406-414. DOI: 10.3350/cmh.2016.0106

[22] Ophir J, Cespedes I, Ponnekanti H, Yazdi Y, Li X. Elastography: A quantitative method for imaging the elasticity of biological tissues. Ultrasonic Imaging. 1991;**13**(2):111-134. DOI: 10.1177/016173469101300201

[23] Sigrist RMS, Liau J, Kaffas AE, Chammas MC, Willmann JK. Ultrasound elastography: Review of techniques and clinical applications. Theranostics. 2017;**7**(5):1303-1329. DOI: 10.7150/thno.18650

[24] Morikawa H, Fukuda K, Kobayashi S, Fujii H, Iwai S, Enomoto M, et al. Real-time tissue elastography as a tool for the noninvasive assessment of liver stiffness in patients with chronic hepatitis C. Journal of Gastroenterology. 2011;**46**(3):350-358. DOI: 10.1007/s00535-010-0301-x

[25] Garra BS. Elastography: History, principles, and technique comparison. Abdominal Imaging. 2015;**40**(4):680-697. DOI: 10.1007/s00261-014-0305-8

[26] Castera L, Forns X, Alberti A. Non-invasive evaluation of liver fibrosis using transient elastography. Journal of Hepatology. 2008;**48**(5):835-847. DOI: 10.1016/j.jhep.2008.02.008

[27] Friedrich-Rust M, Nierhoff J, Lupsor M, Sporea I, Fierbinteanu-Braticevici C, Strobel D, et al. Performance of acoustic radiation force impulse imaging for the staging of liver fibrosis: A pooled meta-analysis. Journal of Viral Hepatitis. 2012;**19**(2):e212-e219. DOI: 10.1111/j.1365-2893.2011.01537.x

[28] Nightingale K. Acoustic radiation force impulse (ARFI) imaging: A review. Current Medical Imaging Reviews. 2011;7(4):328-339. DOI: 10.2174/157340511798038657

[29] Ferraioli G, Filice C, Castera L, Choi BI, Sporea I, Wilson SR, et al. WFUMB guidelines and recommendations for clinical use of ultrasound elastography: Part 3: Liver. Ultrasound in Medicine and Biology. 2015;41(5):1161-1179. DOI: 10.1016/j.ultrasmedbio.2015.03.007

[30] Tang A, Cloutier G, Szeverenyi NM, Sirlin CB. Ultrasound elastography and MR elastography for assessing liver fibrosis: Part 1, principles and techniques. AJR American Journal of Roentgenology. 2015;205(1):22-32. DOI: 10.2214/AJR.15.14552

[31] Bamber J, Cosgrove D, Dietrich CF, Fromageau J, Bojunga J, Calliada F, et al. EFSUMB guidelines and recommendations on the clinical use of ultrasound elastography. Part 1: Basic principles and technology. Ultraschall in der Medizin. 2013;34(2):169-184. DOI: 10.1055/s-0033-1335205

[32] Dietrich CF, Bamber J, Berzigotti A, Bota S, Cantisani V, Castera L, et al. EFSUMB guidelines and recommandations on the clinical use of liver ultrasound elastography, update 2017 (long version). Ultraschall in der Medizin. 2017;38(4):e16-e47. DOI: 10.1055/s-0043-103952

[33] Ferraioli G, Wong VW, Castera L, Berzigotti A, Sporea I, Dietrich CF, et al. Liver ultrasound elastography: An update to the world federation for ultrasound in medicine and biology guidelines and recommendations. Ultrasound in Medicine & Biology. 2018;44(12):2419-2440. DOI: 10.1016/j.ultrasmedbio.2018.07.008

[34] Lee DH, Lee JM, Yoon JH, Kim YJ, Lee JH, Yu SJ, et al. Liver stiffness measured by two-dimensional shear-wave Elastography: Prognostic value after radiofrequency ablation for hepatocellular carcinoma. Liver Cancer. 2018;7(1):65-75. DOI: 10.1159/000484445

[35] Castera L, Foucher J, Bernard PH, Carvalho F, Allaix D, Merrouche W, et al. Pitfalls of liver stiffness measurement: A 5-year prospective study of 13,369 examinations. Hepatology. 2010;51(3):828-835. DOI: 10.1002/hep.23425

[36] Friedrich-Rust M, Hadji-Hosseini H, Kriener S, Herrmann E, Sircar I, Kau A, et al. Transient elastography with a new probe for obese patients for non-invasive staging of non-alcoholic steatohepatitis. European Radiology. 2010;20(10):2390-2396. DOI: 10.1007/s00330-010-1820-9

[37] de Ledinghen V, Wong VW, Vergniol J, Wong GL, Foucher J, Chu SH, et al. Diagnosis of liver fibrosis and cirrhosis using liver stiffness measurement: Comparison between M and XL probe of FibroScan (R). Journal of Hepatology. 2012;56(4):833-839. DOI: 10.1016/j.jhep.2011.10.017

[38] Myers RP, Pomier-Layrargues G, Kirsch R, Pollett A, Duarte-Rojo A, Wong D, et al. Feasibility and diagnostic performance of the FibroScan XL probe for liver stiffness measurement in overweight and obese patients. Hepatology. 2012;55(1):199-208. DOI: 10.1002/hep.24624

[39] Wong VW, Vergniol J, Wong GL, Foucher J, Chan AW, Chermak F, et al. Liver stiffness measurement using XL probe in patients with nonalcoholic fatty liver disease. The American Journal of Gastroenterology. 2012;107(12):1862-1871. DOI: 10.1038/ajg.2012.331

[40] Yoneda M, Thomas E, Sclair SN, Grant TT, Schiff ER. Supersonic shear imaging and transient elastography with the XL probe accurately detect fibrosis in overweight or obese patients with chronic liver disease. Clinical Gastroenterology and Hepatology: The Official Clinical Practice Journal of the American Gastroenterological Association. 2015;**13**(8):1502-1509 e1505. DOI: 10.1016/j.cgh.2015.03.014

[41] Neukam K, Recio E, Camacho A, Macias J, Rivero A, Mira JA, et al. Interobserver concordance in the assessment of liver fibrosis in HIV/HCV-coinfected patients using transient elastometry. European Journal of Gastroenterology & Hepatology. 2010;**22**(7):801-807. DOI: 10.1097/MEG.0b013e328331a5d0

[42] Ferraioli G, Maiocchi L, Lissandrin R, Tinelli C, De Silvestri A, Filice C, et al. Accuracy of the ElastPQ technique for the assessment of liver fibrosis in patients with chronic Hepatitis C: A "real life" single Center study. Journal of Gastrointestinal and Liver Diseases: JGLD. 2016;**25**(3):331-335. DOI: 10.15403/jgld.2014.1121.253.epq

[43] Fang C, Jaffer OS, Yusuf GT, Konstantatou E, Quinlan DJ, Agarwal K, et al. Reducing the number of measurements in liver point shear-wave elastography: Factors that influence the number and reliability of measurements in assessment of liver fibrosis in clinical practice. Radiology. 2018;**287**(3):844-852. DOI: 10.1148/radiol.2018172104

[44] Woo H, Lee JY, Yoon JH, Kim W, Cho B, Choi BI. Comparison of the reliability of acoustic radiation force impulse imaging and supersonic shear imaging in measurement of liver stiffness. Radiology. 2015;**277**(3):881-886. DOI: 10.1148/radiol.2015141975

[45] Ferraioli G, Tinelli C, Zicchetti M, Above E, Poma G, Di Gregorio M, et al. Reproducibility of real-time shear wave elastography in the evaluation of liver elasticity. European Journal of Radiology. 2012;**81**(11):3102-3106. DOI: 10.1016/j.ejrad.2012.05.030

[46] Ferraioli G, Tinelli C, Lissandrin R, Zicchetti M, Bernuzzi S, Salvaneschi L, et al. Ultrasound point shear wave elastography assessment of liver and spleen stiffness: Effect of training on repeatability of measurements. European Radiology. 2014;**24**(6):1283-1289. DOI: 10.1007/s00330-014-3140-y

[47] Anthony PP, Ishak KG, Nayak NC, Poulsen HE, Scheuer PJ, Sobin LH. The morphology of cirrhosis: Definition, nomenclature, and classification. Bulletin of the World Health Organization. 1977;**55**(4):521-540

[48] Suwanthawornkul T, Anothaisintawee T, Sobhonslidsuk A, Thakkinstian A, Teerawattananon Y. Efficacy of second generation direct-acting antiviral agents for treatment naive Hepatitis C genotype 1: A systematic review and network Meta-analysis. PLoS One. 2015;**10**(12):e0145953. DOI: 10.1371/journal.pone.0145953

[49] Terrault NA, Bzowej NH, Chang KM, Hwang JP, Jonas MM, Murad MH. American Association for the Study of liver D. AASLD guidelines for treatment of chronic hepatitis B. Hepatology. 2016;**63**(1):261-283. DOI: 10.1002/hep.28156

[50] Standish RA, Cholongitas E, Dhillon A, Burroughs AK, Dhillon AP. An appraisal of the histopathological assessment of liver fibrosis. Gut. 2006;**55**(4):569-578. DOI: 10.1136/gut.2005.084475

[51] Sandrin L, Fourquet B, Hasquenoph JM, Yon S, Fournier C, Mal F, et al. Transient elastography: A new noninvasive method for assessment of hepatic fibrosis. Ultrasound in Medicine & Biology. 2003;**29**(12):1705-1713. DOI: 10.1016/j.ultrasmedbio.2003.07.001

[52] Castera L, Vergniol J, Foucher J, Le Bail B, Chanteloup E, Haaser M, et al. Prospective comparison of transient elastography, Fibrotest, APRI, and liver biopsy for the assessment of fibrosis in chronic hepatitis C. Gastroenterology. 2005;**128**(2):343-350. DOI: 10.1053/j.gastro.2004.11.018

[53] Ziol M, Handra-Luca A, Kettaneh A, Christidis C, Mal F, Kazemi F, et al. Noninvasive assessment of liver fibrosis by measurement of stiffness in patients with chronic hepatitis C. Hepatology. 2005;**41**(1):48-54. DOI: 10.1002/hep.20506

[54] Marcellin P, Ziol M, Bedossa P, Douvin C, Poupon R, de Ledinghen V, et al. Non-invasive assessment of liver fibrosis by stiffness measurement in patients with chronic hepatitis B. Liver International: Official Journal of the International Association for the Study of the Liver. 2009;**29**(2):242-247. DOI: 10.1111/j.1478-3231.2008.01802.x

[55] Degos F, Perez P, Roche B, Mahmoudi A, Asselineau J, Voitot H, et al. Diagnostic accuracy of FibroScan and comparison to liver fibrosis biomarkers in chronic viral hepatitis: A multicenter prospective study (the FIBROSTIC study). Journal of Hepatology. 2010;**53**(6):1013-1021. DOI: 10.1016/j.jhep.2010.05.035

[56] Castera L, Bernard PH, Le Bail B, Foucher J, Trimoulet P, Merrouche W, et al. Transient elastography and biomarkers for liver fibrosis assessment and follow-up of inactive hepatitis B carriers. Alimentary Pharmacology and Therapeutics. 2011;**33**(4):455-465. DOI: 10.1111/j.1365-2036.2010.04547.x

[57] Castera L. Noninvasive methods to assess liver disease in patients with hepatitis B or C. Gastroenterology. 2012;**142**(6):1293-1302. e 1294. DOI: 10.1053/j.gastro.2012.02.017

[58] Talwalkar JA, Kurtz DM, Schoenleber SJ, West CP, Montori VM. Ultrasound-based transient elastography for the detection of hepatic fibrosis: Systematic review and meta-analysis. Clinical Gastroenterology and Hepatology: The Official Clinical Practice Journal of the American Gastroenterological Association. 2007;**5**(10):1214-1220. DOI: 10.1016/j.cgh.2007.07.020

[59] Friedrich-Rust M, Ong MF, Martens S, Sarrazin C, Bojunga J, Zeuzem S, et al. Performance of transient elastography for the staging of liver fibrosis: A meta-analysis. Gastroenterology. 2008;**134**(4):960-974. DOI: 10.1053/j.gastro.2008.01.034

[60] Tsochatzis EA, Gurusamy KS, Ntaoula S, Cholongitas E, Davidson BR, Burroughs AK. Elastography for the diagnosis of severity of fibrosis in chronic liver disease: A meta-analysis of diagnostic accuracy. Journal of Hepatology. 2011;**54**(4):650-659. DOI: 10.1016/j.jhep.2010.07.033

[61] Li Y, Huang YS, Wang ZZ, Yang ZR, Sun F, Zhan SY, et al. Systematic review with meta-analysis: The diagnostic accuracy of transient elastography for the staging of liver fibrosis in patients with chronic hepatitis B. Alimentary Pharmacology & Therapeutics. 2016;**43**(4):458-469. DOI: 10.1111/apt.13488

[62] Njei B, McCarty TR, Luk J, Ewelukwa O, Ditah I, Lim JK. Use of transient elastography in patients with HIV-HCV coinfection: A systematic review and meta-analysis. Journal of Gastroenterology and Hepatology. 2016;**31**(10):1684-1693. DOI: 10.1111/jgh.13337

[63] Shaheen AA, Wan AF, Myers RP. FibroTest and FibroScan for the prediction of hepatitis C-related fibrosis: A systematic review of diagnostic test accuracy. The American Journal of Gastroenterology. 2007;**102**(11):2589-2600. DOI: 10.1111/j.1572-0241.2007.01466.x

[64] Nobili V, Vizzutti F, Arena U, Abraldes JG, Marra F, Pietrobattista A, et al. Accuracy and reproducibility of transient elastography for the diagnosis of fibrosis in pediatric nonalcoholic steatohepatitis. Hepatology. 2008;**48**(2):442-448. DOI: 10.1002/hep.22376

[65] Loong TC, Wei JL, Leung JC, Wong GL, Shu SS, Chim AM, et al. Application of the combined FibroMeter vibration-controlled transient elastography algorithm in Chinese patients with non-alcoholic fatty liver disease. Journal of Gastroenterology and Hepatology. 2017;**32**(7):1363-1369. DOI: 10.1111/jgh.13671

[66] Kwok R, Tse YK, Wong GL, Ha Y, Lee AU, Ngu MC, et al. Systematic review with meta-analysis: Non-invasive assessment of non-alcoholic fatty liver disease--the role of transient elastography and plasma cytokeratin-18 fragments. Alimentary Pharmacology & Therapeutics. 2014;**39**(3):254-269. DOI: 10.1111/apt.12569

[67] Puigvehi M, Broquetas T, Coll S, Garcia-Retortillo M, Canete N, Fernandez R, et al. Impact of anthropometric features on the applicability and accuracy of FibroScan((R)) (M and XL) in overweight/obese patients. Journal of Gastroenterology and Hepatology. 2017;**32**(10):1746-1753. DOI: 10.1111/jgh.13762

[68] Friedrich-Rust M, Buggisch P, de Knegt RJ, Dries V, Shi Y, Matschenz K, et al. Acoustic radiation force impulse imaging for non-invasive assessment of liver fibrosis in chronic hepatitis B. Journal of Viral Hepatitis. 2013;**20**(4):240-247. DOI: 10.1111/j.1365-2893.2012.01646.x

[69] Liu Y, Dong CF, Yang G, Liu J, Yao S, Li HY, et al. Optimal linear combination of ARFI, transient elastography and APRI for the assessment of fibrosis in chronic hepatitis B. Liver International: Official Journal of the International Association for the Study of the Liver. 2015;**35**(3):816-825. DOI: 10.1111/liv.12564

[70] Zhang D, Chen M, Wang R, Liu Y, Zhang D, Liu L, et al. Comparison of acoustic radiation force impulse imaging and transient elastography for non-invasive assessment of liver fibrosis in patients with chronic hepatitis B. Ultrasound in Medicine & Biology. 2015;**41**(1):7-14. DOI: 10.1016/j.ultrasmedbio.2014.07.018

[71] Park MS, Kim SW, Yoon KT, Kim SU, Park SY, Tak WY, et al. Factors influencing the diagnostic accuracy of acoustic radiation force impulse Elastography in patients with chronic Hepatitis B. Gut and Liver. 2016;**10**(2):275-282. DOI: 10.5009/gnl14391

[72] Sporea I, Sirli R, Bota S, Fierbinteanu-Braticevici C, Petrisor A, Badea R, et al. Is ARFI elastography reliable for predicting fibrosis severity in

chronic HCV hepatitis? World Journal of Radiology. 2011;3(7):188-193. DOI: 10.4329/wjr.v3.i7.188

[73] Takaki S, Kawakami Y, Miyaki D, Nakahara T, Naeshiro N, Murakami E, et al. Non-invasive liver fibrosis score calculated by combination of virtual touch tissue quantification and serum liver functional tests in chronic hepatitis C patients. Hepatology Research : The Official Journal of the Japan Society of Hepatology. 2014;44(3):280-287. DOI: 10.1111/hepr.12129

[74] Friedrich-Rust M, Lupsor M, de Knegt R, Dries V, Buggisch P, Gebel M, et al. Point shear wave elastography by acoustic radiation force impulse quantification in comparison to transient elastography for the noninvasive assessment of liver fibrosis in chronic Hepatitis C: A prospective international multicenter study. Ultraschall in der Medizin. 2015;36(3):239-247. DOI: 10.1055/s-0034-1398987

[75] Conti F, Serra C, Vukotic R, Fiorini E, Felicani C, Mazzotta E, et al. Accuracy of elastography point quantification and steatosis influence on assessing liver fibrosis in patients with chronic hepatitis C. Liver International: Official Journal of the International Association for the Study of the Liver. 2017;37(2):187-195. DOI: 10.1111/liv.13197

[76] Hu X, Qiu L, Liu D, Qian L. Acoustic radiation force impulse (ARFI) Elastography for noninvasive evaluation of hepatic fibrosis in chronic hepatitis B and C patients: A systematic review and meta-analysis. Medical Ultrasonography. 2017;19(1):23-31. DOI: 10.11152/mu-942

[77] Yoneda M, Suzuki K, Kato S, Fujita K, Nozaki Y, Hosono K, et al. Nonalcoholic fatty liver disease: US-based acoustic radiation force

impulse elastography. Radiology. 2010;256(2):640-647. DOI: 10.1148/radiol.10091662

[78] Palmeri ML, Wang MH, Rouze NC, Abdelmalek MF, Guy CD, Moser B, et al. Noninvasive evaluation of hepatic fibrosis using acoustic radiation force-based shear stiffness in patients with nonalcoholic fatty liver disease. Journal of Hepatology. 2011;55(3):666-672. DOI: 10.1016/j.jhep.2010.12.019

[79] Guzman-Aroca F, Frutos-Bernal MD, Bas A, Lujan-Mompean JA, Reus M, Berna-Serna Jde D, et al. Detection of non-alcoholic steatohepatitis in patients with morbid obesity before bariatric surgery: Preliminary evaluation with acoustic radiation force impulse imaging. European Radiology. 2012;22(11):2525-2532. DOI: 10.1007/s00330-012-2505-3

[80] Fierbinteanu Braticevici C, Sporea I, Panaitescu E, Tribus L. Value of acoustic radiation force impulse imaging elastography for non-invasive evaluation of patients with nonalcoholic fatty liver disease. Ultrasound in Medicine & Biology. 2013;39(11):1942-1950. DOI: 10.1016/j.ultrasmedbio.2013.04.019

[81] Friedrich-Rust M, Romen D, Vermehren J, Kriener S, Sadet D, Herrmann E, et al. Acoustic radiation force impulse-imaging and transient elastography for non-invasive assessment of liver fibrosis and steatosis in NAFLD. European Journal of Radiology. 2012;81(3):e325-e331. DOI: 10.1016/j.ejrad.2011.10.029

[82] Leung VY, Shen J, Wong VW, Abrigo J, Wong GL, Chim AM, et al. Quantitative elastography of liver fibrosis and spleen stiffness in chronic hepatitis B carriers: Comparison of shear-wave elastography and transient elastography with liver biopsy correlation. Radiology. 2013;269(3):910-918. DOI: 10.1148/radiol.13130128

[83] Zeng J, Liu GJ, Huang ZP, Zheng J, Wu T, Zheng RQ, et al. Diagnostic accuracy of two-dimensional shear wave elastography for the non-invasive staging of hepatic fibrosis in chronic hepatitis B: A cohort study with internal validation. European Radiology. 2014;**24**(10):2572-2581. DOI: 10.1007/s00330-014-3292-9

[84] Verlinden W, Bourgeois S, Gigase P, Thienpont C, Vonghia L, Vanwolleghem T, et al. Liver fibrosis evaluation using real-time shear wave elastography in Hepatitis C-Monoinfected and human immunodeficiency virus/Hepatitis C-Coinfected patients. Journal of Ultrasound in Medicine : Official Journal of the American Institute of Ultrasound in Medicine. 2016;**35**(6):1299-1308. DOI: 10.7863/ultra.15.08066

[85] Jiang T, Tian G, Zhao Q, Kong D, Cheng C, Zhong L, et al. Diagnostic accuracy of 2D-shear wave Elastography for liver fibrosis severity: A Meta-analysis. PLoS One. 2016;**11**(6):e0157219. DOI: 10.1371/journal.pone.0157219

[86] Herrmann E, de Ledinghen V, Cassinotto C, Chu WC, Leung VY, Ferraioli G, et al. Assessment of biopsy-proven liver fibrosis by two-dimensional shear wave elastography: An individual patient data-based meta-analysis. Hepatology. 2018;**67**(1):260-272. DOI: 10.1002/hep.29179

[87] Lee DH, Lee ES, Bae JS, Lee JY, Han JK, Yi NJ, et al. 2D shear wave elastography is better than transient elastography in predicting post-hepatectomy complication after resection. European Radiology. 2021;**31**(8):5802-5811. DOI: 10.1007/s00330-020-07662-3

[88] Cassinotto C, Boursier J, de Ledinghen V, Lebigot J, Lapuyade B, Cales P, et al. Liver stiffness in nonalcoholic fatty liver disease: A comparison of supersonic shear imaging, FibroScan, and ARFI with liver biopsy. Hepatology. 2016;**63**(6):1817-1827. DOI: 10.1002/hep.28394

[89] Sugimoto K, Moriyasu F, Oshiro H, Takeuchi H, Abe M, Yoshimasu Y, et al. The role of multiparametric US of the liver for the evaluation of nonalcoholic Steatohepatitis. Radiology. 2020;**296**(3):532-540. DOI: 10.1148/radiol.2020192665

[90] Lee DH, Cho EJ, Bae JS, Lee JY, Yu SJ, Kim H, et al. Accuracy of two-dimensional shear wave elastography and attenuation imaging for evaluation of patients with nonalcoholic Steatohepatitis. Clinical Gastroenterology and Hepatology: The Official Clinical Practice Journal of the American Gastroenterological Association. 2021;**19**(4):797-805 e797. DOI: 10.1016/j.cgh.2020.05.034

[91] Palmeri ML, Nightingale KR. What challenges must be overcome before ultrasound elasticity imaging is ready for the clinic? Imaging in Medicine. 2011;**3**(4):433-444. DOI: 10.2217/iim.11.41

[92] Cosgrove D, Piscaglia F, Bamber J, Bojunga J, Correas JM, Gilja OH, et al. EFSUMB guidelines and recommendations on the clinical use of ultrasound elastography. Part 2: Clinical applications. Ultraschall in der Medizin. 2013;**34**(3):238-253. DOI: 10.1055/s-0033-1335375

[93] Ferraioli G, De Silvestri A, Lissandrin R, Maiocchi L, Tinelli C, Filice C, et al. Evaluation of inter-system variability in liver stiffness measurements. Ultraschall in der Medizin. 2019;**40**(1):64-75. DOI: 10.1055/s-0043-124184

[94] Vigano M, Massironi S, Lampertico P, Iavarone M, Paggi S, Pozzi R, et al. Transient elastography assessment of the liver stiffness dynamics during acute hepatitis B. European Journal of Gastroenterology and Hepatology. 2010;**22**(2):180-184. DOI: 10.1097/MEG.0b013e328332d2fa

[95] Shiina T, Nightingale KR, Palmeri ML, Hall TJ, Bamber JC, Barr RG, et al. WFUMB guidelines and recommendations for clinical use of ultrasound elastography: Part 1: Basic principles and terminology. Ultrasound in Medicine and Biology. 2015;**41**(5):1126-1147. DOI: 10.1016/j.ultrasmedbio.2015.03.009

Chapter 5

Noninvasive Assessment of HCV Patients Using Ultrasound Elastography

Monica Lupsor-Platon, Teodora Serban
and Alexandra Iulia Silion

Abstract

Among patients with chronic hepatitis C (CHC) infection, extensive research showed that fibrosis progression is a proper surrogate marker for advanced liver disease, eventually leading to dramatic endpoints such as cirrhosis and hepatocellular carcinoma. Therefore, there is growing interest in the use of noninvasive methods for fibrosis assessment in order to replace liver biopsy (LB) in clinical practice and provide optimal risk stratification. Elastographic techniques, such as Vibration Controlled Transient Elastography (VCTE), point-shear wave elastography (p-SWE), and 2D-SWE have shown promising results in this regard, with excellent performance in diagnosing hepatic cirrhosis, and great accuracy for steatosis detection through the Controlled Attenuation Parameter embedded on the VCTE device. In addition, the recent introduction of highly efficient direct-acting antivirals (DAAs) led to viral eradication and a significant decrease in liver damage, lowering the risk of hepatic decompensation, and HCC. Therefore, CHC patients need proper noninvasive and repeatable methods for adequate surveillance, even after treatment, as there still remains a risk of portal hypertension and HCC. However, the usefulness for monitoring fibrosis after the sustained virological response (SVR) needs further research.

Keywords: chronic hepatitis C, fibrosis, Vibration Controlled Transient Elastography, point-shear wave elastography, 2D shear wave elastography

1. Introduction

Hepatitis C virus (HCV) infection is a major causative agent of chronic liver disease (CLD) and liver-related death worldwide. Approximately 4 out of 5 infected individuals develop chronic hepatitis C (CHC) and nearly 20% of them insidiously progress to cirrhosis, hepatocellular carcinoma (HCC), and end-stage liver disease [1]. It is estimated that 71.1 people were infected in 2015 worldwide, making it a global public health issue due to its substantial prevalence and effect on overall morbidity and mortality [2].

It has been shown that the accumulation of liver fibrosis has a great impact on the evolution of CHC. Fibrosis is the hallmark of progressive disease, eventually leading to cirrhosis and end-stage liver complications [3]. As highlighted by a prospective study conducted by Yano et al. [4], relatively few patients with absent or low-grade fibrosis develop cirrhosis over the next 20 years (25–30%). However, portal and septal fibrosis were followed by cirrhosis in all cases with a progression rate of 18–20 years for portal fibrosis and 8–10 years for septal fibrosis. Furthermore, the advent of direct-acting antivirals (DAAs) has changed the perspective of CHC therapy, being both well-tolerated and highly efficient in achieving sustained virologic response (SVR) [5]. Therefore, staging liver fibrosis as a triage for starting therapy may no longer be as decisive as before. Rather, prompt diagnosis and management of advanced stages of fibrosis can prevent complications and death through comprehensive preventive and management strategies [6].

Liver biopsy (LB) is traditionally considered the gold standard evaluation for necroinflammatory activity, steatosis, and fibrosis in CHC [7]. However, the method has several drawbacks. Firstly, the result of the histopathological examination is significantly affected by the specimen's quality and the pathologist's experience [8–11]. Secondly, it is an invasive procedure, implies high costs, and might lead to several complications. Noninvasive methods are therefore necessary for optimal risk stratification in order to avoid the use of LB. Even if conventional imaging techniques are noninvasive, they require absolute signs of severe fibrosis or cirrhosis. Therefore, the latest studies focused on noninvasive elastographic techniques, which have shown promising results for the appraisal of liver fibrosis and steatosis in CHC patients.

2. Fibrosis assessment in HCV patients using noninvasive elastographic methods: a classification

Elastography-based imaging techniques quantify tissue stiffness, defined as the resistance of a material in response to an applied mechanical force [12]. Fibrosis modifies the elastic properties of liver tissue so that new techniques have been developed in the past two decades to grade liver fibrosis according to tissue stiffness.

Ultrasonographic (US) and magnetic resonance-based elastographic techniques are available, of which we will focus on US methods. Several guidelines classify elastographic techniques in two main categories: quantitative ("Shear Wave Elastography", SWE) and qualitative ("Strain Elastography) [13–15]. Regarding CHC, quantitative methods are most frequently used to evaluate liver stiffness (LS). Currently, three main quantitative techniques showed promising results in this pathology: Vibration Controlled Transient Elastography (VCTE; FibroScan®, Echosens, Paris, France) point-shear wave elastography (pSWE), and 2D- shear wave elastography (2DSWE). For integrative purposes, we decided to summarize the specific advantages and limitations of each technique in HCV patients.

3. Confounders: pathological changes influencing liver stiffness in HCV patients

Several technical and biological factors affect the performance of elastographic techniques due to an increase in LS unrelated to fibrosis. The former includes shear wave frequencies, location and depth of measurements, and device dependencies. The latter include ingestion of food prior to the examination, inflammation, cholestasis, hepatic venous congestion, and amyloid deposits [16, 17]. Inflammation in acute hepatitis might increase LS up to mimicking cirrhosis, returning to normal simultaneously with the decrease of liver transaminases. A study of 112 CHC patients found a higher value for LS in the case of F3-F4 stages of fibrosis and necroinflammatory activity of at least A2 compared to A0-A1 (14.6 and 6.2 kPa, p = 0.04) [18]. Therefore, it is recommended to consider transaminases' value before interpreting LS in order to avoid overestimation [19]. If ALT levels are 3 times the normal value, there is a risk of overestimating the fibrosis stage and this should be mentioned with the results [20].

Concerning cholestasis and heart failure with hepatic congestion, LS decreases after proper treatment, hence the effect on shear wave propagation [21, 22]. Of note, a study suggests FibroScan as a potential tool to reveal heart decompensation [23]. In addition, waist circumference may lead to both technical failure and higher LS, but studies show various results and are mainly referring to body mass index (BMI). This is common because central obesity is associated with low-grade inflammation, insulin resistance, and liver steatosis, increasing LS. Furthermore, male gender, dyslipidemia and statins are debated in this regard, with different results (**Table 1**) [29].

	Advantages	Disadvantages
Vibration Controlled Transient Elastography (VCTE)	Widely used, less expensive, easy to learn [24] Can be easily repeated overtime Can provide steatosis assessment through CAP measurement Great reproducibility (>90 interclass correlation coefficients) [15] Point-of-care method [6] Good diagnostic accuracy for fibrosis stages and high performance for cirrhosis (AUROC>0.9) [6]	It cannot be performed in subjects with ascites [6] Obesity increases LSM (the use of XL probe reduces the limits among these subjects) [24] Affected by acute hepatitis, food intake, liver congestion, cholestasis, and alcohol consumption [6]
Point-shear Wave Elastography (p-SWE)	Can be easily executed on modified commercial US devices (if the machine is provided with adequate software) [6, 14] Offers the possibility of choosing the ROI in real-time [14, 25] Enables entire liver parenchyma examination under B-mode visualization [26] Avoids masses or large vessels [26] Can evaluate focal liver lesions' stiffness, discriminating between malignant and benign lesions [24] Good applicability: practicable among patients with ascites and obesity [6, 15, 25, 27] Excellent diagnostic accuracy for advanced fibrosis and cirrhosis [6, 25] Enables spleen stiffness measurement [6]	Narrow range (0.5–4.4 m/s), making it difficult to set proper cut-off values [14] Affected by acute hepatitis, food intake, liver congestion, cholestasis, and alcohol consumption [6]
2D-shear Wave Elastography (2D-SW)	Can be easily executed on modified commercial US devices (if the machine is provided with adequate software) [6, 14] Offers the possibility of choosing a large and adjustable ROI in real-time [14, 25, 28] Good applicability: practicable among patients with ascites and obesity [6, 28] Excellent diagnostic accuracy for advanced fibrosis and cirrhosis [6, 28]	Affected by acute hepatitis, food intake, liver congestion, cholestasis, and alcohol consumption [6]

Table 1.
Advantages and disadvantages of noninvasive elastographic techniques.

4. Vibration controlled transient elastography performance for fibrosis staging in HCV-infected patients

As already mentioned, staging fibrosis is beneficial to determine the prognosis and follow-up of patients with chronic HCV infection. VCTE is the most validated elastographic modality in this regard. Several meta-analysis found an excellent diagnostic performance of VCTE in diagnosing hepatic cirrhosis, with an AUROC exceeding 0.90. However, the technique is less accurate in case of significant fibrosis ($\geq$F2), with an AUROC ranging between 0.80 and 0.90 with overlapping cutoff values, so that the method is facing difficulties in distinguishing different stages of fibrosis [30–34]. Concerning CHC, two of these meta-analysis reported AUROC values of 0.83–0.85 and 0.96 for diagnosing significant fibrosis and cirrhosis, respectively [31, 33]. EASL guidelines suggest combining VCTE with serological markers for the assessment of moderate fibrosis (F2-F4) in patients with CHC [6].

A recent meta-analysis counting 24 articles evaluated the performance of VCTE for diagnosing liver cirrhosis in CHC patients. It estimated a sensitivity (Se) of 84% and a specificity (Sp) of 90%, with AUROC 0.95 [35]. Ganne-Carrié suggests in a study with 775 patients that VCTE should be particularly used for ruling out cirrhosis, given its high negative predictive value (NPV) (96%), rather than ruling it in, since the positive predictive value (PPV) was only 74%. Nevertheless, the excellent diagnostic performance for cirrhosis is hereby confirmed [36].

A recent study [37] compares the performance of VCTE with conventional B-mode ultrasound (US). VCTE is clearly superior in diagnosing severe fibrosis and subclinical cirrhosis, with an AUROC of 0.95 for severe fibrosis and 0.96 for cirrhosis versus 0.76 and 0.71, respectively, in the case of US ($p < 0.001$). Furthermore, combining the two methods does not significantly improve diagnostic accuracy compared with VCTE alone. The two would improve Sp (95.7% versus 76.7; $p < 0.001$) and PPV (94.3% versus 77.1%; $p = 0.002$) [37]. Another study by Berzigotti et al. [38] suggests that the two methods work complementary so that US is the preferred technique for ruling in cirrhosis, while VCTE should be used for ruling out the disease. Contrary to the first example, Benzigotti claims a better performance when the two are combined.

The diagnostic performance of VCTE in staging fibrosis is exemplified in **Table 2**, in reliance to our previous research [50]. Cutoff values range from 4.5 to 9.5 kPa for significant fibrosis ($\geq$F2) and from 11.3 to 16.9 kPa for diagnosing cirrhosis (F4). These values vary considerably mainly according to the prevalence of fibrosis in each study group and the expected outcome [51].

5. Liver fibrosis assessment through point-shear wave elastography in HCV patients

Point-shear wave elastography (p-SWE) is incorporated into devices such as Virtual Touch Tissue Quantification (VTTQ®) (Siemens Healthcare, Erlangen, Germany) and Elastography Point Quantification (ElastPQ®) (EPIQ7 ultrasound system, Philips Healthcare, Bothell, WE, USA). Under B-mode visualization, p-SWE enables the precise acquisition of shear wave speed (SWS) in a small ROI (around 1 cm³). After 10 valid measurements in the right hepatic lobe, the median of SWS is reported and interpreted [15, 52]. Results are expressed in m/s for VTTQ or in m/s and kPa for ElastPQ [13]. However, its narrow range (0.5–4.4 m/s) restricts the

Fibrosis stage	≥ F1			≥ F2			≥ F3			= F4		
Study	Cut-off (kPa)	AUROC	Se/Sp (%)	Cut-off (kPa)	AUROC	Se/Sp (%)	Cut-off (kPa)	AUROC	Se/Sp (%)	Cut-off (m/s)	AUROC	Se/Sp (%)
Njei (n = 756) [39]*	N/S	N/S	N/S	N/S	N/S	97/64	N/S	N/S	N/S	11.8–14.6	N/S	90/87
Lupsor (n = 1202) [20]	5.3	0.879	84.99/73.21	7.4	0.889	80.32/83.97	9.1	0.941	88.8/88.3	13.2	0.970	93.75/93.31
Castera (n = 183) [40]	N/S	N/S	N/S	7.1	0.83	67/89	9.5	0.90	73/91	12.5	0.95	87/91
Afdhal (n = 560) [41][1]	N/S	N/S	N/S	8.4	0.73	58/75	9.6	0.83	71.8/80	12.8	0.90	76/85
Degos (n = 913) [42]	N/S	N/S	N/S	5.2	0.75	90/32	N/S	N/S	N/S	12.9	0.90	72/89
Ziol (n = 251) [43]	N/S	N/S	N/S	8.80	0.79/0.81	56/91	9.6	0.91/0.95	86/85	14.6	0.95	87/91
Carrion (n = 169) [44]	8.5	N/S	N/S	N/S	0.90	90/81	N/S	0.93	N/S	12.5	0.95	87/91
Arena (n = 150) [19]	N/S	N/S	N/S	7.8	0.91	83/82	10.8	0.99	91/94	14.8	0.98	94/92
Sporea (n = 191) [45]	N/S	N/S	N/S	6.8	0.733	59.6/93.3	N/S	N/S	NS	N/S	N/S	N/S
Nitta (n = 165) [46]	N/S	N/S	N/S	7.1	0.87	80.8/80.3	9.6	0.91	87.7/82.4	11.6	0.93	62.5–91.7/ 78.9–91.5
Zarski (n = 382) [47]	N/S	N/S	N/S	5.2	0.82	93.6/34.8	N/S	N/S	N/S	12.9	0.93	76.8/89.6
Wang (n = 214) [48]	6.5	0.86	75/78	9.5	0.82	69/81	N/S	0.87	N/S	12	0.93	89/84
Yoneda (n = 102) [49][2]	N/S	N/S	N/S	7.8	0.91	78/90	10.4	0.95	88/91	11.3	0.91	90/84

Abbreviations: N/S – not specified; AUROC – area under ROC curve; Se – sensibility; Sp – specificity
*meta-analysis.
[1]HCV 92%, HBV 8%.
[2]vXL probe.

Table 2.
Performance of VCTE for detecting different stages of fibrosis in HCV-infected patients.

Fibrosis stage Study	Technology	[≥ F1] Cut-off (m/s)	ROC	Se/Sp (%)	≥ F2 Cut-off (m/s)	ROC	Se/Sp (%)	≥ F3 Cut-off (m/s)	ROC	Se/Sp (%)	= F4 Cut-off (m/s)	ROC	Se/Sp (%)
Lupsor (n = 112) [53]	VTTQ	1.19	0.725	62.07/85.71	1.34	0.869	67.8/92.86	1.61	0.9	79.07/94.83	2.0	0.936	80/95.45
Fierbinteanu-Braticevici (n = 74) [54]	VTTQ	1.185	N/S	89/87	1.215	90.2	100/71	1.54	99.3	97/100	1.94	99.3	100/98.1
Friedrich-Rust (n = 64) [55]	VTTQ	N/S	N/S	N/S	1.35	0.86	72.9/93.8	1.55	0.93	81.5/91.9	1.75	0.95	88.9/89.1
Rizzo (n = 139) [56]	VTTQ	N/S	N/S	N/S	1.3	0.86	81/70	1.7	0.94	91/86	2.0	0.89	83/86
Sporea (n = 274) [57]	VTTQ	1.19	0.880	73/93	1.21	0.893	84/91	1.58	0.908	84/94	1.82	0.937	91/90
Friedrich-Rust (n = 380) [58]*	VTTQ	N/S	N/S	N/S	N/S	0.88	N/S	N/S	0.90	N/S	N/S	0.92	N/S
Sporea (n = 911) [59]	VTTQ	1.19	0.779	69.9/80	1.33	0.792	69.1/79.8	1.43	0.829	74.8/81.5	1.55	0.842	84.3/76.3
Chen (n = 127) [60]	VTTQ	N/S	N/S	N/S	1.55	0.847	74.1/87	1.81	0.902	90.2/89.5	1.98	0.831	88.9/79.8
Zhang (n = 108) [61]	N/S	N/S	N/S	N/S	1.529	0.779	56.9/88.9	1.78	0.863	73.2/92.5	1.797	0.79	78.6/74.5
Nishikawa (n = 108) [62]	VTTQ	1.28	0.810	69.1/85.7	1.28	0.909	81.8/87.1	1.44	0.869	88.9/82.5	1.73	0.885	85.7/86.2
Yamada (n = 124) [63]	VTTQ	N/S	N/S	N/S	1.26	0.890	92.5/76.2	1.46	0.943	84.6/87.8	N/S	N/S	N/S
Li (n = 128) [64]	ElastPQ	N/S	N/S	N/S	1.53	0.775	57.6/89.5	1.79	0.901	76.4/96.5	1.789	0.792	78.9/75.4
Takaki (n = 176)[1] [65]	VTTQ	N/S	N/S	N/S	1.25 / 1.205	0.773 / 0.882	75/78.1 / 75/90.9	1.595 / 1.595	0.863 / 0.858	84.9/81.5 / 94.3/81.8	1.775 / 1.775	0.915 / 1.000	85.6/88.9 / 100/40

Fibrosis stage	Technology	[≥ F1]			≥ F2			≥ F3			= F4		
Study		Cut-off (m/s)	ROC	Se/Sp (%)	Cut-off (m/s)	ROC	Se/Sp (%)	Cut-off (m/s)	ROC	Se/Sp (%)	Cut-off (m/s)	ROC	Se/Sp (%)
Silva Junior (n = 51) [66]	VTTQ	1.19	0.88	88.4/75	1.31	0.90	89.3/87	1.68	0.97	94.4/90.9	1.95	0.98	100/95.2
Tai (n = 83) [67]	VTTQ	N/S	N/S	N/S	N/S	N/S	N/S	N/S	N/S	N/S	1.41	0.802	70.6/80.3
Chen (n = 137) [68]	VTTQ	N/S	N/S	N/S	1.59	0.8434	72.8/79.4	1.73	0.8997	91.4/77.2	1.96	0.9036	100/68.1
Joo (n = 101) [69]	VTTQ	1.190	0.872	84/85.7	1.335	0.853	83.8/75.8	1.645	0.840	79.5/75.8	1.665	0.828	85/69.1
Mare (n = 168)[2,3] [70]	ElastPQ	N/S	N/S	N/S	6.4	0.96	92/100	6.7	0.97	88.4/100	8.9	0.83	90.9
Gani (n = 29) [71]	N/S	N/S	N/S	N/S	1.32	0.802	79/75	1.48	0.802	78/80	1.79	0.802	72/82
Ragazzo (n = 107) [72]	VTTQ	N/S	N/S	N/S	1.22	0.67	64/69	1.41	0.74	57/84	2.37	0.96	100/94
Alem (n = 2103) [73][3]	VTTQ	N/S	N/S	N/S	1.36	0.89	87.5/80.6	1.45	0.94	97.5/90.3	1.7	0.95	90.3/90.9
Hsu (n = 63) [74]	N/S	N/S	N/S	N/S	1.225	0.786	65/70.9	1.370	0.857	73.1/78.4	1.710	0.937	81.8/86.5
Ueda (n = 108) [75]	VTTQ	N/S	N/S	N/S	1.26	0.93	N/S	1.78	0.83	N/S	1.94	0.86	N/S
Baldea (N = 176)[2,3] [76]	ElastPQ	N/S	N/S	N/S	6.51	0.92	96.6/76.4	8.73	0.94	88/85.4	11.1	0.95	86.8/96.7

Abbreviations: N/S – not specified; ROC – receiver operating characteristics curve; Se – sensibility; Sp – specificity
*meta-analysis.
[1]The Takaki study used two groups: the training set (n = 120) the validation set of VIA index (n = 56); for integrative purposes, we presented in our table only the values of p-SWE measurement (SWV), omitting the VIA index' ones.
[2]The Mare and Baldea studies used kPa for ElastPQ cut-off values.
[3]VCTE as reference method.

Table 3.
Performance of p-SWE for detecting different stages of fibrosis in HCV-infected patients.

demarcation of proper cutoff values for discriminating between certain fibrosis stages, making management decisions difficult [14].

We identified several studies that evaluate p-SWE in HCV-infected patients [53–76]. A 2011 pooled meta-analysis by Friedrich-Rust et al. [58] with 380 CHC patients, found AUROC values of 0.88, 0.90, and 0.92 for diagnosing moderate fibrosis (≥ F2), severe fibrosis (≥ F3), and cirrhosis (= F4), respectively. Subsequently, an international multicenter study with 911 HCV-infected patients offered cut-off values of 1.19, 1.33, 1.43, respectively 1.55 m/s for ≥ F1, ≥ F2, ≥ F3 respectively F4, with AUROC values of 0.779, 0.792, 0.829 and 0.842, respectively [59]. Off note is the Takaki study [65] which elaborated the VIA index, a formula that increases the diagnostic accuracy of SWV alone, from 0.882, 0.858 and 1.000 to 0.917, 0.906, and 1.000 for moderate fibrosis, severe fibrosis, and cirrhosis, respectively in the validation set. In 2019, Hsu et al. [74] propound different SWV cutoff values in various diseases. For CHC patients, a SWV cut-off value of 1.225, 1.370 and 1.710 m/s predicts fibrosis stages ≥ F2, ≥ F3 and F4 with AUROC values of 0.786, 0.857 and 0.937, respectively. Overall, in our considered studies presented in **Table 3**, the AUROC ranged from 0.725 to 0.88 for ≥F1, 0.67 to 0.93 for ≥F2, 0.74 to 0.97 for ≥F3 and 0.79 to 1 for F4 prediction. Nonetheless, the EFSUMB Clinical Practice Guidelines suggest that pSWE can be the first-line assessment in HCV-infected patients for fibrosis evaluation, performing best at ruling out cirrhosis [15].

6. Appraisal of liver fibrosis by 2D shear wave elastography in HCV-infected patients

2D shear wave elastography, a novel US-based technique, allows the estimation of tissue dynamics using focused ultrasonic beams in a certain ROI. This technique has the advantage of displaying a real-time color-coded map overlaid on a B-mode image. Furthermore, 2D-SWE estimates LS expressed in kPa or m/s [28, 77]. It should be executed in a well-visualized area of the right hepatic lobe, clear of large vessels, ligaments, gallbladder, and the liver capsule, with the patient situated in a supine position with breathing suspension [15].

As exemplified in **Table 4**, several studies reported the diagnostic accuracy of 2D-SWE for fibrosis assessment among HCV-infected patients [76, 78–86, 88]. In 2017, Herrmann et al. [81] performed a meta-analysis including 13 studies, gathering 379 patients with CHC, that evaluated the diagnostic performance of 2D-SWE for the noninvasive staging of liver fibrosis. They found AUROC values of 0.863, 0.915, and 0.929 for diagnosing significant fibrosis, severe fibrosis, and cirrhosis, respectively. In our analysis, the AUROC values range from 0.82 to 0.888 for ≥ F1, 0.783 to 0.97 for ≥ F2, 0.877 to 0.97 for ≥ F3 and 0.893 to 0.98 for ≥ F4, respectively (**Table 4**).

7. HCV post-sustained virological response/antiviral therapy appraised by liver stiffness

Due to their potency, ease of use, tolerability, and safety, DAA regiments are the recommended choice in subjects with compensated advanced chronic liver disease (cACLD). Their introduction resulted in increasing rates of SVR, reducing LS among these patients. Nonetheless, most of the studies concerning interferon-free treatments are retrospective, with small sample sizes, with short follow-up after SVR, and

Fibrosis stage	≥ F1			≥ F2			≥ F3			= F4		
Study	Cut-off (kPa)	ROC	Se/Sp (%)	Cut-off (kPa)	ROC	Se/Sp (%)	Cut-off (kPa)	ROC	Se/Sp (%)	Cut-off (kPa)	ROC	Se/Sp (%)
Bavu (n=113) [78]	N/S	N/S	N/S	9.12	0.948	72/81	10.08	0.962	0.968	13.3	0.968	87/80
Ferraioli (n = 121) [79]	N/S	N/S	N/S	7.1	0.92	90/87.5	8.7	0.99	97.3/95.1	10.4	0.98	87.5/96.8
Tada (n = 55) [80]	N/S	N/S	N/S	8.8	0.940	88.9/91.9	N/S	N/S	N/S	N/S	N/S	N/S
Herrmann (n = 379) [81]*	N/S	N/S	N/S	7.1	0.864	94.7/52	9.2	0.915	90.3/76.8	13.0	0.929	85.8/87.8
Abe (n = 233)[1] [82]	1.480	0.888	75.9/88.2	1.560	0.915	85.3/85.5	1.720	0.940	88.8/83.8	1.930	0.949	91.4/90.8
Serra (n = 51) [83]	N/S	N/S	N/S	9.225	0.783	59.1/86.2	10.695	0.877	72.7/90	11.525	0.893	85.7/88.6
Villani (n = 178) [84][2,3]	N/S	N/S	N/S	8.15	0.899	87.1/73	10.31	0.900	77.2/85.4	12.65	0.899	73.3/88.5
Baldea (n = 176) [76]	N/S	N/S	N/S	6.5	0.92	84.1/88.2	8.19	0.93	96.7/77.4	11.3	0.96	95.7/92.7
Baldea (n = 208) [85][3,4]	N/S	N/S	N/S	7.7 8.5	0.97 0.96	86.3/96.9 87.6/100	8.3 11.1	0.97 0.95	94.8/90.3 89.7/95.1	9.7 12.3	0.97 0.96	92.6/91.6 92.5/94
Aksakal (n = 43) [86]	6.09	0.82	86/70	7.81	0.97	84/96	9.00	0.97	90/97	12.47	0.98	85/98
Numao (n = 141) [87]	N/S	N/S	N/S	N/S	0.86	N/S	N/S	0.97	N/S	N/S	0.91	N/S

Abbreviations: N/S – not specified; ROC – receiver operating characteristics curve; Se – sensibility; Sp – specificity.
*meta-analysis.
[1]The Abe study used SWV, expressed in m/s.
[2]The Villani study used the novel EPIQ 7 US system (ElastQ).
[3]These studies used VCTE as reference standard for fibrosis evaluation.
[4]The Baldea study offered result two 2D-SWE techniques: General Electric and SuperSonic Imagine, respectively.

Table 4.
Performance of 2D-SWE for detecting different stages of fibrosis in patients with CHC.

lacking post-SVR LB [6, 89, 90]. A recent prospective longitudinal study by Knop et al. [91] sought to elucidate the dynamics of liver and spleen stiffness in cirrhotic patients through VCTE and p-SWE, 3 years post-treatment. Even if their analysis showed that LS decreases in a significant proportion of patients with CHC, spleen stiffness, a non-invasive marker for portal hypertension, remained unchanged. Similarly, other research found lower LS values by p-SWE (VTTQ) in HCV-infected patients who achieved SVR [92, 93].

In addition, the diagnostic accuracy of VCTE for SVR prediction remains controversial, since the improvement of LS post-DAA treatment may be overrated by elastography in contrast with histological staging [94]. In fact, a recent prospective multicenter study comprising of 746 HCV-infected patients with CHC with SVR evaluated 3 years post-DAA therapy, discovered cirrhosis by LB in more than half of cACLD patients, in spite of normal VCTE values or liver function parameters. Due to its poor diagnostic accuracy (AUROC = 0.75), VCTE turned out to be an unreliable method for the accurate identification of the fibrosis stage in HCV-infected patients who acquired SVR [95].

Latest EASL guidelines conclude that neither noninvasive elastographic techniques are appropriate enough to detect fibrosis regression after SVR in CHC patients. Additionally, cut-off values of LS by VCTE used in untreated HCV patients should not be utilized for liver fibrosis staging after SVR. Therefore, the appraisal of liver disease severity and prognosis remains an unmet need in this field, requiring larger cohort sizes and extended follow-up in order to establish the role of noninvasive techniques in treating HCV-infected patients [6].

8. The prognostic value of elastography for the prediction of clinical outcomes (decompensation; HCC) in patients with HCV-related cACLD who achieved sustained virological response

In HCV-infected patients, the risk of all-cause mortality and the incidence of HCC diminished in subjects who achieved SVR after interferon-based antiviral therapy, regardless of the grade of fibrosis [96, 97]. In addition, the introduction of novel highly efficient DAAs improved the capability of decreasing the HCC risk, even among patients with advanced liver disease [50]. Nonetheless, a relevant risk of 1.5% remains, requiring proper and cost-effective surveillance methods for these patients [98, 99]. Evidence shows that clinically significant portal hypertension (CSPH), defined as hepatic venous pressure gradient (HVPG) $\geq$10 mmHg, is the strongest predictor for hepatic decompensation [6]. For these patients, compensated advanced CLD (cACLD) is the proposed term by the Baveno VI consensus [100]. However, HVPG is an invasive and expensive method, requiring reliable noninvasive alternatives [50].

Being a noninvasive, low-cost, and easy to perform method, VCTE turned out to be an outstanding diagnostic instrument for CSPH, with a hierarchical summary ROC of 0.93 [101]. A recent multicenter study of 5648 patients, found that lowering the dual-threshold to <7 kPa and > 12 kPa, provided excellent Se of 91% for excluding and great Sp of 92% for diagnosing cACLD, respectively [100]. In addition, elastography might enable the dynamic appraisal of the HCC risk, especially before and after antiviral treatment. Several studies aimed to elucidate whether VCTE, p-SWE, and 2D-SWE may facilitate HCC surveillance in HCV-infected patients [102–105]. A recent meta-analysis, comprising 3398 patients, found a pooled HR for HCC development of 3.43 (95% CI, 1.63–7.19) between positive and negative LSM, indicating that

VCTE is a trustworthy procedure for HCC prediction in CHC patients treated with DAAs [106]. In a multicenter cohort study, Alonso et al. [107] provided two easy and broadly applicable models for the estimation of HCC risk after SVR. Their model, including baseline albumin ($\geq$ or < 4.2 g/dl), baseline LS (> or $\leq$ 17.3 KPa), and LS after 1 year ($\geq$ or < 25.5%), increased HCC surveillance efforts (Harrell's C: 0.77). In 2018, Ioannou et al. [108] internally validated models that calculate the HCC risk following antiviral treatment. However, current EASL clinical practice guidelines recommend that patients with cACLD before antiviral therapy should be continuously supervised for HCC and portal hypertensions, regardless of measurement values of noninvasive tests post-SVR.

9. Controlled attenuation parameter (CAP) for the noninvasive estimation of steatosis in HCV-infected patients

Steatosis is a common histological feature and has an important role in the evolution of CHC, in particular in HCV genotype 3 infections [109, 110]. According to a meta-analysis counting 25 studies and 6400 patients, the prevalence of steatosis in CHC patients is estimated at 55.54%, in most cases affecting less than 33% of hepatocytes [111, 112].

Steatosis seems to accelerate fibrosis in the early stages of the disease, reduce treatment response and promote oncogenesis [2, 113, 114]. A recent retrospective study with 515 CHC patients undergoing DAA treatment found a significant correlation between the grade of steatosis and mortality of any cause or HCC development. Furthermore, steatosis surpasses advanced fibrosis regarding the prediction of a poor response to treatment [115]. Steatosis is thus a simple and important predictor of progression in chronic HCV patients.

US is the commonest imaging technique used in clinical practice to diagnose steatosis due to its high accessibility and low cost. However, it is operator- and machine-dependent and the performance is questionable [116, 117]. There is an increasing interest in developing novel tools for steatosis evaluation. At present, the non-invasive parameter, called controlled attenuation parameter (CAP), available on the FibroScan system, is the most validated one. Using the postulate that fat content is directly related to US beam attenuation, CAP enables the diagnosis and quantification of steatosis [118]. Results are expressed in decibels per meter (dB/m), with values ranging from 100 to 400 dB/m.

Several meta-analysis assessed the CAP performance for detecting and grading hepatic steatosis using LB as reference standard [119, 120]. One of the most important meta-analysis dates from 2017 and includes 2735 patients (36.5% with HCV infection) [119]. Results are consistent, so that CAP provided an AUROC of 0.823 (Se = 68.8%, Sp = 82.2%) for detecting mild steatosis ($\geq$S1), 0.865 (Se = 77.3%, Sp = 81.2%) for moderate steatosis ($\geq$S2) and 0.882 (Se = 88.2%, Sp = 77.6%) for severe steatosis ($\geq$S3) [119].

Concerning CHC, we cite 3 studies, one with 854 CHC patients, the other with 115 patients with chronic hepatitis, 76% of them being infected with HCV, and the latter with 201 patients with 118 (58.7%) subjects with HCV infection [121–123]. CAP had good diagnostic accuracy for detecting steatosis and for differentiating between different grades at least two grades apart, independently of fibrosis stage or activity grade. Optimal cutoff values were similar and are presented in **Table 5**. Further validation in large cohorts is however needed in order to validate proper cutoff values. CAP could be ideal as a screening test, as the NPV was high, 0.89–0.87 for $\geq$S1.

		Sasso et al. [121]	Ferraioli [122]	Lupsor-Platon [123]
	Patients number	854	115 (76% HCV pts)	201 (58.7% HCV pts)
≥S1	Optimal cutoff (dB/m)	222	219	260
	AUROC	0.80	0.76	0.813
≥S2	Optimal cutoff (dB/m)	233	296	285
	AUROC	0.86	0.82	0.822
≥S3	Optimal cutoff (dB/m)	290	N/S	294
	AUROC	0.88	N/S	0.838

Table 5.
Diagnostic performance of CAP in HCV-infected patients.

10. Perspectives

Since shear wave propagation spectroscopy can also provide additional mechanical information on soft tissues, such as viscosity, it might be possible to achieve additional data regarding the utility of 2D-SWE (SSI) for viscosity quantification, a potential marker for necroinflammatory activity [124]. Nonetheless, large cohort prospective studies are required in order to assess the performance of such parameters in biopsied HCV-infected patients.

11. Conclusions

Elastography-based imaging methods are of high interest nowadays. HCV patients can greatly benefit from VCTE due to its numerous qualities- rapid, noninvasive, repeatable for longitudinal evaluation, and cost-effectiveness. It has great discriminative power for fibrosis assessment, performing better at ruling out cirrhosis rather than diagnosing it, because of high specificity and negative predictive value. In addition, CAP is a precious tool for the noninvasive quantification of steatosis. Further validation in large cohorts is still needed in order to validate cutoff values in CHC patients. Among other elastographic techniques, pSWE and 2D-SWE proved to have the similar diagnostic performance to VCTE for the prediction of fibrosis severity in HCV-infected patients. One of the main advantages of non-invasive techniques is that they opened a new era in HCV management, since it can be easily executed when deemed necessary before antiviral therapy and after HCV eradication, as a repeatable surveillance method. Since the introduction of DAAs in HCV therapy, many patients achieve SVR, which is associated with a reduction in fibrosis. However, clinical practice guidelines do not currently recommend using elastography for the assessment of fibrosis decrease after treatment. Moreover, patients should continue surveillance for decompensation and HCC after SVR, regardless of the result of noninvasive methods.

It is essential that further studies focus on establishing standardized cutoff values of LS for adequate prediction of HCC risk in HCV patients, which is considered to be of great importance in current clinical practice.

Conflict of interest

The authors declare no conflict of interest.

Author details

Monica Lupsor-Platon[1,2]*, Teodora Serban[1] and Alexandra Iulia Silion[1]

1 Medical Imaging Department, Iuliu Hatieganu University of Medicine and Pharmacy, Cluj-Napoca, Romania

2 Regional Institute of Gastroenterology and Hepatology "Prof. Dr. Octavian Fodor", Cluj-Napoca, Romania

*Address all correspondence to: monica.lupsor@umfcluj.ro

IntechOpen

References

[1] Chen SL, Morgan TR. The natural history of hepatitis C virus (HCV) infection. International Journal of Medical Sciences. 2006;**3**(2):47-52

[2] Blach S, Zeuzem S, Manns M, et al. Global prevalence and genotype distribution of hepatitis C virus infection in 2015: A modelling study. The Lancet Gastroenterology & Hepatology. 2017;**2**(3):161-176

[3] Sebastiani G, Alberti A. How far is noninvasive assessment of liver fibrosis from replacing liver biopsy in hepatitis C? Journal of Viral Hepatitis. 2012;**19**(Suppl 1):18-32

[4] Yano M, Kumada H, Kage M, Ikeda K, Shimamatsu K, Inoue O, et al. The long-term pathological evolution of chronic hepatitis C. Hepatology. 1996;**23**(6):1334-1340

[5] Banerjee D, Reddy KR. Review article: Safety and tolerability of direct-acting anti-viral agents in the new era of hepatitis C therapy. Alimentary Pharmacology & Therapeutics. 2016;**43**(6):674-696

[6] European Association for the Study of the Liver. Electronic address eee, Clinical Practice Guideline P, Chair, representative EGB, Panel m. EASL Clinical Practice Guidelines on non-invasive tests for evaluation of liver disease severity and prognosis - 2021 update. Journal of Hepatology. 2021;**75**(3):659-689

[7] Bedossa P, Carrat F. Liver biopsy: The best, not the gold standard. Journal of Hepatology. 2009;**50**(1):1-3

[8] Colloredo G, Guido M, Sonzogni A, Leandro G. Impact of liver biopsy size on histological evaluation of chronic viral hepatitis: The smaller the sample, the milder the disease. Journal of Hepatology. 2003;**39**(2):239-244

[9] Pagliaro L, Rinaldi F, Craxi A, Di Piazza S, Filippazzo G, Gatto G, et al. Percutaneous blind biopsy versus laparoscopy with guided biopsy in diagnosis of cirrhosis. A prospective, randomized trial. Digestive Diseases and Sciences. 1983;**28**(1):39-43

[10] Poniachik J, Bernstein DE, Reddy KR, Jeffers LJ, Coelho-Little ME, Civantos F, et al. The role of laparoscopy in the diagnosis of cirrhosis. Gastrointestinal Endoscopy. 1996;**43**(6): 568-571

[11] Regev A, Berho M, Jeffers LJ, Milikowski C, Molina EG, Pyrsopoulos NT, et al. Sampling error and intraobserver variation in liver biopsy in patients with chronic HCV infection. The American Journal of Gastroenterology. 2002;**97**(10):2614-2618

[12] Wells RG. Tissue mechanics and fibrosis. Biochimica et Biophysica Acta. 2013;**1832**(7):884-890

[13] Ferraioli G, Filice C, Castera L, Choi BI, Sporea I, Wilson SR, et al. WFUMB guidelines and recommendations for clinical use of ultrasound elastography: Part 3: liver. Ultrasound in Medicine & Biology. 2015;**41**(5):1161-1179

[14] European Association for Study of L, Asociacion Latinoamericana para el Estudio del H. EASL-ALEH clinical practice guidelines: Non-invasive tests for evaluation of liver disease severity and prognosis. Journal of Hepatology. 2015;**63**(1):237-264

[15] Dietrich CF, Bamber J, Berzigotti A, Bota S, Cantisani V, Castera L, et al. EFSUMB guidelines and recommendations on the clinical use of liver ultrasound elastography, update 2017 (Long Version). Ultraschall in der Medizin (Stuttgart, Germany : 1980). 2017;**38**(4):e16-e47

[16] Tang A, Cloutier G, Szeverenyi NM, Sirlin CB. Ultrasound elastography and mr elastography for assessing liver fibrosis: Part 2, diagnostic performance, confounders, and future directions. AJR. American Journal of Roentgenology. 2015;**205**(1):33-40

[17] Mueller S, Sandrin L. Liver stiffness: A novel parameter for the diagnosis of liver disease. Hepatic Medicine : Evidence And Research. 2010;**2**:49-67

[18] Vispo E, Barreiro P, Del Valle J, Maida I, de Ledinghen V, Quereda C, et al. Overestimation of liver fibrosis staging using transient elastography in patients with chronic hepatitis C and significant liver inflammation. Antiviral Therapy. 2009;**14**(2):187-193

[19] Arena U, Vizzutti F, Corti G, Ambu S, Stasi C, Bresci S, et al. Acute viral hepatitis increases liver stiffness values measured by transient elastography. Hepatology. 2008;**47**(2):380-384

[20] Lupsor Platon M, Stefanescu H, Feier D, Maniu A, Badea R. Performance of unidimensional transient elastography in staging chronic hepatitis C. Results from a cohort of 1,202 biopsied patients from one single center. Journal of Gastrointestinal and Liver Diseases. 2013;**22**(2):157-166

[21] Millonig G, Reimann FM, Friedrich S, Fonouni H, Mehrabi A, Buchler MW, et al. Extrahepatic cholestasis increases liver stiffness (FibroScan) irrespective of fibrosis. Hepatology. 2008;**48**(5): 1718-1723

[22] Trifan A, Sfarti C, Cojocariu C, Dimache M, Cretu M, Hutanasu C, et al. Increased liver stiffness in extrahepatic cholestasis caused by choledocholithiasis. Hepatitis Monthly. 2011;**11**(5):372-375

[23] Colli A, Pozzoni P, Berzuini A, Gerosa A, Canovi C, Molteni EE, et al. Decompensated chronic heart failure: Increased liver stiffness measured by means of transient elastography. Radiology. 2010;**257**(3):872-878

[24] Lupsor-Platon M, Serban T, Silion AI, Tirpe A, Florea M. Hepatocellular carcinoma and non-alcoholic fatty liver disease: A step forward for better evaluation using ultrasound elastography. Cancers (Basel). 2020;**12**(10):2778

[25] Berzigotti A, Ferraioli G, Bota S, Gilja OH, Dietrich CF. Novel ultrasound-based methods to assess liver disease: The game has just begun. Digestive and Liver Disease. 2018;**50**(2):107-112

[26] Barr RG. Shear wave liver elastography. Abdominal Radiology (NY). 2018;**43**(4):800-807

[27] Ferraioli G, Wong VW, Castera L, Berzigotti A, Sporea I, Dietrich CF, et al. Liver ultrasound elastography: An update to the world federation for ultrasound in medicine and biology guidelines and recommendations. Ultrasound in Medicine & Biology. 2018;**44**(12):2419-2440

[28] Popescu A, Sirli R, Sporea I. 2D shear wave elastography for liver fibrosis evaluation. In: Lupsor-Platon M, editor. Ultrasound Elastography. London, United Kingdom: IntechOpen; 2019. pp. 37-48

[29] Bazerbachi F, Haffar S, Wang Z, Cabezas J, Arias-Loste MT, Crespo J, et al. Range of normal liver stiffness and factors associated with increased

stiffness measurements in apparently healthy individuals. Clinical Gastroenterology and Hepatology. 2019;**17**(1):54-64

[30] Stebbing J, Farouk L, Panos G, Anderson M, Jiao LR, Mandalia S, et al. A meta-analysis of transient elastography for the detection of hepatic fibrosis. Journal of Clinical Gastroenterology 2010;**44**(3):214-219

[31] Friedrich-Rust M, Ong MF, Martens S, Sarrazin C, Bojunga J, Zeuzem S, et al. Performance of transient elastography for the staging of liver fibrosis: A meta-analysis. Gastroenterology. Apr 2008;**134**(4):960-974

[32] Talwalkar JA, Kurtz DM, Schoenleber SJ, West CP, Montori VM. Ultrasound-based transient elastography for the detection of hepatic fibrosis: Systematic review and meta-analysis. Clinical Gastroenterology and Hepatology. Oct 2007;**5**(10):1214-1220

[33] Shaheen AA, Wan AF, Myers RP. FibroTest and FibroScan for the prediction of hepatitis C-related fibrosis: A systematic review of diagnostic test accuracy. The American Journal of Gastroenterology. 2007;**102**(11):2589-2600

[34] Abd El Rihim AY, Omar RF, Fathalah W, El Attar I, Hafez HA, Ibrahim W. Role of fibroscan and APRI in detection of liver fibrosis: A systematic review and meta-analysis. Arab Journal of Gastroenterology. 2013;**14**(2):44-50

[35] Ying HY, Lu LG, Jing DD, Ni XS. Accuracy of transient elastography in the assessment of chronic hepatitis C-related liver cirrhosis. Clinical and Investigative Medicine. 2016;**39**(5):E150-EE60

[36] Ganne-Carrie N, Ziol M, de Ledinghen V, Douvin C, Marcellin P,

Castera L, et al. Accuracy of liver stiffness measurement for the diagnosis of cirrhosis in patients with chronic liver diseases. Hepatology. 2006;**44**(6):1511-1517

[37] Zhang GL, Zhao QY, Lin CS, Hu ZX, Zhang T, Gao ZL. Transient elastography and ultrasonography: Optimal evaluation of liver fibrosis and cirrhosis in patients with chronic hepatitis B concurrent with nonalcoholic fatty liver disease. BioMed Research International. 2019;**2019**:3951574

[38] Berzigotti A, Abraldes JG, Tandon P, Erice E, Gilabert R, Garcia-Pagan JC, et al. Ultrasonographic evaluation of liver surface and transient elastography in clinically doubtful cirrhosis. Journal of Hepatology. 2010;**52**(6):846-853

[39] Njei B, McCarty TR, Luk J, Ewelukwa O, Ditah I, Lim JK. Use of transient elastography in patients with HIV-HCV coinfection: A systematic review and meta-analysis. Journal of Gastroenterology and Hepatology. 2016;**31**(10):1684-1693

[40] Castera L, Vergniol J, Foucher J, Le Bail B, Chanteloup E, Haaser M, et al. Prospective comparison of transient elastography, fibrotest, APRI, and liver biopsy for the assessment of fibrosis in chronic hepatitis C. Gastroenterology. 2005;**128**(2):343-350

[41] Afdhal NH, Bacon BR, Patel K, Lawitz EJ, Gordon SC, Nelson DR, et al. Accuracy of fibroscan, compared with histology, in analysis of liver fibrosis in patients with hepatitis B or C: A United States multicenter study. Clinical Gastroenterology and Hepatology. 2015;**13**(4):772-779

[42] Degos F, Perez P, Roche B, Mahmoudi A, Asselineau J, Voitot H, et al. Diagnostic accuracy of FibroScan

and comparison to liver fibrosis biomarkers in chronic viral hepatitis: A multicenter prospective study (the FIBROSTIC study). Journal of Hepatology. 2010;**53**(6):1013-1021

[43] Ziol M, Handra-Luca A, Kettaneh A, Christidis C, Mal F, Kazemi F, et al. Noninvasive assessment of liver fibrosis by measurement of stiffness in patients with chronic hepatitis C. Hepatology. 2005;**41**(1):48-54

[44] Carrion JA, Navasa M, Bosch J, Bruguera M, Gilabert R, Forns X. Transient elastography for diagnosis of advanced fibrosis and portal hypertension in patients with hepatitis C recurrence after liver transplantation. Liver Transplantation. 2006;**12**(12):1791-1798

[45] Sporea I, Sirli R, Deleanu A, Tudora A, Curescu M, Cornianu M, et al. Comparison of the liver stiffness measurement by transient elastography with the liver biopsy. World Journal of Gastroenterology. 2008;**14**(42): 6513-6517

[46] Nitta Y, Kawabe N, Hashimoto S, Harata M, Komura N, Kobayashi K, et al. Liver stiffness measured by transient elastography correlates with fibrosis area in liver biopsy in patients with chronic hepatitis C. Hepatology Research. 2009;**39**(7):675-684

[47] Zarski JP, Sturm N, Guechot J, Paris A, Zafrani ES, Asselah T, et al. Comparison of nine blood tests and transient elastography for liver fibrosis in chronic hepatitis C: The ANRS HCEP-23 study. Journal of Hepatology. 2012;**56**(1):55-62

[48] Wang JH, Changchien CS, Hung CH, Eng HL, Tung WC, Kee KM, et al. FibroScan and ultrasonography in the prediction of hepatic fibrosis in patients

with chronic viral hepatitis. Journal of Gastroenterology. 2009;**44**(5):439-446

[49] Yoneda M, Thomas E, Sclair SN, Grant TT, Schiff ER. Supersonic shear imaging and transient elastography with the XL probe accurately detect fibrosis in overweight or obese patients with chronic liver disease. Clinical Gastroenterology and Hepatology. 2015;**13**(8):1502-1509

[50] Florea M, Serban T, Tirpe GR, Tirpe A, Lupsor-Platon M. Noninvasive assessment of hepatitis C virus infected patients using vibration-controlled transient elastography. Journal of Clinical Medicine. 2021;**10**(12):2575

[51] Poynard T, Halfon P, Castera L, Munteanu M, Imbert-Bismut F, Ratziu V, et al. Standardization of ROC curve areas for diagnostic evaluation of liver fibrosis markers based on prevalences of fibrosis stages. Clinical Chemistry. 2007;**53**(9):1615-1622

[52] Karlas T, Pfrepper C, Wiegand J, Wittekind C, Neuschulz M, Mossner J, et al. Acoustic radiation force impulse imaging (ARFI) for non-invasive detection of liver fibrosis: Examination standards and evaluation of interlobe differences in healthy subjects and chronic liver disease. Scandinavian Journal of Gastroenterology. 2011;**46**(12):1458-1467

[53] Lupsor M, Badea R, Stefanescu H, Sparchez Z, Branda H, Serban A, et al. Performance of a new elastographic method (ARFI technology) compared to unidimensional transient elastography in the noninvasive assessment of chronic hepatitis C preliminary results. Journal of Gastrointestinal and Liver Diseases. 2009;**18**(3):303-310

[54] Fierbinteanu-Braticevici C, Andronescu D, Usvat R, Cretoiu D,

Baicus C, Marinoschi G. Acoustic radiation force imaging sonoelastography for noninvasive staging of liver fibrosis. World Journal of Gastroenterology. 2009;15(44):5525-5532

[55] Friedrich-Rust M, Wunder K, Kriener S, Sotoudeh F, Richter S, Bojunga J, et al. Liver fibrosis in viral hepatitis: Noninvasive assessment with acoustic radiation force impulse imaging versus transient elastography. Radiology. 2009;252(2):595-604

[56] Rizzo L, Calvaruso V, Cacopardo B, Alessi N, Attanasio M, Petta S, et al. Comparison of transient elastography and acoustic radiation force impulse for non-invasive staging of liver fibrosis in patients with chronic hepatitis C. The American Journal of Gastroenterology. 2011;106(12):2112-2120

[57] Sporea I, Sirli R, Bota S, Fierbinteanu-Braticevici C, Petrisor A, Badea R, et al. Is ARFI elastography reliable for predicting fibrosis severity in chronic HCV hepatitis? World Journal of Radiology. 2011;3(7):188-193

[58] Friedrich-Rust M, Nierhoff J, Lupsor M, Sporea I, Fierbinteanu-Braticevici C, Strobel D, et al. Performance of acoustic radiation force impulse imaging for the staging of liver fibrosis: A pooled meta-analysis. Journal of Viral Hepatitis. 2012;19(2):e212-e219

[59] Sporea I, Bota S, Peck-Radosavljevic M, Sirli R, Tanaka H, Iijima H, et al. Acoustic radiation force impulse elastography for fibrosis evaluation in patients with chronic hepatitis C: An international multicenter study. European Journal of Radiology. 2012;81(12):4112-4118

[60] Chen SH, Li YF, Lai HC, Kao JT, Peng CY, Chuang PH, et al. Effects of patient factors on noninvasive liver stiffness measurement using acoustic radiation force impulse elastography in patients with chronic hepatitis C. BMC Gastroenterology. 2012;12:105

[61] Zhang DK, Chen M, Liu Y, Wang RF, Dong XY, Li ZY, et al. Clinical value of acoustic radiation force impulse imaging for quantitative evaluation of degree of liver fibrosis in chronic hepatitis C patients. Zhonghua Gan Zang Bing Za Zhi. 2013;21(8):599-603

[62] Nishikawa T, Hashimoto S, Kawabe N, Harata M, Nitta Y, Murao M, et al. Factors correlating with acoustic radiation force impulse elastography in chronic hepatitis C. World Journal of Gastroenterology. 2014;20(5):1289-1297

[63] Yamada R, Hiramatsu N, Oze T, Morishita N, Harada N, Miyazaki M, et al. Significance of liver stiffness measurement by acoustic radiation force impulse (ARFI) among hepatitis C patients. Journal of Medical Virology. 2014;86(2):241-247

[64] Li SM, Li GX, Fu DM, Wang Y, Dang LQ. Liver fibrosis evaluation by ARFI and APRI in chronic hepatitis C. World Journal of Gastroenterology. 2014;20(28):9528-9533

[65] Takaki S, Kawakami Y, Miyaki D, Nakahara T, Naeshiro N, Murakami E, et al. Non-invasive liver fibrosis score calculated by combination of virtual touch tissue quantification and serum liver functional tests in chronic hepatitis C patients. Hepatology Research. 2014;44(3):280-287

[66] Silva Junior RG, Schmillevitch J, Nascimento Mde F, Miranda ML, Brant PE, Schulz PO, et al. Acoustic radiation force impulse elastography and serum fibrosis markers in chronic hepatitis C. Scandinavian Journal of Gastroenterology. 2014;49(8):986-992

[67] Tai DI, Tsay PK, Jeng WJ, Weng CC, Huang SF, Huang CH, et al. Differences in liver fibrosis between patients with chronic hepatitis B and C: Evaluation by acoustic radiation force impulse measurements at 2 locations. Journal of Ultrasound in Medicine. 2015;**34**(5):813-821

[68] Chen SH, Peng CY, Lai HC, Chang IP, Lee CJ, Su WP, et al. Head-to-head comparison between collagen proportionate area and acoustic radiation force impulse elastography in liver fibrosis quantification in chronic hepatitis C. PLoS One. 2015;**10**(10): e0140554

[69] Joo SK, Kim JH, Oh S, Kim BG, Lee KL, Kim HY, et al. Prospective comparison of noninvasive fibrosis assessment to predict advanced fibrosis or cirrhosis in asian patients with hepatitis C. Journal of Clinical Gastroenterology. 2015;**49**(8):697-704

[70] Mare R, Sporea I, Lupusoru R, Sirli R, Popescu A, Danila M, et al. The value of ElastPQ for the evaluation of liver stiffness in patients with B and C chronic hepatopathies. Ultrasonics. 2017;**77**:144-151

[71] Gani RA, Hasan I, Sanityoso A, Lesmana CRA, Kurniawan J, Jasirwan COM, et al. Evaluation of acoustic radiation force impulse (ARFI) for fibrosis staging in chronic liver diseases. Acta Medica Indonesiana. 2017;**49**(2):128-135

[72] Ragazzo TG, Paranagua-Vezozzo D, Lima FR, de Campos Mazo DF, Pessoa MG, Oliveira CP, et al. Accuracy of transient elastography-FibroScan(R), acoustic radiation force impulse (ARFI) imaging, the enhanced liver fibrosis (ELF) test, APRI, and the FIB-4 index compared with liver biopsy in patients with chronic hepatitis C. Clinics (São Paulo, Brazil). 2017;**72**(9):516-525

[73] Alem SA, Abdellatif Z, Mabrouk M, Zayed N, Elsharkawy A, Khairy M, et al. Diagnostic accuracy of acoustic radiation force impulse elastography (ARFI) in comparison to other non-invasive modalities in staging of liver fibrosis in chronic HCV patients: Single-center experience. Abdominal Radiology (NY). 2019;**44**(8):2751-2758

[74] Hsu TH, Tsui PH, Yu WT, Huang SF, Tai J, Wan YL, et al. Cutoff values of acoustic radiation force impulse two-location measurements in different etiologies of liver fibrosis. Journal of Medical Ultrasound. 2019;**27**(3):130-134

[75] Ueda N, Kawaoka T, Imamura M, Aikata H, Nakahara T, Murakami E, et al. Liver fibrosis assessments using FibroScan, virtual-touch tissue quantification, the FIB-4 index, and mac-2 binding protein glycosylation isomer levels compared with pathological findings of liver resection specimens in patients with hepatitis C infection. BMC Gastroenterology. 2020;**20**(1):314

[76] Baldea V, Sporea I, Lupusoru R, Bende F, Mare R, Popescu A, et al. Comparative study between the diagnostic performance of point and 2-D shear-wave elastography for the non-invasive assessment of liver fibrosis in patients with chronic hepatitis C using transient elastography as reference. Ultrasound in Medicine & Biology. 2020;**46**(11):2979-2988

[77] Lupsor-Platon M, Badea R, Gersak M, Maniu A, Rusu I, Suciu A, et al. Noninvasive assessment of liver diseases using 2D shear wave elastography. Journal of Gastrointestinal and Liver Diseases. 2016;**25**(4):525-532

[78] Bavu E, Gennisson JL, Couade M, Bercoff J, Mallet V, Fink M, et al. Noninvasive in vivo liver fibrosis evaluation using supersonic shear

imaging: A clinical study on 113 hepatitis C virus patients. Ultrasound in Medicine & Biology. 2011;**37**(9):1361-1373

[79] Ferraioli G, Tinelli C, Dal Bello B, Zicchetti M, Filice G, Filice C, et al. Accuracy of real-time shear wave elastography for assessing liver fibrosis in chronic hepatitis C: A pilot study. Hepatology. 2012;**56**(6):2125-2133

[80] Tada T, Kumada T, Toyoda H, Ito T, Sone Y, Okuda S, et al. Utility of real-time shear wave elastography for assessing liver fibrosis in patients with chronic hepatitis C infection without cirrhosis: Comparison of liver fibrosis indices. Hepatology Research. 2015;**45**(10):E122-E129

[81] Herrmann E, de Ledinghen V, Cassinotto C, Chu WC, Leung VY, Ferraioli G, et al. Assessment of biopsy-proven liver fibrosis by two-dimensional shear wave elastography: An individual patient data-based meta-analysis. Hepatology. 2018;**67**(1):260-272

[82] Abe T, Kuroda H, Fujiwara Y, Yoshida Y, Miyasaka A, Kamiyama N, et al. Accuracy of 2D shear wave elastography in the diagnosis of liver fibrosis in patients with chronic hepatitis C. Journal of Clinical Ultrasound. 2018;**46**(5):319-327

[83] Serra C, Grasso V, Conti F, Felicani C, Mazzotta E, Lenzi M, et al. A new two-dimensional shear wave elastography for noninvasive assessment of liver fibrosis in healthy subjects and in patients with chronic liver disease. Ultraschall in der Medizin (Stuttgart, Germany: 1980). 2018;**39**(4):432-439

[84] Villani R, Cavallone F, Romano AD, Bellanti F, Serviddio G. Two-dimensional shear wave elastography versus transient elastography: A non-invasive comparison for the assessment of liver fibrosis

in patients with chronic hepatitis C. Diagnostics (Basel). 2020;**10**(5)

[85] Baldea V, Bende F, Popescu A, Sirli R, Sporea I. Comparative study between two 2D-shear waves elastography techniques for the non-invasive assessment of liver fibrosis in patients with chronic hepatitis C virus (HCV) infection. Medical Ultrasonography. 2021;**23**(3):257-264

[86] Aksakal M, Oktar SO, Sendur HN, Esendagli G, Ozenirler S, Cindoruk M, et al. Diagnostic performance of 2D shear wave elastography in predicting liver fibrosis in patients with chronic hepatitis B and C: a histopathological correlation study. Abdominal Radiology (NY). 2021;**46**(7):3238-3244

[87] Numao H, Shimaya K, Kakuta A, Shibutani K, Igarashi S, Hasui K, et al. The utility of two-dimensional real-time shear wave elastography for assessing liver fibrosis in patients with chronic hepatitis C virus infection. European Journal of Gastroenterology & Hepatology. 2021;**33**(11):1400-1407

[88] Matos J, Paparo F, Bacigalupo L, Cenderello G, Mussetto I, De Cesari M, et al. Noninvasive liver fibrosis assessment in chronic viral hepatitis C: Agreement among 1D transient elastography, 2D shear wave elastography, and magnetic resonance elastography. Abdominal Radiology (NY). 2019;**44**(12):4011-4021

[89] Persico M, Rosato V, Aglitti A, Precone D, Corrado M, De Luna A, et al. Sustained virological response by direct antiviral agents in HCV leads to an early and significant improvement of liver fibrosis. Antiviral Therapy. 2018;**23**(2):129-138

[90] Singh S, Facciorusso A, Loomba R, Falck-Ytter YT. Magnitude and kinetics of decrease in liver stiffness after antiviral therapy in patients with chronic hepatitis

C: A systematic review and meta-analysis. Clinical Gastroenterology and Hepatology. 2018;**16**(1):27-38

[91] Knop V, Hoppe D, Vermehren J, Troetschler S, Herrmann E, Vermehren A, et al. Non-invasive assessment of fibrosis regression and portal hypertension in patients with advanced chronic hepatitis C virus (HCV)-associated liver disease and sustained virologic response (SVR): 3 years follow-up of a prospective longitudinal study. Journal of Viral Hepatitis. 2021;**28**(11):1604-1613

[92] Tachi Y, Hirai T, Kojima Y, Miyata A, Ohara K, Ishizu Y, et al. Liver stiffness measurement using acoustic radiation force impulse elastography in hepatitis C virus-infected patients with a sustained virological response. Alimentary Pharmacology & Therapeutics. 2016;**44**(4):346-355

[93] Chen SH, Lai HC, Chiang IP, Su WP, Lin CH, Kao JT, et al. Performance of acoustic radiation force impulse elastography for staging liver fibrosis in patients with chronic hepatitis C after viral eradication. Clinical Infectious Diseases. 2020;**70**(1):114-122

[94] Pan JJ, Bao F, Du E, Skillin C, Frenette CT, Waalen J, et al. Morphometry confirms fibrosis regression from sustained virologic response to direct-acting antivirals for hepatitis C. Hepatology Communications. 2018;**2**(11):1320-1330

[95] Broquetas T, Herruzo-Pino P, Marino Z, Naranjo D, Vergara M, Morillas RM, et al. Elastography is unable to exclude cirrhosis after sustained virological response in HCV-infected patients with advanced chronic liver disease. Liver International. 2021;**41**(11):2733-2746

[96] van der Meer AJ, Veldt BJ, Feld JJ, Wedemeyer H, Dufour JF, Lammert F, et al. Association between sustained virological response and all-cause mortality among patients with chronic hepatitis C and advanced hepatic fibrosis. JAMA. 2012;**308**(24):2584-2593

[97] Morgan RL, Baack B, Smith BD, Yartel A, Pitasi M, Falck-Ytter Y. Eradication of hepatitis C virus infection and the development of hepatocellular carcinoma: A meta-analysis of observational studies. Annals of Internal Medicine. 2013;**158**(5 Pt 1):329-337

[98] European Association for the Study of the Liver. Electronic address eee, European Association for the Study of the L. EASL Clinical Practice Guidelines: Management of hepatocellular carcinoma. Journal of Hepatology. 2018;**69**(1):182-236

[99] Kanwal F, Kramer JR, Asch SM, Cao Y, Li L, El-Serag HB. Long-term risk of hepatocellular carcinoma in HCV patients treated with direct acting antiviral agents. Hepatology. 2020;**71**(1):44-55

[100] Papatheodoridi M, Hiriart JB, Lupsor-Platon M, Bronte F, Boursier J, Elshaarawy O, et al. Refining the Baveno VI elastography criteria for the definition of compensated advanced chronic liver disease. Journal of Hepatology. 2021;**74**(5):1109-1116

[101] Shi KQ, Fan YC, Pan ZZ, Lin XF, Liu WY, Chen YP, et al. Transient elastography: A meta-analysis of diagnostic accuracy in evaluation of portal hypertension in chronic liver disease. Liver International. 2013;**33**(1):62-71

[102] Lee HW, Chon YE, Kim SU, Kim BK, Park JY, Kim DY, et al. Predicting liver-related events using transient elastography in chronic hepatitis c

patients with sustained virological response. Gut Liver. 2016;**10**(3):429-436

[103] Hamada K, Saitoh S, Nishino N, Fukushima D, Horikawa Y, Nishida S, et al. Shear wave elastography predicts hepatocellular carcinoma risk in hepatitis C patients after sustained virological response. PLoS One. 2018;**13**(4):e0195173

[104] Fernandes FF, Piedade J, Guimaraes L, Nunes EP, Chaves U, Goldenzon RV, et al. Effectiveness of direct-acting agents for hepatitis C and liver stiffness changing after sustained virological response. Journal of Gastroenterology and Hepatology. 2019;**34**(12):2187-2195

[105] Tachi Y, Hirai T, Kojima Y, Tachino H, Hosokawa C, Ohya T, et al. Diagnostic performance of real-time tissue elastography in chronic hepatitis C patients with sustained virological response. European Journal of Gastroenterology & Hepatology. 2020;**32**(5):609-615

[106] You MW, Kim KW, Shim JJ, Pyo J. Impact of liver-stiffness measurement on hepatocellular carcinoma development in chronic hepatitis C patients treated with direct-acting antivirals: A systematic review and time-to-event meta-analysis. Journal of Gastroenterology and Hepatology. 2021;**36**(3):601-608

[107] Alonso Lopez S, Manzano ML, Gea F, Gutierrez ML, Ahumada AM, Devesa MJ, et al. A model based on noninvasive markers predicts very low hepatocellular carcinoma risk after viral response in hepatitis C virus-advanced fibrosis. Hepatology. 2020;**72**(6):1924-1934

[108] Ioannou GN, Green PK, Beste LA, Mun EJ, Kerr KF, Berry K. Development of models estimating the risk of hepatocellular carcinoma after antiviral treatment for hepatitis C. Journal of Hepatology. 2018;**69**(5):1088-1098

[109] Modaresi Esfeh J, Ansari-Gilani K. Steatosis and hepatitis C. Gastroenterology Report (Oxford). 2016;**4**(1):24-29

[110] Mazhar SM, Shiehmorteza M, Sirlin CB. Noninvasive assessment of hepatic steatosis. Clinical Gastroenterology and Hepatology. 2009;**7**(2):135-140

[111] El-Zayadi AR. Hepatic steatosis: a benign disease or a silent killer. World Journal of Gastroenterology. 2008;**14**(26):4120-4126

[112] Lonardo A, Loria P, Adinolfi LE, Carulli N, Ruggiero G. Hepatitis C and steatosis: A reappraisal. Journal of Viral Hepatitis. 2006;**13**(2):73-80

[113] Kurosaki M, Hosokawa T, Matsunaga K, Hirayama I, Tanaka T, Sato M, et al. Hepatic steatosis in chronic hepatitis C is a significant risk factor for developing hepatocellular carcinoma independent of age, sex, obesity, fibrosis stage and response to interferon therapy. Hepatology Research. 2010;**40**(9):870-877

[114] Castera L, Hezode C, Roudot-Thoraval F, Bastie A, Zafrani ES, Pawlotsky JM, et al. Worsening of steatosis is an independent factor of fibrosis progression in untreated patients with chronic hepatitis C and paired liver biopsies. Gut. 2003;**52**(2):288-292

[115] Peleg N, Issachar A, Sneh Arbib O, Cohen-Naftaly M, Harif Y, Oxtrud E, et al. Liver steatosis is a major predictor of poor outcomes in chronic hepatitis C patients with sustained virological response. Journal of Viral Hepatitis. 2019;**26**(11):1257-1265

[116] Stauber RE, Lackner C. Noninvasive diagnosis of hepatic fibrosis in chronic hepatitis C. World Journal of Gastroenterology. 2007;**13**(32):4287-4294

[117] Hepburn MJ, Vos JA, Fillman EP, Lawitz EJ. The accuracy of the report of hepatic steatosis on ultrasonography in patients infected with hepatitis C in a clinical setting: A retrospective observational study. BMC Gastroenterology. 2005;**5**:14

[118] Sasso M, Beaugrand M, de Ledinghen V, Douvin C, Marcellin P, Poupon R, et al. Controlled attenuation parameter (CAP): A novel VCTE guided ultrasonic attenuation measurement for the evaluation of hepatic steatosis: preliminary study and validation in a cohort of patients with chronic liver disease from various causes. Ultrasound in Medicine & Biology. 2010;**36**(11):1825-1835

[119] Karlas T, Petroff D, Sasso M, Fan JG, Mi YQ, de Lédinghen V, et al. Individual patient data meta-analysis of controlled attenuation parameter (CAP) technology for assessing steatosis. Journal of Hepatology. 2017;**66**(5):1022-1030

[120] Wang Y, Fan Q, Wang T, Wen J, Wang H, Zhang T. Controlled attenuation parameter for assessment of hepatic steatosis grades: A diagnostic meta-analysis. International Journal of Clinical and Experimental Medicine. 2015;**8**(10):17654-17663

[121] Sasso M, Tengher-Barna I, Ziol M, Miette V, Fournier C, Sandrin L, et al. Novel controlled attenuation parameter for noninvasive assessment of steatosis using Fibroscan((R)): Validation in chronic hepatitis C. Journal of Viral Hepatitis. 2012;**19**(4):244-253

[122] Ferraioli G, Tinelli C, Lissandrin R, Zicchetti M, Dal Bello B, Filice G, et al. Controlled attenuation parameter for evaluating liver steatosis in chronic viral hepatitis. World Journal of Gastroenterology. 2014;**20**(21): 6626-6631

[123] Lupșor-Platon M, Feier D, Stefănescu H, Tamas A, Botan E, Sparchez Z, et al. Diagnostic accuracy of controlled attenuation parameter measured by transient elastography for the non-invasive assessment of liver steatosis: A prospective study. Journal of Gastrointestinal and Liver Diseases. 2015;**24**(1):35-42

[124] Deffieux T, Gennisson JL, Bousquet L, Corouge M, Cosconea S, Amroun D, et al. Investigating liver stiffness and viscosity for fibrosis, steatosis and activity staging using shear wave elastography. Journal of Hepatology. 2015;**62**(2):317-324

Chapter 6

Shear Wave Elastography in the Assessment of Liver Changes in Children with Cystic Fibrosis

Mikhail Pykov, Natalia Kuzmina and Nikolay Rostovtsev

Abstract

A standard ultrasound examination of the liver was performed in 232 children. It was supplemented by a two-dimensional shear wave elastography. There were 200 healthy children aged 3 to 18 years (control group) and 32 patients with cystic fibrosis aged 2 to 17 years (study group) among them. The procedure was carried out by means of Aixplorer device (Supersonic Imagine, France) using a convex sensor operating in the 1–6 MHz frequency range. Ten measurements of Young modulus values were carried out in different segments of the right lobe of the liver followed by data averaging. In patients with cystic fibrosis, the values of Young modulus were significantly higher than in healthy children (Emean median: 6.50 and 5.00 kPa, interquartile range: 5.62–7.52 and 4.70–5.38 kPa, respectively ($p < 0.001$). In patients with severe cystic fibrosis, the values of Young modulus were significantly higher compared to patients suffering from moderate disease (Emean median: 7.30 and 5.90 kPa, interquartile range: 6.20–10.70 and 5.20–6.75 kPa, respectively ($p < 0.002$). Shear wave elastography is a non-invasive technique that can be successfully used in a comprehensive ultrasound assessment of the liver in children with cystic fibrosis to facilitate the diagnosis and monitoring of fibrous changes.

Keywords: ultrasound elastography, shear wave elastography, stiffness, young modulus, cystic fibrosis, fibrosis, liver, children

1. Introduction

Recently, ultrasound elastography has become perhaps the most important achievement in the evolution of non-invasive techniques, particularly ultrasound examination, to assess the condition of the liver in general. This is a method of qualitative and quantitative analysis of elastic properties of tissues, which makes it possible to evaluate the elastic properties of tissues during a conventional ultrasound examination by measuring the values of shear wave velocity (m/s) or Young modulus (kPa) in the organs and tissues of interest [1].

As a rule, the stiffness in pathological tissues is more pronounced compared to the adjacent healthy tissues, and this fact is registered by ultrasound elastography of different types. According to the international guidelines, ultrasound elastography methods are divided into compressive elastography (SE) and shear wave elastography (SWE) [2–5]. SWE methods measure the velocity of shear waves generated in the tissues by an external mechanical shock (transient elastography, TE) or an electronic impulse (ARFI). The advantages of ARFI-based elastography methods (point elastography, pSWE and two-dimensional elastography, 2D-SWE) are that they are fast and integrated into the ultrasound diagnostic system, which enables to perform grayscale navigation. When conducting 2D-SWE, we get not only quantitative data in the form of digital values of the shear wave velocity but also qualitative information, since the areas with different values of the Young modulus are mapped in different colours. It is the digital values of indicated parameters that determine the colour in the area of interest [1, 6].

Most guidelines and recommendations for the clinical use of elastography (EFSUMB, WFUMB) focus on the assessment of diffuse liver disease in adults [2–9]. However, recommendations for adult patients cannot be immediately used in paediatric practice, taking into account the peculiarities of paediatric patients, i.e., restless behaviour during the examination of young children, small intervals between meals in infants, difficulties with breath-holding. These factors can affect the reproducibility of measurements and the accuracy of diagnostics in paediatrics. Psychological, anatomical and morphological features of children make the technique of elastography even more complex than a conventional ultrasound examination. Therefore, ultrasound elastography is less studied in children than in adults. Nevertheless, there are more and more reports from different research groups about the use of elastography to assess liver stiffness in healthy children. Special attention is paid to the age and gender characteristics of stiffness, the dependence of values on body mass index, use of sedatives and food intake. The technique of the procedure is discussed concerning the position of the patient during the examination, the choice of the sensor, the zone and the number of measurements, the ambient conditions during the procedure. There are also works where elastography is used in the assessment of the spleen, thyroid gland, renal parenchyma, intestines and muscles [6, 10–13].

Numerous studies in adult patients have demonstrated that ultrasound elastography is a useful non-invasive method for diagnosing liver fibrosis. Preliminary findings using TE, pSWE and 2D-SWE have also shown that they are all feasible and can be used to assess liver fibrosis of various aetiology in children [6, 10, 11, 13]. Various infectious agents can act as an etiological factor causing fibrosis and cirrhosis of the liver in children, such as hepatitis B, C, D, G viruses, cytomegalovirus, Epstein-Barr virus, as well as autoimmune liver diseases, cystic fibrosis, metabolic diseases and others. Regardless of the aetiology, cirrhosis results in lethal outcome of patients due to the development of complications, i.e., bleeding from the oesophageal varices, ascites, encephalopathy, hemorrhagic syndrome.

Liver biopsy, being an invasive procedure, is less acceptable for children due to the need for general anaesthesia, as well as physical and emotional impact on the child. This procedure can cause a number of complications, such as pain syndrome, profuse bleeding, formation of subcapsular hematomas of the liver, development of biliary peritonitis, etc. [14, 15]. Non-invasive methods are extremely important in paediatrics, especially when repeated examinations are necessary, for example, during follow-up of patients with chronic liver diseases, when elastography can be used additionally to ultrasound examination and laboratory data facilitating observation of children with chronic liver diseases [10, 11, 13].

2. Pathophysiology of fibrotic changes in the liver in cystic fibrosis

Cystic fibrosis is one of the most common monogenic diseases with an autosomal recessive type of inheritance and multiple organ manifestations. In most countries of

Europe and North America, cystic fibrosis prevalence ranges from 1:2,000 to 1:4,000 newborns, in Russia, it is 1:8000–1:10,000 newborns. The disease is caused by the gene mutation of the transmembrane regulator of cystic fibrosis and is characterised by damage to the external secretion glands and severe respiratory disorders. However, due to the increased life expectancy of patients with cystic fibrosis, liver damage becomes an important clinical manifestation that determines the prognosis and quality of life [16–18].

Cystic fibrosis is no longer considered exclusively a childhood disease since the current life expectancy of such patients is more than 35 years [19]. According to different authors, the incidence of clinically apparent liver lesions in cystic fibrosis (cystic fibrosis-associated liver disease – CFLD) varies from 27 to 35% [18]. Symptoms of liver fibrosis of varying degrees are revealed in almost all patients with cystic fibrosis, and 5–10% of patients develop biliary cirrhosis of the liver with portal hypertension syndrome requiring surgical intervention [20, 21]. In the general list of causes of death in cystic fibrosis, liver cirrhosis is in the second place after bronchopulmonary complications and is 2.3–2.5% [20, 22].

The hepatobiliary system failure in cystic fibrosis is a direct consequence of a basic genetic defect. The CFTR protein is responsible for the pathogenesis functions as a channel of chloride ions [20, 23]. Insufficiency of the function of the channel of chlorine ions of cells lining the intrahepatic and extrahepatic bile ducts and gallbladder results in dehydration of hepatic secretions, i.e., they become adherent and poorly soluble [24]. Consequently, hepatocellular and canalicular cholestasis develops, which leads to a number of undesirable reactions, namely, delay of hepatotoxic bile acids, production of inflammatory mediators, cytokines and free radicals, increased lipid peroxidation and damage to cellular membranes, an excessive inflow of bile into the blood and tissues [25]. According to the clinical and morphological principle, liver cirrhosis in cystic fibrosis refers to biliary cirrhosis with obstruction of the intrahepatic biliary tract; microscopically – to multilobular cirrhosis; according to etiological characteristic – to cirrhosis caused by genetic metabolic disorders. Liver damage is characterized by chronic inflammatory cell infiltration and bile duct proliferation. These alterations are initially of a limited focal nature, but then they progress and lead to multilobular cirrhosis and portal hypertension. The process can slowly develop without pronounced clinical and biochemical manifestations, but it is irreversibly progressing [21–23, 26].

To date, there is no consensus on the risk factors and the rate of development of fibrotic liver changes in cystic fibrosis. Prematurity, low birth weight and prolonged parenteral nutrition are indicated as the causes of cystic fibrosis progression. Also, the severity of liver damage is associated with recurrent sepsis (including catheter sepsis) and bacterial load. Although it is believed that liver damage is more common in patients with severe mutations pertaining to classes I–III, genotype-phenotype correlation, which predicts the effect of mutation on the clinical expression of CFLD, is not possible at this stage. So, the clinical course in patients with diagnosed cystic fibrosis and the same mutation of the CFTR gene may be different [27]. It is still unclear why only a small number of patients with the same severe mutations develop CFLD symptoms. Some authors consider age at the time of diagnosis, male gender, intestinal obstruction of meconium in the anamnesis, external secretory insufficiency of the pancreas to be important factors [28, 29].

Early diagnosis of liver damage is complicated by a prolonged subclinical phase and lack of a reliable diagnostic technique: biochemical indices of liver failure (increased bilirubin level, decreased albumin concentration and increased pro-thrombin time) appear late, when severe liver failure has developed. Therefore, all patients with cystic fibrosis should be carefully monitored for the occurrence of this complication in the first decade of their life [18, 25, 26]. Regular examination of patients, biochemical tests and imaging methods of examination are of utmost importance. At the same time, a normal ultrasound picture cannot exclude the presence of fibrosis [30].

Despite the high informativeness of morphological methods, diagnostic liver biopsy for all patients with cystic fibrosis, and especially performed repeatedly, cannot be justified, primarily because of its traumatic nature. In addition, due to inhomogeneous liver damage, a biopsy may underestimate the severity of the lesion. The procedure is indicated when the diagnosis is doubtful or to confirm the findings before liver transplantation [17, 20].

That is why the efforts of researchers are aimed at finding such diagnostic non-invasive methods (especially important in paediatric practice), which will be informative, accessible, capable of detecting liver changes and carrying out dynamic monitoring of the fibrous process. The use of shear wave elastography in the early diagnosis of liver diseases in patients with cystic fibrosis becomes particularly relevant since a number of authors point to the reversible nature of such conditions as fatty hepatosis and cholestasis following treatment [17, 25]. The aim of our investigation was to study the stiffness of the liver using shear wave elastography in children suffering from cystic fibrosis.

3. Materials and methods

The study was approved by the Ethics Committee of 'The Russian Medical Academy of Continuing Professional Education' of the Health Ministry of the Russian Federation and the Ethics Committee of the Chelyabinsk Regional Children Clinical Hospital. Written informed consent of legal representatives was obtained for all patients. Liver biopsy was not included in the algorithm of examination of patients with cystic fibrosis. Ultrasound examination was performed by an Aixplorer device (Supersonic Imagine, France) with a broadband convex sensor operating in the frequency range of 1–6 MHz. A standard ultrasound examination of the liver, supplemented by two-dimensional shear wave elastography, was performed in 232 children. There were 200 healthy children aged 3 to 18 years (control group) and 32 patients with cystic fibrosis aged 2 to 17 years (study group) among them.

The control group included healthy children. The following criteria were taken into account:

- height and weight of each child in the range from the 5th to the 95th percentile of the age norm [31];

- absence of liver disease and (or) congestive heart failure in the history;

- absence of inflammatory changes according to general and biochemical blood tests (signs of cholestasis, cytolysis);

- absence of pathology of the liver, biliary tract, pancreas and spleen according to ultrasound in grayscale and Doppler exam (colour Doppler mapping, pulse-wave Doppler) modes;

- calm behaviour of a child during the study.

The diagnosis of cystic fibrosis was established on the basis of a comprehensive clinical and laboratory examination with history data analysis, DNA diagnostics with genotype specification, and it was confirmed by a positive sweat test. The course of the disease in 17 (53.1%) children was regarded as moderate (subgroup I), in 15 (46.9%) children – as severe (subgroup II). The severity of the disease course was assessed by the Schwachman-Brasfield scale, modified by S.V. Rachinsky and N.I. Kapranov. This scale takes into account the general activity of the patient, state of his nutrition and physical development, clinical manifestations of the disease, as well as the results of X-ray examination [32].

After a standard ultrasound examination of the abdominal organs in the grayscale mode, the stiffness of different segments of the right liver lobe was measured in the areas free of vascular structures at a depth of 3–5 cm from the capsule. The study was performed fasting, the patients breathing calmly, the older children holding breath for no more than 10 seconds or during shallow inhalation, in a supine position. The sensor was positioned perpendicular to the body surface with minimal manual pressure, using subcostal, intercostal and epigastric approaches. The area of interest (colour window) was selected, the image stabilization was set, the measurement was considered successful if more than 90% of the colour window was filled with colour. Ten measurements of the average value of the Young modulus (Emean) (kPa) were performed, and according to the results, the arithmetic mean value of Emean was calculated. Examples of liver stiffness assessment in patients of both groups are shown in **Figures 1–4**.

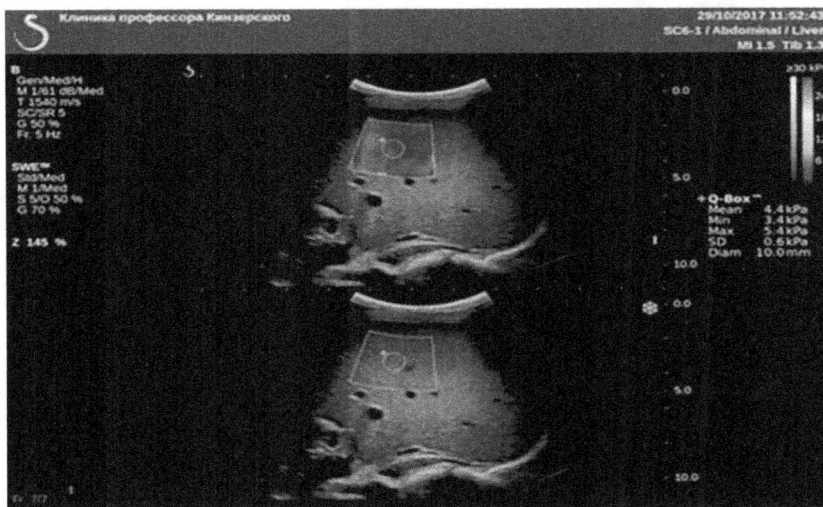

Figure 1.
An example of stiffness assessment of unchanged liver parenchyma in a healthy child: B-mode and two-dimensional shear wave elastography mode. The results of one of 10 measurements. Emean = 4.4 kPa. The child is 10 years old.

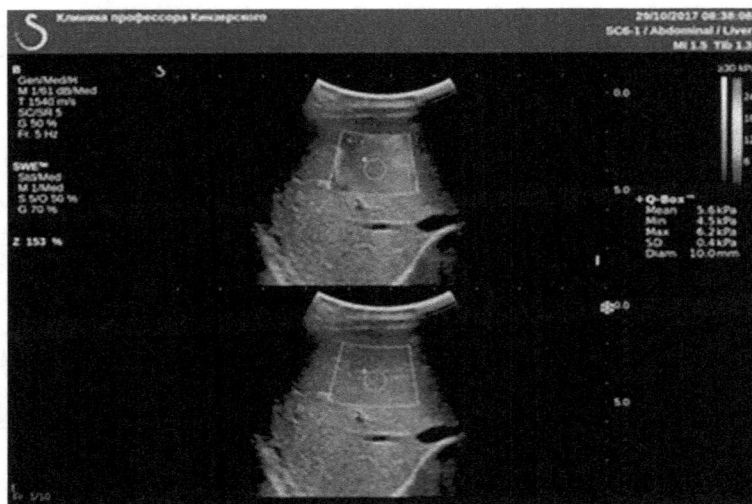

Figure 2.
An example of liver stiffness assessment in a child with cystic fibrosis: B-mode and two-dimensional shear wave elastography mode. The results of one of 10 measurements. Emean = 5.6 kPa. The child is 13 years old.

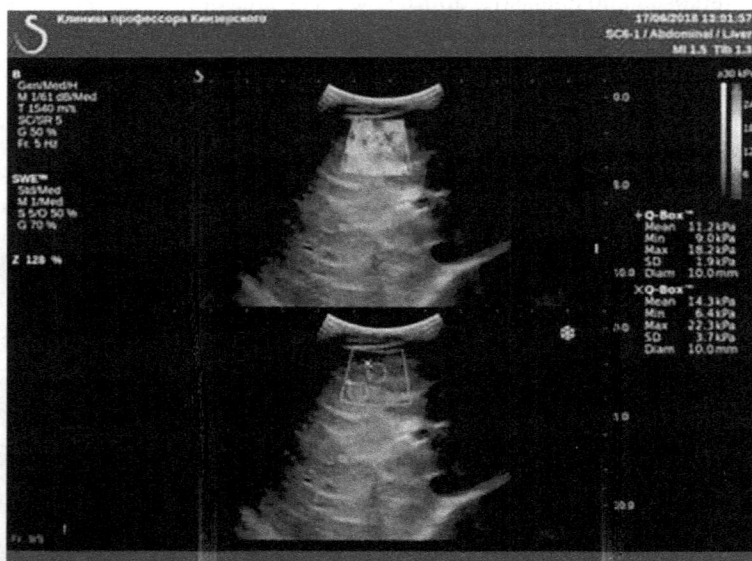

Figure 3.
An example of liver stiffness assessment in a child with cystic fibrosis: B-mode and two-dimensional shear wave elastography mode. Emean = 11.2 kPa. The child is 11 years old.

4. Statistical analysis

Statistical data processing was performed by the IBM SPSS Statistics 19 pack. Most quantitative values were not within the normal distribution, so nonparametric statistic methods were applied. All quantitative data were presented as M (mean),

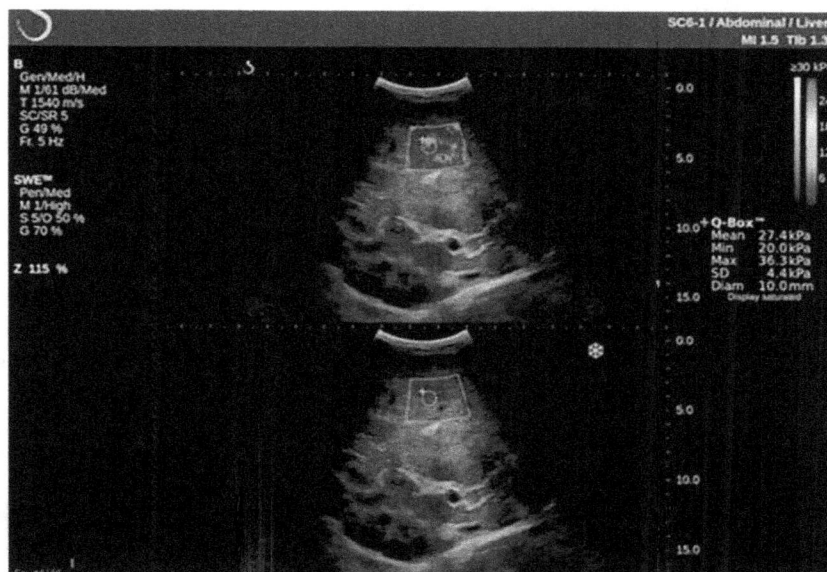

Figure 4.
An example of liver stiffness assessment in a child with cystic fibrosis: B-mode and two-dimensional shear wave elastography mode. The results of one of 10 measurements. Emean = 27.4 kPa. The child is 12 years old.

m (standard error of the mean), σ (standard deviation), median (50th percentile), 25th–75th percentiles and minimum and maximum values. Quantitative parameters were compared using Mann–Whitney criterion, qualitative ones were compared using Fisher criterion of accuracy. The differences were considered significant at $P \leq 0.05$.

5. Results

Two-dimensional shear wave elastography was performed in 200 (control group) conditionally healthy children aged 3 to 18 years who underwent ultrasound examination for reasons unrelated to hepatobiliary diseases. Routine ultrasound examination did not reveal any changes in the liver, spleen and gallbladder in children of the control group. The technique and results of two-dimensional liver elastography performed in healthy children of different age groups had been published by us earlier [33, 34]. Statistical processing of the results of the previous study allowed to establish the mean value of Young modulus in the group of healthy children, i.e., 5.01 ± 0.03 kPa, the median of the average Emean value was 5.00 kPa (4.70–5.38). We did not find statistically significant gender differences in liver stiffness in children of the control group [33, 34].

In the group of children with cystic fibrosis, hepatomegaly was revealed in the vast majority of children – 31 patients (96.9%), splenomegaly – in 10 patients (31.3%). In 13 children (40.6%), changes in the gallbladder were detected in the form of a wall thickening of more than 4 mm, or its decreased size. Six children had signs of portal hypertension (18.8%), which was manifested by hepatosplenomegaly, portal vein dilation with decreased linear blood flow velocity and oesophageal varices according to gastroduodenoscopy. The ultrasound picture of the liver was presented as unchanged parenchyma. Also, a diffuse or inhomogeneous increase of echogenicity, heterogeneity of the parenchyma with a pronounced vascular pattern, cirrhotic nodes with depletion and deformation of a typical vascular tree, pronounced periportal fibrosis were determined. The elastography picture of the liver in children with cystic fibrosis was various. It was represented both by homogeneous colouring of the colour window in dark blue or blue tones, with the absence of areas of increased stiffness, in that case, the qualitative characteristics did not differ from the control group of healthy children (**Figures 1** and **2**), and also, blue-green with yellow areas, as well as red-orange colouring of the area of interest in children with pronounced ultrasound signs of cirrhotic liver changes (**Figures 3–5**).

The values of the liver parenchyma stiffness in the studied groups and subgroups are shown in **Tables 1** and **2**.

Significant differences in the values of Young modulus (Emean) were obtained when comparing the values of the study and control groups: median Emean – 6.50

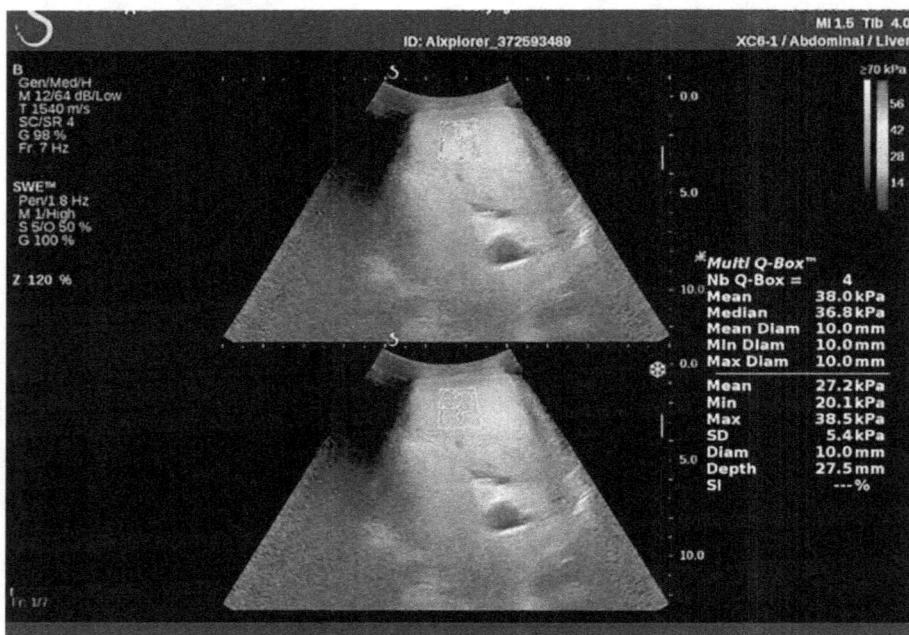

Figure 5.
An example of liver stiffness assessment in a child with cystic fibrosis: B-mode and two-dimensional shear wave elastography mode. The results of 4 measurements. Emean = 38.0 kPa. Median – 36.8 kPa. The child is 14 years old.

Groups	M ± m	σ	Median	25th–75th percentile	Minimum – maximum values
Control group (n = 200)	5.01 ± 0.03	0.49	5.00	4.70–5.38	3.00–6.30
Study group (n = 32)	7.11 ± 0.44	2.48	6.50	5.62–7.52	4.30–16.90

Note: Comparison of two groups, $p < 0.001$.

Table 1.
Stiffness (Emean, kPa) of liver parenchyma in children of the studied groups: healthy children and children with cystic fibrosis.

Subgroups	M ± m	σ	Median	25th–75th percentile	Minimum – maximum values
Moderate course (n = 17)	5.98 ± 0.23	0.94	5.90	5.20–6.75	4.30–7.90
Severe course (n = 15)	8.39 ± .79	3.05	7.30	6.20–10.70	5.60–16.90

Note: Comparison of two subgroups, p < 0.002.

Table 2.
Stiffness (Emean, kPa) of liver parenchyma in children with cystic fibrosis of various severity (n = 32).

and 5.00 kPa, interquartile range – 5.62–7.52 and 4.70–5.38 kPa, respectively (P< 0.001). Most children suffering from cystic fibrosis had some degree of change in liver stiffness. In the group of patients with cystic fibrosis, only 9 (28.1%) children had Young modulus values that did not exceed those in healthy children. Analysis of the data obtained showed that the values of Young modulus in the group of patients with a severe course of the disease was significantly higher than in patients with a moderate course of cystic fibrosis: median Emean – 7.30 and 5.90 kPa, interquartile range – 6.20–10.70 and 5.20–6.75 kPa, respectively (P< 0.002).

6. Discussion

In the available publications, we were able to find only a few works devoted to the shear wave elastography assessment of liver stiffness in a group of children suffering from cystic fibrosis. It should be noted that the paediatric age group is the most interesting for assessing liver changes since cystic fibrosis-associated liver diseases develop in early childhood, and new cases are rare after the age of 20. In 2009, P. Witters et al. [35] used transient elastography to study liver stiffness in 66 patients with cystic fibrosis [35]. The obtained elastometry findings were compared with those of a control group consisting of 59 people (98th percentile (or M + 2σ), Young modulus for children under 12 years of age was 5.63 kPa, 12 years and older – 6.50 kPa). In our study, the maximum value of 6.30 kPa (with a median of 5.00 kPa) in the control group was used as a threshold. Such clinical manifestations as hepato-splenomegaly and changes in biochemical parameters were taken into consideration in the patients of the study group. Only one patient underwent a liver biopsy. The study showed an increase in stiffness in patients with clinical manifestations, such as palpable hepatosplenomegaly (11.07 ± 5.51 kPa (n = 6) vs. 5.08 ± 3.45 kPa (n = 60), P < 0.0001), biochemical (7.40 ± 3.10 kPa (n = 7) vs. 5.42 ± 4.08 kPa (n = 59), P = 0.013) and ultrasound (8.19 ± 5.96 kPa (n = 23) vs. 4.27 ± 0.94 kPa (n = 41), P = 0.0001) signs of liver damage. The mean value of liver stiffness in children with cystic fibrosis was 5.63 ± 4.02 kPa [35]. In our study, the median of Young modulus was 6.50 kPa in patients with cystic fibrosis. We got fairly close values, although the two studies were conducted on different devices. The stage of liver fibrosis during puncture biopsy was not evaluated in both studies.

In 2012, the research group of L. Monti et al. [36] evaluated liver stiffness using shear wave point elastography in the group of 75 children with cystic fibrosis. Measurements of the shear wave velocity were carried out in the right liver lobe, followed by averaging of 10 indices. The patients underwent ultrasound examination, gastroscopy and analysis of biochemical parameters. Liver biopsy was not performed. The study found that the median shear wave velocity was significantly higher in patients with clinical, biochemical and ultrasound signs of liver damage, than in patients with their absence. The velocity increased as the signs of decompensation of portal hypertension increased, that is, with the progression of fibrous changes. The median in patients with portal hypertension, splenomegaly and oesophageal varices was 1.30, 1.54 and 1.63 m/s, respectively (P < 0.001) [36].

A study by T. Canas et al conducted in 2015 [37] included 72 patients with cystic fibrosis aged 9 months to 18 years. The stiffness of the liver and spleen was assessed using shear wave point elastography after the routine ultrasound examination. The biopsy was not included in the protocol. As in our study, a convex sensor was used, five measurements of the shear wave velocity were carried out in the right and left liver lobes (intercostal and subcostal access) and in the spleen. The obtained data were compared with the results of the control group (n = 60). The shear wave point elastography revealed a significant increase in the shear wave velocity in patients with cystic fibrosis-associated liver disease compared with healthy children and patients with cystic fibrosis without liver involvement (P = 0.003). The diagnosis of 'cystic fibrosis-associated liver disease' was made using non-invasive Colombo criteria [18]. The threshold value of the shear wave velocity for the diagnosis of cystic fibrosis-associated liver disease was 1.27 cm/s (measurement in the right liver lobe) with 56.5 % sensitivity, 90.5% specificity, AUC 0.746 [37].

Reports on the study of liver stiffness by two-dimensional shear wave elastography using the Aixplorer device (Supersonic Imagine, France) in children suffering from cystic fibrosis could not be found. We carried out measurements on segments of the right liver lobe using a convex sensor to standardise the study protocol as the linear sensor measurements were not always considered technically possible in older children. The analysis of the data obtained by us, as well as other research groups, revealed that the indices of hepatic tissue stiffness in patients with cystic fibrosis had significantly higher values than in healthy children. Liver stiffness in children with a severe course of the disease was more apparent than in children with a moderately severe course. As the clinical, biochemical and ultrasound signs of liver damage increased, the stiffness indices accordingly increased. A clear insight into the degree of damage, stage and rate of fibrosis progression in chronic liver disease in children is important when making a comprehensive decision when to resort to surgical methods of treatment and to liver transplantation. Taking into consideration the above mentioned and based on the results of our study, we consider it appropriate to monitor the indices of Young modulus in patients with cystic fibrosis, as it enables to identify a group of children with high rates of fibrosis.

7. Conclusions

Shear wave elastography can be successfully used in the comprehensive assessment of liver damage in children with cystic fibrosis to facilitate diagnosis and dynamic monitoring of the severity of fibrous degenerations in the parenchyma and sampling of patients in need of liver transplantation.

Author details

Mikhail Pykov[1*], Natalia Kuzmina[2] and Nikolay Rostovtsev[3]

1 Division of Pediatric Radiology, Russian Medical Academy of Postgraduate Education, Moscow, Russia

2 Department of Radiation Diagnostics, Chelyabinsk Regional Children Clinical Hospital, Chelyabinsk, Russia

3 Department of Pediatric Surgery, Federal State Budgetary Institution of Higher Education "South Ural State Medical University", Chelyabinsk, Russia

*Address all correspondence to: pykov@yandex.ru

IntechOpen

References

[1] Mitkov VV, Mitkova MD. Ultrasonic shear wave elastography. Ultrasound and Functional Diagnostics. 2015;2:94-108

[2] Dietrich CF, Bamber J, Berzigotti A, Bota S, Cantisani V, Castera L, et al. EFSUMBguidelinesandrecommendations on the clinical use of liver ultrasound elastography, update 2017 (long version). Ultraschall in der Medizin-European Journal of Ultrasound. 2017;38:e16-e47

[3] Dietrich CF, Bamber J, Berzigotti A, Bota S, Cantisani V, Castera L, et al. EFSUMBguidelinesandrecommendations on the clinical use of liver ultrasound elastography, update 2017 (short version). Ultraschall in der Medizin-European Journal of Ultrasound. 2017;38:377-394

[4] Bamber J, Cosgrove D, Dietrich CF, Fromageau J, Bojunga J, Calliada F, et al. Efsumb guidelines and recommendations on the clinical use of ultrasound elastography. Part 1: Basic principles and technology. Ultraschall in der Medizin-European Journal of Ultrasound. 2013;34:169-184

[5] Shiina T, Nightingale KR, Palmeri ML, Hall TJ, Bamber JC, Barr RG, et al. Wfumb guidelines and recommendations for clinical use of ultrasound elastography: Part 1: Basic principles and terminology. Ultrasound in Medicine & Biology. 2015;41:1126-1147

[6] Pawluś A, Sokołowska-Dąbek D, Szymańska K, Inglot MS, Zaleska-Dorobisz U. Ultrasound elastography – Review of techniques and its clinical applications in pediatrics – Part 1. Advances in Clinical and Experimental Medicine: Official Organ Wrocław Medical University. 2015;24(3):537-543

[7] Cosgrove D, Piscaglia F, Bamber J, et al. EFSUMB guidelines and recommendations on the clinical use of ultrasound elastography. Part 2: Clinical applications. Ultraschall in der Medizin-European Journal of Ultrasound. 2013;34:238-253

[8] Ferraioli G, Filice C, Castera L, et al. WFUMB guidelines and recommendations for clinical use of ultrasound elastography: Part 3: Liver. Ultrasound in Medicine & Biology. 2015;41:1161-1179

[9] Ferraioli G, Wong VW, Castera L, et al. Liver ultrasound elastography: An update to the world federation for ultrasound in medicine and biology guidelines and recommendations. Ultrasound in Medicine & Biology. 2018;44:2419-2440

[10] Dietrich CF, Sirli R, Ferraioli G, Popescu A, Sporea I, Pienar C, et al. Current knowledge in ultrasound-based liver elastography of pediatric patients. Applied Sciences. 2018;8:944. DOI: 10.3390/app8060944

[11] Dietrich CF, Ferraioli G, Sirli R, Popescu A, Sporea I, Pienar C, et al. General advice in ultrasound based elastography of pediatric patients. Medical Ultrasonography. 2019;21(3): 315-326. DOI: 10.11152/mu-2063

[12] Zaleska-Dorobisz U, Pawluś A, Szymańska K, Łasecki M, Ziajkiewicz M. Ultrasound elastography—Review of techniques and its clinical applications in pediatrics—Part 2. Advances in Clinical and Experimental Medicine. 2015;24(4):725-730. DOI: 10.17219/acem/34581

[13] Andersen SB, Ewertsen C, Carlsen JF, Henriksen BM, Nielsen MB. Ultrasound

elastography is useful for evaluation
of liver fibrosis in children—A
systematic review. Journal of Pediatric
Gastroenterology and Nutrition.
2016;**63**(4):389-399. DOI: 10.1097/
MPG.0000000000001171

[14] Dezsofi A, Baumann U, Dhawan A,
Durmaz O, Fischler B, Hadzic N, et al.
Liver biopsy in children: Position paper
of the ESPGHAN hepatology committee.
JPGN. 2015;**60**(3):408-420

[15] Potter C, Hogan MJ, Henry-
Kendjorsky K, et al. Safety of pediatric
percutaneous liver biopsy performed
by interventional radiologists. Journal
of Pediatric Gastroenterology and
Nutrition. 2011;**53**:202-206

[16] Kapranov NI, Radionovich AM,
Kashirskaya NY, Tolstova VD. Cystic
fibrosis: Modern aspects of diagnosis and
treatment. Clinician. 2006;**(4)**:42-51.
(Article in Russian)

[17] Kashirskaya NY, Kapranov NI,
Kusova ZA, Asherova IK, Voronkov AY.
Multi-function of the gastrointestinal
tract and hepatobiliary system in cystic
fibrosis. Journal of Pediatrics named
after G.N. Speransky. 2012;**91**(4):
106-115. (Article in Russian)

[18] Kobelska-Dubel N, Klintsevich B,
Tsikhi V. Liver disease in cystic fibrosis.
Psheglad Gastroenterological.
2014;**9**(3):136-141. DOI: 10.5114/
p.2014.43574

[19] Parisi GF, Di Dio G, Franzonello S,
Gennaro A, Rotolo N, etc. Liver disease
in cystic fibrosis. Update. Hepatitis
Monthly. 2013;**13**(8):e11215.
DOI: 10.5812/hepatitis.11215

[20] Debray D, Kelly D, Howen R,
Strandwick B, Colombo S. Best practice
guidance for the diagnosis and
management of cystic fibrosis-associated

liver diseases. Journal of Cystic Fibrosis.
2011;**10**(2):29-36. DOI: 10.1016/
S1569-1993(11)60006-4

[21] Lamireau T, Monnereau S.
Epidemiology of liver diseases in cystic
fibrosis: A longitudinal study. Journal of
Hepatology. 2004;**41**:920-925

[22] Hodson M. Cystic Fibrosis, Liver
and Biliary Disease in Cystic Fibrosis.
Third edition by M. Hodson, G. Duncan,
A. Bush. London: Edward Arnold
(Publishers) Ltd; 2007. p. 477

[23] Colombo S, Apostolo MG, Ferrari M,
et al. Analysis of risk factors for the
development of liver disease associated
with cystic fibrosis. The Journal of
Pediatrics. 1994;**124**(3):393-399

[24] Marino SR, Gorelik FS.
Scientific advances in cystic fibrosis.
Gastroenterology. 1992;**103**(2):681-693

[25] Strandvik B. In: Kelly DA, editor.
Hepatobiliary disease in cystic fibrosis.
Diseases of the liver and biliary system in
children. London, UK: Blackwell Science
Ltd.; 1999. pp. 141-156

[26] Lenaerts C, Lapierre C, Patriquin H,
et al. Surveillance for cystic fibrosis –
associated hepatobiliary disease: Early
ultrasound changes and predisposing
factors. The Journal of Pediatrics.
2003;**143**:343-350

[27] Vicek S. Liver changes in the course
of cystic fibrosis, cystic fibrosis –
heterogeneity and personalized
treatment, Dennis Wat and Dilip
Nazareth. Rijeka: IntechOpen; 2019.
DOI: 10.5772/intechopen.89306

[28] Lindblad A, Glaumann H,
Strandvik B. Natural history of liver
disease in cystic fibrosis. Hepatology.
1999;**30**:1151-1158

[29] Colombo C, Battezzati PM, Crosignani A, et al. Liver disease in cystic fibrosis: A prospective study on incidence, risk factors and outcome. Hepatology. 2002;**36**:1374-1382

[30] Mueller-Abt PR, Frawley KJ, Greer RM, et al. Comparison of ultrasound and biopsy findings in children with cystic fibrosis related liver disease. Journal of Cystic Fibrosis. 2008;7:215-221

[31] Baranov AA. Pediatrics. National Guidance. Vol. 1. Moscow: GEOTAR-Media; 2009. p. 1024. (Book in Russian)

[32] Kapranov NI, Kashirskaya NY, Tolstova VD. Cystic Fibrosis. Early Diagnosis and Treatment. Moscow: GEOTAR-Media; 2008. p. 104. (Book in Russian)

[33] Pykov MI, Kuzmina NE, Kinzersky AY. Study of normal parameters of liver stiffness in children using shear wave elastometry. Pediatrics Journal named after G.N. Speransky. 2017;4:63-69

[34] Pykov M, Kuzmina N, Rostovtsev N, Kinzersky A. Elastometry Indices of Unchanged Liver in Healthy Children. Rijeka: IntechOpen. DOI: 10.5772/intechopen.88004

[35] Witters P, De Boeck K, Dupont L, Proesmans M, Vermeulen F, Servaes R, et al. Non-invasive liver elastography (Fibroscan) for detection of cystic fibrosis-associated liver disease. Journal of Cystic Fibrosis. 2009;**8**(6):392-399. DOI: 10.1016/j.jcf.2009.08.001

[36] Monti L, Manco M, Lo ZC, Latini A, D'Andrea ML, Alghisi F, et al. Acoustic radiation force impulse (ARFI) imaging with virtual touch tissue quantification in liver disease associated with cystic fibrosis in children. La Radiologia Medica. 2012;**117**(8):1408-1418. DOI: 10.1007/s11547-012-0874-y

[37] Cañas T, Maciá A, Muñoz-Codoceo RA, Fontanilla T, González-Rios P, Miralles M, et al. Hepatic and splenic acoustic radiation force impulse shear wave velocity elastography in children with liver disease associated with cystic fibrosis. BioMed Research International. 2015;**2015**:7. Article ID 517369. DOI: 10.1155/2015/517369

Chapter 7

Elastography for the Evaluation of Portal Hypertension

Roxana Şirli, Iulia Rațiu and Ioan Sporea

Abstract

Liver cirrhosis, regardless of its etiology, is an important health problem with a chronic evolution, characterized by the possibility of developing several important complications. The best management of these patients implies the correct and early diagnosis of the disease and of its complications. A major complication of cirrhosis is portal hypertension. The reference method for its diagnosis is the direct measurement of hepatic vein portal gradient, an invasive procedure. In the last years, several noninvasive techniques for the evaluation of liver fibrosis were developed, such as biological tests and elastographic methods. Ultrasound-based and MRI-based elastographic techniques have been assessed as predictive tools for the presence and severity of portal hypertension. This paper reviews published data regarding the value of ultrasound and MRI-based elastography (liver, spleen, or both) for the evaluation of portal hypertension.

Keywords: portal hypertension, clinically significant portal hypertension (CSPH), elastography, liver stiffness, spleen stiffness

1. Introduction

The prevalence of chronic hepatopathies in daily practice is increasing due to their multiple causes, such as chronic viral infections, alcoholic or non-alcoholic steato-hepatitis, cholestatic or autoimmune chronic liver disease. Evaluation of such patients is important for therapeutical decisions, follow-up, and for prognosis assessment.

One main complication of advanced chronic liver disease is portal hypertension (PHT), and the exact evaluation of this entity is crucial for further steps. The direct measurement of hepatic vein portal gradient (HVPG) is the "gold standard" for portal hypertension assessment, but this procedure is invasive, and it is not available in all centers of hepatology. Upper endoscopy for the evaluation of possible esophageal varices or portal gastropathy is a surrogate used in daily practice. Ultrasound and other imaging methods that can reveal collateral circulation in the abdomen can be used to suggest portal hypertension.

Elastography techniques developed in the last 10–15 years mainly evaluate liver stiffness as a marker of fibrosis severity and, lately of portal hypertension. More recently, spleen stiffness was used for the assessment of liver disease severity and evaluation of portal hypertension. Ultrasound-based elastography techniques are the most used in practice, but some studies also evaluated magnetic resonance elastography (MR-E).

2. Portal hypertension: definition and standard method of diagnosis

The main consequence of fibrosis during chronic liver disease, regardless of the etiology, is a perturbation of the sinusoidal blood flow in the liver that leads to increased pressure in the portal venous system, namely portal hypertension (PHT). Additionally, as a compensatory reaction, splanchnic vasodilatation further aggravates the PHT, this mechanism contributing 25–30% to the portal vein pressure [1].

The standard method to diagnose PHT is by measurement of the hepatic venous pressure gradient (HVPG). It is an invasive method that implies catheterization with a balloon catheter of one of the hepatic veins, via the jugular or via a cubital vein. The balloon catheter, with a pressure transducer at the tip, is inflated as to totally occlude the hepatic outflow, thus measuring the wedge hepatic venous pressure (WHVP) [2]. With the balloon deflated free hepatic venous pressure (FHVP) is measured. The hepatic venous pressure gradient (HVPG) is calculated as the difference between WHVP and FHVP [3].

Normal values of HVPG are ≤5 mmHg. As liver injury and fibrosis progress, the HVPG increases progressively. HVPG between 5 and 10 mmHg represents subclinical PHT while HVPG ≥10 mmHg represents the threshold from where PHT-related complications may occur and thus is known as clinically significant PHT (CSPH) [3, 4].

Upper endoscopy is the standard diagnostic method for the presence and severity of esophageal varices (EV), the most visible and severe consequence of PHT. To diagnose clinically significant EV (large-grade 2, or 3 EV), a screening program with periodic upper digestive endoscopy should be implemented. However, it is an invasive procedure and numerous endoscopies are performed in patients with advanced liver disease without finding EV, thus raising questions regarding cost-efficiency and patients' acceptance.

Considering the invasiveness of these methods, their availability, and also patients' acceptance, effective noninvasive methods are needed to assess the presence and progression of PHT, as well as the occurrence of EV and their bleeding risk [5].

3. Ultrasound-based elastographic techniques in the liver

According to international guidelines [6, 7], elastography techniques can be classified into Strain Elastography (used mostly for breast, thyroid, and prostate) and Shear Waves Elastography (SWE). In SWE, an external impulse generates shear waves inside the examined organ. The shear waves speed is subsequently measured by ultrasound. Based on the type of external impulse and measurement technique of the shear-waves speed, SWE elastography is subdivided into Transient Elastography (mechanic external impulse); Point SWE (pSWE)—in which an Acoustic Radiation Force Impulse (ARFI) is used as stimulus and the shear-waves speed is measured in a point; and real-time elastography which includes 2D-SWE and 3D-SWE (ARFI used as a stimulus, the shear-waves speed is measured in an area of interest and, in the same time, a color-coded elastogram is generated) [6, 7]. It must be noted that cut-off values proposed for various stages of fibrosis are system-specific.

3.1 Transient elastography (TE)

Transient Elastography was the first elastographic method developed for the evaluation of liver stiffness (LS) [8] and it is not integrated into a standard ultrasound system. It uses a FibroScan device (Echosens, Paris, France) that includes a special ultrasound probe (3.5 MHz for the standard M probe) integrated into a piston that "punches" the body surface. The "punch" generates shear waves that propagate into the liver. Their velocity is measured by pulse-echo ultrasound acquisition and is proportional to LS, increasing in parallel with LS. Increased BMI decreases the feasibility, an inconvenience partially solved by using an XL probe. The FibroScan device displays Young's modulus, expressed in kilopascals (kPa), which is proportional to the shear-wave velocity [6, 7, 9, 10].

Several published meta-analyses have demonstrated that LS measurement by TE is a reliable method for diagnosing cirrhosis, with a pooled sensitivity ranging from 84.4 to 87% and a pooled specificity ranging from 91 to 94.69% [11, 12]. Liver stiffness measured by TE showed a good correlation with HVPG and the presence of EV; as a result, it has been evaluated as a noninvasive tool for portal hypertension quantification. The first studies were performed in rather small numbers of patients. In an Italian study, the AUROC for predicting HVPG $\geq$10 mmHg was 0.99 with 97% sensitivity (Se), while for predicting HVPG$\geq$12 mmHg the calculated AUROC was 0.92 with 94% Se. The calculated cut-offs were 13.6 kPa for HVPG $\geq$10 mmHg and 17.6 kPa for HVPG $\geq$12 mmHg. The cut-off for predicting any EV was 17.6 kPa (AUROC 0.76, Se-90%) [13]. In a French study, TE predicted HVPG $\geq$10 mmHg with AUROC 0.945 (cut-off 21 kPa) [14]. In a study that followed up 100 patients for 2 years, none of the patients who initially had LS measurements (LSM) values <21.1 kPa (the calculated cut-off) had PHT complications, vs. 47.5% of those with higher values [15].

Finally, a method's value is demonstrated by meta-analyses. Regarding TE and portal hypertension, a meta-analysis that included 18 studies with more than 3500 patients was published in 2013 [16]. The conclusion was that, due to the low specificity of this method, TE cannot replace upper gastrointestinal endoscopy for EV screening. However, in 2017 another meta-analysis on 11 studies was published [17]. The summary correlation coefficient was 0.783. Summary Se, Sp, and area under the hierarchical summary receiver operating characteristic curve (AUC) were 87.5%, 85.3%, and 0.9 respectively. In summary, LS correlated well with HVPG and had a good diagnostic performance in diagnosing CSPH. Low cut-off values of 13.6–18 kPa were proposed to ensure a good sensitivity for screening purposes.

The latest EASL guidelines on noninvasive tests for the evaluation of liver disease severity and prognosis proposed an algorithm for risk stratification in compensated advanced chronic liver disease (cACLD) using the Baveno VI criteria [4, 18]: patients with LSM <20 kPa and PLT >150 × 10^9/L should be considered to have a very low risk of having CSPH. These criteria [4] have been well validated for the identification of patients with cACLD who are unlikely to have varices needing treatment and can safely avoid variceal screening endoscopy, while those not meeting these criteria are at an increased risk of clinical decompensation. Numerous studies validated these criteria [19–23]. However, in the latest update of the EASL and AASLD guidelines on noninvasive tests for liver fibrosis severity, no clear recommendation was given on whether 20 kPa or 25 kPa is better to rule in the risk of clinical decompensation [18, 24]. A very recently published study demonstrated that patients not meeting the Baveno VI criteria were indeed at a significantly higher risk of liver decompensation. More importantly, the patients with LSMs ranging from 20 to 25 kPa, regardless of the platelet count, might be classified as having a medium risk of clinical decompensation, while those with LSM higher than 25 kPa could be classified as having a high risk of clinical decompensation [25].

In a meta-analysis performed exclusively in patients with chronic viral hepatitis, it was suggested that two cut-offs can be used, namely, $\leq$13.6 kPa to rule out CSPH (pooled Se 96%), and $\geq$ 22 kPa to rule in CSPH (pooled Sp 94%), thus confirming Baveno VI consensus recommendations [26]. Another systematic review and meta-analysis of 30 studies, including 8469 participants, assessed the accuracy of Baveno VI criteria (LSM <20 kPa and platelet count >150 x 10^9cells/L) and Expanded Baveno criteria (LSM <25 kPa and platelet count >110 x 10^9cells/L) to identify high-risk varices (HRVs) in patients with cACLD were published in 2019 [27]. This meta-analysis concluded that the Baveno criteria and expanded criteria can identify patients with HRVs with high sensitivity but with low specificity. The Expanded Baveno criteria reduce the proportion of unnecessary endoscopies, with a higher rate of missed HRVs [27].

3.2 Shear-wave elastography techniques using acoustic radiation force impulse (ARFI)

In this type of elastography, the shear waves are generated into the tissue by acoustic impulses. It is divided into point Shear-Waves elastography (pSWE) and real-time elastography (2D-SWE and 3D-SWE).

3.2.1 Point shear-waves elastography (pSWE)

In pSWE, the shear-waves speed is measured in a small, fixed-size region of interest (ROI), at the focal point of the US beam, the results being expressed either in m/s, or converted into kPa [6, 7]. pSWE technology is used by several vendors, using proprietary techniques implemented on standard US machines. The first one that appeared on the market and was studied the most is Virtual Touch Tissue Quantification (VTQ) by Siemens, followed by ElastPQ from Philips, and later by techniques by Hitachi, Esaote, Samsung, and others.

Several studies demonstrated the value of VTQ elastography to predict cirrhosis when compared to liver biopsy, the cut-offs ranging from 1.55 to 2 m/s and AUROCS ranging from 0.89 to 0.937 [28, 29], with similar performance to TE in diagnosing cirrhosis [30, 31]. These results were confirmed by several meta-analyses [32–34].

Regarding VTQ measurements as a predictor of PHT, the published studies had shown controversial results. In European studies, VTQ had poor results in predicting large EV, with AUROCs 0.596 [35] and 0.580 [36]. A Japanese study had shown much better results: for a cut-off of 2.05 m/s, VTQ had 83% Se, 76% Sp, and an AUROC of 0.89 to predict any grade EV; while a cut-off of 2.39 m/s had 81% Se, 82% Sp and an AUROC of 0.868 to predict HRVs [37].

3.2.2 Real-time shear-wave elastography (2D-SWE and 3D-SWE)

Two-dimensional Shear-Wave Elastography (2D-SWE) also uses Acoustic Radiation Force Impulse technology (ARFI) to generate shear waves into the tissue. As opposed to pSWE, in 2D-SWE multiple ARFI impulses evaluate a large field of view, inside which a ROI can be selected. Thus, tissue elasticity is displayed in a "real-time" color map (elastogram) superimposed on a B-mode image (red for stiff tissues and blue for soft ones), and also a numerical value is displayed. LS measured in the user-adjustable ROI is expressed in kPa or m/s at the operator's decision [6, 7]. 2D-SWE technology is used by several vendors, using proprietary techniques implemented on standard US machines. The first 2D-SWE that appeared on the market was developed by SuperSonic Imagine and integrated into the Aixplorer™ system, followed by other vendors (General Electric, Canon/Toshiba, Philips, Samsung, etc.).

Liver 2D-SWE has proven to be an accurate method for diagnosing cirrhosis, with AUROCs ranging from 0.94 to 0.98, for cut-off values ranging from 10.4 to 11.7 kPa (lower than those of TE) [38–42].

There are promising results regarding the predictive value of 2D-SWE for predicting CSPH. Studies evaluating 2D-SWE from Supersonic Imagine (2D-SWE.SSI) reported cut-offs of 15.2 kPa to predict CSPH, with AUROC 0.819 (85.7% Se and 80% Sp) and 15.4 kPa [43], with AUROC 0.948 (Se and Sp > 90%) [44]. Similar good results have been obtained using 2D-SWE from General Electric (2D-SWE.GE) [45].

An individual patient data meta-analysis was published in 2020 regarding the performance of 2D-SWE.SSI to identify CSPH, severe PHT, and large varices in cirrhotic patients, using HVPG and upper endoscopy as reference. The study included data of 519 patients from seven centers. A cut-off of 2D-SWE.SSI < 14 kPa ruled out CSPH with 85% accuracy (summary AUROC (sROC)—0.88, 91% Se and 37% Sp) [46]. 2D-SWE.SSI ≥ 32 kPa ruled in CSPH with 55% accuracy (sROC—0.83, 47% Se, 89% Sp). The authors concluded that LS values by 2D-SWE.SSI below 14 kPa may be used to rule out SCPH, however, 2D-SWE.SSI cannot predict varices needing treatment [46].

The consensus panel on Ultrasound Liver Elastography of the Society of Radiologists proposes a vendor-neutral "rule of four" (5, 9, 13, 17 kPa) regarding LSM by ARFI techniques (pSWE and 2D-SWE) for viral etiologies and NAFLD: LS ≤ 5 kPa (1.3 m/sec) has a high probability of being normal; LS ≤ 9 kPa (1.7 m/sec), in the absence of clinical signs, rules out cACLD; values between 9 kPa (1.7 m/sec) and 13 kPa (2.1 m/sec) are suggestive of cACLD but need further tests for confirmation; LS ≥ 13 kPa (2.1 m/sec) are highly suggestive of cACLD. There is a probability of CSPH with LS ≥ 17 kPa (2.4 m/sec) [47].

4. Ultrasound-based elastographic techniques in the spleen

Portal hypertension leads to splenic congestion, which induces architectural changes in the splenic arteries and veins, resulting in fibrosis and an increase in spleen stiffness (SS). Recently, noninvasive techniques that measure spleen stiffness to identify CSPH are gaining more and more interest [48, 49]. SS can be evaluated through elastography techniques, such as TE and ARFI based technologies (pSWE and 2D-SWE) [6, 7, 50, 51].

4.1 Transient elastography

Since TE is the oldest ultrasound-based elastographic technique, it was the first used to assess SS as a predictor of PHT, based on the idea that splenomegaly is one of the clinical signs of cirrhosis. Several studies found a good correlation between SS and LS by TE in patients with cirrhosis and between SS and the presence of EV or HVPG.

The first study that evaluated SS measurement (SSM) by TE showed that SS values become higher as the liver disease is more advanced, correlating well with LS, the association being stronger (r = 0.587) in patients with varices [52]. The SS value was also higher in patients with EV, the best cut-off to predict the presence of EV was ≥46.4 kPa (AUROC = 0.781, PPV = 93.4%). If LS and SS are combined, using LSM ≥ 19 kPa for high Se and SSM ≥ 55 kPa for high Sp, the diagnostic accuracy increased to 88.5%. In an Italian study on 100 patients with HCV cirrhosis, SS correlated better with HVPG than LS (r2 = 0.78 vs. r2 = 0.7) [53]. For the same specificity, SS has a better sensitivity than LS to rule in the presence of EV and both HVPG >10 mmHg and HVPG >12 mmHg).

In another study on 498 patients, the authors developed a prediction model combining SS with Baveno VI criteria, useful to rule out HRVs, that could make it possible to avoid a significantly larger number of unnecessary upper endoscopies as compared to Baveno VI criteria only. Applying the newly identified SSM cut-off (≤46 kPa) to exclude HRVs, or Baveno VI criteria, 35.8 and 21.7% of patients in the internal validation cohort could have avoided upper digestive endoscopy, with only 2% of HRVs being missed with either model. By combining SSM with Baveno VI criteria an additional 22.5% endoscopies could be avoided, reaching a final value of 43.8% spared EGDs, with <5% missed HRVs [54]. Results were confirmed in a prospective external validation cohort, as the combined Baveno VI and SSM ≤46 kPa model would have safely spared 37.4% endoscopies, as compared to 16.5% when using the Baveno VI criteria alone, with 0 HRVs missed [54].

Initial studies regarding SSM were made using the standard FibroScan® device (SSM@50 Hz), with a ceiling threshold of 75 kPa, which could lead to underestimating EV severity. Therefore, EchoSens developed a novel spleen dedicated FibroScan® (SSM@100 Hz), in which the vibrator has a higher frequency (100 Hz) than the standard machine (50 Hz). In a study comparing the two techniques, Stefanescu et al. found out that valid measurements could be obtained in a significantly higher proportion by patients by SSM@100 Hz than by SSM@50 Hz (92.5% vs. 76.0%, p < 0.001) [55]. The accuracy of SSM@100 Hz to predict the presence of EV (AUC = 0.728) and HRVs (AUC = 0.756) was higher than that of other noninvasive tests, including LSM. The proportion of spared endoscopies using Baveno VI criteria (8.1%) significantly increased if combined with SSM@50 Hz (26.5%) or SSM@100 Hz (38.9%, p < 0.001 vs. others). The proportions of missed HRVs were 0% for Baveno VI criteria and 4.7% for combinations [55].

4.2 Shear-wave elastography techniques using acoustic radiation force impulse (ARFI)

4.2.1 Point shear-waves elastography

There are several studies that evaluated VTQ for the assessment of SS, alone [35, 56, 57] or in comparison with TE [58]. Studies considering HVPG as a reference for evaluating SSM performance revealed a remarkable accuracy of SSM in predicting CSPH [59, 60]. A study published in 2019 found out that VTQ is an excellent method of predicting HRVs. Patients with EV of any grade had significantly higher average SS values as compared to those without EVs (3.37 m/s vs. 2.79 m/s, p < 0.001), while patients with HRVs had even higher SS values (3.96 m/s vs. 2.93 m/s, p < 0.001) [61].

4.2.2 Real time shear-wave Elastography

A prospective multicentric study evaluated LS and SS by 2D-SWE.SSI as predictor of CSPH considering HVPG as a reference in 158 subjects, with valid measurements obtained in 109 patients [62]. LS > 29.5 kPa and SS > 35.6 kPa were able to "rule-in" CSPH, with a specificity >92%. LS ≤ 16.0 kPa and SS ≤ 21.7 kPa were able to "rule-out" CSPH. Patients with a LS >38.0 kPa had a substantial risk of having CSPH. In patients with LS ≤ 38.0 kPa, a SS >27.9 kPa ruled in CSPH. This algorithm has 89.2% Se and 91.4% Sp to rule-in CSPH [62].

A recent study evaluated SSM by 2D-SWE.GE to predict the presence of HRVs and compared it to VTQ (a pSWE technique). The optimal SS cut-off value by 2D-SWE was 13.2 kPa (AUROC–0.84), while for VTQ it was 2.91 m/s (AUROC–0.90), with no significant performance difference between the two techniques (p = 0.1606) [63].

A meta-analysis published in 2016, including 12 studies (5 regarding SSM by TE, 5 SSM by pSWE, and 2 SSM by strain elastography) evaluated SS as a predictor of the presence of EV. SS detected the presence of any EV with 78% Se, 76% Sp, 3.4 positive likelihood ratio (LR), 0.2 negative LR, and a diagnostic odds ratio (DOR) of 19.3 [64]. In a subsequent meta-analysis of nine studies, SS predicted the presence HRVs with 81% Se, 66% Sp, 2.5 positive LR, 0.2 negative LR, and 12.6 DOR [64].

A meta-analysis published in 2018, including 9 studies (3 regarding SSM by TE, 2 SSM by pSWE, and 4 SSM by 2D-SWE) showed a good correlation between SS and HVPG, the summary correlation coefficient was 0.72 [65]. In detection of CSPH, the sensitivity, specificity, AUC and DOR were: 88%, 84%, 0.92 and 38 respectively; while for severe PHT they were 92%, 79%, 0.79 and 41 respectively [65].

5. Magnetic resonance elastography (MRE)

The predictive value of MRE for liver fibrosis severity was evaluated by several meta-analyses, which found diagnostic accuracies higher than 90% for the diagnosis of advanced fibrosis and cirrhosis [66–68]. Among its advantages are that it is evaluating the whole liver at the same time, the possibility of steatosis quantification and also of possible focal liver lesions, as well as the fact that the presence of obesity does not decrease feasibility or accuracy [18]. The main limitations of MRE include its prohibitive costs, limited availability, and the need for specialized infrastructure, equipment, and considerable need for radiological expertise.

A preliminary study on 34 patients regarding the value of liver MRE to predict PHT evaluated by HVPG shoved a significant but weak correlation of LS with HVPG (r = 0.478, p = 0.016). ROC analysis provided significant AUROCs for LS to predict PHT (0.809), and CSPH (0.742) [69]. In another study on 263 patients, LS and SS by MRE were evaluated as predictors of the presence of EV. SS was higher in patients with EV and, in multivariate analysis, there was a significant association of SS with EV, but not of LS and EV. The AUROC of MRE-SS for EV was 0.853. A cut-off value of 9.53 kPa had 84.4% Se and 73.7% Sp to predict EV [70]. Similar satisfactory results have been obtained by two other studies [71, 72].

In a recently published meta-analysis, LS and SS by MRE were evaluated as predictors of PHT. Fourteen studies were included (12 evaluating LS and 8 evaluating SS). The pooled and weighted Se, Sp, and AUROC for LS were 83%, 80% and 0.88 respectively, while for SS they were 79%, 90% and 0.92 respectively [73]. The conclusion of this meta-analysis was that SS may be more specific and accurate than LS for detecting PHT.

6. Conclusions

Numerous studies on the diagnostic performance of elastography-based methods to predict the presence of CSPH have been published, mostly reporting data on liver and spleen stiffness measurements by means of TE, pSWE, and 2D-SWE, which represent promising tools for portal hypertension screening.

According to international guidelines, patients with NASH cirrhosis and those with viral etiology who have LS by TE ≥20–25 kPa should be considered at elevated risk of having endoscopic signs of PH. Patients with LS by TE < 20 kPa and with a platelet count >150 x 10^9cells/L have a very low risk of having varices requiring treatment and can avoid screening endoscopy.

Patients with LS values evaluated by pSWE and 2D-SWE higher than 17 kPa (2.4 m/sec) are likely to have CSPH.

Spleen stiffness using TE, pSWE or 2D-SWE can be used for PH evaluation.

Author details

Roxana Şirli[1,2*], Iulia Raţiu[1,2] and Ioan Sporea[2]

1 Department of Internal Medicine II, Division of Gastroenterology and Hepatology, Center for Advanced Research in Gastroenterology and Hepatology, "Victor Babeş" University of Medicine and Pharmacy Timişoara, Romania

2 Regional Center of Research in Advanced Hepatology, Academy of Medical Sciences, Timişoara, Romania

*Address all correspondence to: roxanasirli@gmail.com

IntechOpen

References

[1] Bosch J, Berzigotti A, Garcia-Pagan JC, Abraldes JG. The management of portal hypertension: Rational basis, available treatments and future options. Journal of Hepatology. 2008;**48**(Suppl 1):S68-S92

[2] Perello A, Escorsell A, Bru C, Gilabert R, Moitinho E, Garcia-Pagan JC, et al. Wedged hepatic venous pressure adequately reflects portal pressure in hepatitis C virus-related cirrhosis. Hepatology. 1999;**30**(6):1393-1397

[3] Bosch J, Abraldes JG, Berzigotti A, Garcia-Pagan JC. The clinical use of HVPG measurements in chronic liver disease. Nature Reviews. Gastroenterology & Hepatology. 2009;**6**(10):573-582

[4] de Franchis R, Baveno VIF. Expanding consensus in portal hypertension: Report of the Baveno VI consensus workshop: Stratifying risk and individualizing care for portal hypertension. Journal of Hepatology. 2015;**63**(3):743-752

[5] Bari K, Garcia-Tsao G. Treatment of portal hypertension. World Journal of Gastroenterology. 2012;**18**(11):1166-1175

[6] Bamber J, Cosgrove D, Dietrich CF, Fromageau J, Bojunga J, Calliada F, et al. EFSUMB guidelines and recommendations on the clinical use of ultrasound elastography. Part 1: Basic principles and technology. Ultraschall in der Medizin—European Journal of Ultrasound. 2013;**34**(2):169-184

[7] Shiina T, Nightingale KR, Palmeri ML, Hall TJ, Bamber JC, Barr RG, et al. WFUMB guidelines and recommendations for clinical use of ultrasound elastography: Part 1: Basic principles and terminology. Ultrasound in Medicine & Biology. 2015;**41**(5):1126-1147

[8] Sandrin L, Fourquet B, Hasquenoph JM, Yon S, Fournier C, Mal F, et al. Transient elastography: A new noninvasive method for assessment of hepatic fibrosis. Ultrasound in Medicine & Biology. 2003;**29**(12):1705-1713

[9] Cosgrove D, Piscaglia F, Bamber J, Bojunga J, Correas JM, Gilja OH, et al. EFSUMB guidelines and recommendations on the clinical use of ultrasound elastography. Part 2: Clinical applications. Ultraschall in der Medizin—European Journal of Ultrasound. 2013;**34**(3):238-253

[10] Sporea I, Bota S, Saftoiu A, Sirli R, Gradinaru-Tascau O, Popescu A, et al. Romanian national guidelines and practical recommendations on liver elastography. Medical Ultrasonography. 2014;**16**(2):123-138

[11] Stebbing J, Farouk L, Panos G, Anderson M, Jiao LR, Mandalia S, et al. A meta-analysis of transient elastography for the detection of hepatic fibrosis. Journal of Clinical Gastroenterology. 2010;**44**(3):214-219

[12] Talwalkar JA, Kurtz DM, Schoenleber SJ, West CP, Montori VM. Ultrasound-based transient elastography for the detection of hepatic fibrosis: Systematic review and meta-analysis. Clinical Gastroenterology and Hepatology. 2007;**5**(10):1214-1220

[13] Vizzutti F, Arena U, Romanelli RG, Rega L, Foschi M, Colagrande S, et al. Liver stiffness measurement predicts severe portal hypertension in patients with HCV-related cirrhosis. Hepatology. 2007;**45**(5):1290-1297

[14] Bureau C, Metivier S, Peron JM, Selves J, Robic MA, Gourraud PA,

et al. Transient elastography accurately predicts presence of significant portal hypertension in patients with chronic liver disease. Alimentary Pharmacology & Therapeutics. 2008;**27**(12):1261-1268

[15] Robic MA, Procopet B, Metivier S, Peron JM, Selves J, Vinel JP, et al. Liver stiffness accurately predicts portal hypertension related complications in patients with chronic liver disease: A prospective study. Journal of Hepatology. 2011;**55**(5):1017-1024

[16] Shi KQ, Fan YC, Pan ZZ, Lin XF, Liu WY, Chen YP, et al. Transient elastography: A meta-analysis of diagnostic accuracy in evaluation of portal hypertension in chronic liver disease. Liver International. 2013;**33**(1):62-71

[17] You MW, Kim KW, Pyo J, Huh J, Kim HJ, Lee SJ, et al. A Meta-analysis for the diagnostic performance of transient Elastography for clinically significant portal hypertension. Ultrasound in Medicine & Biology. 2017;**43**(1):59-68

[18] European Association for the Study of the Liver. EASL clinical practice guidelines on non-invasive tests for evaluation of liver disease severity and prognosis. Journal of Hepatology. 2021;**75**(3):659-689

[19] Nawalerspanya S, Sripongpun P, Chamroonkul N, Kongkamol C, Piratvisuth T. Validation of original, expanded Baveno VI, and stepwise & platelet-MELD criteria to rule out varices needing treatment in compensated cirrhosis from various etiologies. Annals of Hepatology. 2020;**19**(2):209-213

[20] Perazzo H, Fernandes FF, Castro Filho EC, Perez RM. Points to be considered when using transient elastography for diagnosis of portal

hypertension according to the Baveno's VI consensus. Journal of Hepatology. 2015;**63**(4):1048-1049

[21] Thabut D, Bureau C, Layese R, Bourcier V, Hammouche M, Cagnot C, et al. Validation of Baveno VI criteria for screening and surveillance of esophageal Varices in patients with compensated cirrhosis and a sustained response to antiviral therapy. Gastroenterology. 2019;**156**(4):997-1009e5

[22] Bae J, Sinn DH, Kang W, Gwak GY, Choi MS, Paik YH, et al. Validation of the Baveno VI and the expanded Baveno VI criteria to identify patients who could avoid screening endoscopy. Liver International. 2018;**38**(8):1442-1448

[23] Maurice JB, Brodkin E, Arnold F, Navaratnam A, Paine H, Khawar S, et al. Validation of the Baveno VI criteria to identify low risk cirrhotic patients not requiring endoscopic surveillance for varices. Journal of Hepatology. 2016;**65**(5):899-905

[24] Qi X, Berzigotti A, Cardenas A, Sarin SK. Emerging non-invasive approaches for diagnosis and monitoring of portal hypertension. The Lancet Gastroenterology & Hepatology. 2018;**3**(10):708-719

[25] Liu Y, Liu C, Li J, Kim TH, Enomoto H, Qi X. Risk stratification of decompensation using liver stiffness and platelet counts in compensated advanced chronic liver disease (CHESS2102). Journal of Hepatology. 2022;**76**(1):248-250

[26] Song J, Ma Z, Huang J, Liu S, Luo Y, Lu Q, et al. Comparison of three cut-offs to diagnose clinically significant portal hypertension by liver stiffness in chronic viral liver diseases: A meta-analysis. European Radiology. 2018;**28**(12):5221-5230

[27] Stafylidou M, Paschos P, Katsoula A, Malandris K, Ioakim K, Bekiari E, et al. Performance of Baveno VI and Expanded Baveno VI criteria for excluding high-risk Varices in patients with chronic liver diseases: A systematic review and Meta-analysis. Clinical Gastroenterology and Hepatology. 2019;**17**(9):1744-55e11

[28] Lupsor M, Badea R, Stefanescu H, Sparchez Z, Branda H, Serban A, et al. Performance of a new elastographic method (ARFI technology) compared to unidimensional transient elastography in the noninvasive assessment of chronic hepatitis C. Preliminary results. Journal of Gastrointestinal and Liver Diseases. 2009;**18**(3):303-310

[29] Sporea I, Sirli R, Bota S, Fierbinteanu-Braticevici C, Petrisor A, Badea R, et al. Is ARFI elastography reliable for predicting fibrosis severity in chronic HCV hepatitis? World Journal of Radiology. 2011;**3**(7):188-193

[30] Rizzo L, Calvaruso V, Cacopardo B, Alessi N, Attanasio M, Petta S, et al. Comparison of transient elastography and acoustic radiation force impulse for non-invasive staging of liver fibrosis in patients with chronic hepatitis C. The American Journal of Gastroenterology. 2011;**106**(12):2112-2120

[31] Sporea I, Badea R, Sirli R, Lupsor M, Popescu A, Danila M, et al. How efficient is acoustic radiation force impulse elastography for the evaluation of liver stiffness? Hepatitis Monthly. 2011;**11**(7):532-538

[32] Bota S, Herkner H, Sporea I, Salzl P, Sirli R, Neghina AM, et al. Meta-analysis: ARFI elastography versus transient elastography for the evaluation of liver fibrosis. Liver International. 2013;**33**(8):1138-1147

[33] Friedrich-Rust M, Nierhoff J, Lupsor M, Sporea I, Fierbinteanu-Braticevici C, Strobel D, et al. Performance of acoustic radiation force impulse imaging for the staging of liver fibrosis: A pooled meta-analysis. Journal of Viral Hepatitis. 2012;**19**(2):e212-e219

[34] Nierhoff J, Chavez Ortiz AA, Herrmann E, Zeuzem S, Friedrich-Rust M. The efficiency of acoustic radiation force impulse imaging for the staging of liver fibrosis: A meta-analysis. European Radiology. 2013;**23**(11):3040-3053

[35] Bota S, Sporea I, Sirli R, Focsa M, Popescu A, Danila M, et al. Can ARFI elastography predict the presence of significant esophageal varices in newly diagnosed cirrhotic patients? Annals of Hepatology. 2012;**11**(4):519-525

[36] Vermehren J, Polta A, Zimmermann O, Herrmann E, Poynard T, Hofmann WP, et al. Comparison of acoustic radiation force impulse imaging with transient elastography for the detection of complications in patients with cirrhosis. Liver International. 2012;**32**(5):852-858

[37] Morishita N, Hiramatsu N, Oze T, Harada N, Yamada R, Miyazaki M, et al. Liver stiffness measurement by acoustic radiation force impulse is useful in predicting the presence of esophageal varices or high-risk esophageal varices among patients with HCV-related cirrhosis. Journal of Gastroenterology. 2014;**49**(7):1175-1182

[38] Bavu E, Gennisson JL, Couade M, Bercoff J, Mallet V, Fink M, et al. Noninvasive in vivo liver fibrosis evaluation using supersonic shear imaging: A clinical study on 113 hepatitis C virus patients. Ultrasound in Medicine & Biology. 2011;**37**(9):1361-1373

[39] Ferraioli G, Tinelli C, Dal Bello B, Zicchetti M, Filice G, Filice C, et al. Accuracy of real-time shear wave elastography for assessing liver fibrosis in chronic hepatitis C: A pilot study. Hepatology. 2012;**56**(6):2125-2133

[40] Leung VY, Shen J, Wong VW, Abrigo J, Wong GL, Chim AM, et al. Quantitative elastography of liver fibrosis and spleen stiffness in chronic hepatitis B carriers: Comparison of shear-wave elastography and transient elastography with liver biopsy correlation. Radiology. 2013;**269**(3):910-918

[41] Sporea I, Bota S, Gradinaru-Tascau O, Sirli R, Popescu A, Jurchis A. Which are the cut-off values of 2D-shear wave Elastography (2D-SWE) liver stiffness measurements predicting different stages of liver fibrosis, considering transient Elastography (TE) as the reference method? European Journal of Radiology. 2014;**83**(3):e118-e122

[42] Zeng J, Liu GJ, Huang ZP, Zheng J, Wu T, Zheng RQ, et al. Diagnostic accuracy of two-dimensional shear wave elastography for the non-invasive staging of hepatic fibrosis in chronic hepatitis B: A cohort study with internal validation. European Radiology. 2014;**24**(10):2572-2581

[43] Kim TY, Jeong WK, Sohn JH, Kim J, Kim MY, Kim Y. Evaluation of portal hypertension by real-time shear wave elastography in cirrhotic patients. Liver International. 2015;**35**(11):2416-2424

[44] Procopet B, Berzigotti A, Abraldes JG, Turon F, Hernandez-Gea V, Garcia-Pagan JC, et al. Real-time shear-wave elastography: Applicability, reliability and accuracy for clinically significant portal hypertension. Journal of Hepatology. 2015;**62**(5):1068-1075

[45] Stefanescu H, Rusu C, Lupsor-Platon M, Nicoara Farcau O, Fischer P, Grigoras C, et al. Liver stiffness assessed by ultrasound shear wave Elastography from General Electric accurately predicts clinically significant portal hypertension in patients with advanced chronic liver disease. Ultraschall in der Medizin—European Journal of Ultrasound. 2020;**41**(5):526-533

[46] Thiele M, Hugger MB, Kim Y, Rautou PE, Elkrief L, Jansen C, et al. 2D shear wave liver elastography by Aixplorer to detect portal hypertension in cirrhosis: An individual patient data meta-analysis. Liver International. 2020;**40**(6):1435-1446

[47] Barr RG, Wilson SR, Rubens D, Garcia-Tsao G, Ferraioli G. Update to the society of radiologists in ultrasound liver Elastography consensus statement. Radiology. 2020;**296**(2):263-274

[48] Roccarina D, Rosselli M, Genesca J, Tsochatzis EA. Elastography methods for the non-invasive assessment of portal hypertension. Expert Review of Gastroenterology & Hepatology. 2018;**12**(2):155-164

[49] Takuma Y, Nouso K, Morimoto Y, Tomokuni J, Sahara A, Takabatake H, et al. Portal hypertension in patients with liver cirrhosis: Diagnostic accuracy of spleen stiffness. Radiology. 2016;**279**(2):609-619

[50] Ferraioli G, Wong VW, Castera L, Berzigotti A, Sporea I, Dietrich CF, et al. Liver ultrasound elastography: An update to the world federation for ultrasound in medicine and biology guidelines and recommendations. Ultrasound in Medicine & Biology. 2018;**44**(12):2419-2440

[51] Saftoiu A, Gilja OH, Sidhu PS, Dietrich CF, Cantisani V, Amy D, et al. The EFSUMB guidelines and

recommendations for the clinical practice of elastography in non-hepatic applications: Update 2018. Ultraschall in der Medizin—European Journal of Ultrasound. 2019;**40**(4):425-453

[52] Stefanescu H, Grigorescu M, Lupsor M, Procopet B, Maniu A, Badea R. Spleen stiffness measurement using Fibroscan for the noninvasive assessment of esophageal varices in liver cirrhosis patients. Journal of Gastroenterology and Hepatology. 2011;**26**(1):164-170

[53] Colecchia A, Montrone L, Scaioli E, Bacchi-Reggiani ML, Colli A, Casazza G, et al. Measurement of spleen stiffness to evaluate portal hypertension and the presence of esophageal varices in patients with HCV-related cirrhosis. Gastroenterology. 2012;**143**(3):646-654

[54] Colecchia A, Ravaioli F, Marasco G, Colli A, Dajti E, Di Biase AR, et al. A combined model based on spleen stiffness measurement and Baveno VI criteria to rule out high-risk varices in advanced chronic liver disease. Journal of Hepatology. 2018;**69**(2):308-317

[55] Stefanescu H, Marasco G, Cales P, Fraquelli M, Rosselli M, Ganne-Carrie N, et al. A novel spleen-dedicated stiffness measurement by FibroScan(R) improves the screening of high-risk oesophageal varices. Liver International. 2020;**40**(1):175-185

[56] Park J, Kwon H, Cho J, Oh J, Lee S, Han S, et al. Is the spleen stiffness value acquired using acoustic radiation force impulse (ARFI) technology predictive of the presence of esophageal varices in patients with cirrhosis of various etiologies? Medical Ultrasonography. 2016;**18**(1):11-17

[57] Rizzo L, Attanasio M, Pinzone MR, Berretta M, Malaguarnera M, Morra A,

et al. A new sampling method for spleen stiffness measurement based on quantitative acoustic radiation force impulse elastography for noninvasive assessment of esophageal varices in newly diagnosed HCV-related cirrhosis. BioMed Research International. 2014;**2014**:365982

[58] Kim HY, Jin EH, Kim W, Lee JY, Woo H, Oh S, et al. The role of spleen stiffness in determining the severity and bleeding risk of esophageal varices in cirrhotic patients. Medicine (Baltimore). 2015;**94**(24):e1031

[59] Takuma Y, Nouso K, Morimoto Y, Tomokuni J, Sahara A, Toshikuni N, et al. Measurement of spleen stiffness by acoustic radiation force impulse imaging identifies cirrhotic patients with esophageal varices. Gastroenterology. 2013;**144**(1):92-101e2

[60] Attia D, Schoenemeier B, Rodt T, Negm AA, Lenzen H, Lankisch TO, et al. Evaluation of liver and spleen stiffness with acoustic radiation force impulse quantification Elastography for diagnosing clinically significant portal hypertension. Ultraschall in der Medizin—European Journal of Ultrasound. 2015;**36**(6):603-610

[61] Fierbinteanu-Braticevici C, Tribus L, Peagu R, Petrisor A, Baicus C, Cretoiu D, et al. Spleen stiffness as predictor of esophageal varices in cirrhosis of different etiologies. Scientific Reports. 2019;**9**(1):16190

[62] Jansen C, Bogs C, Verlinden W, Thiele M, Moller P, Gortzen J, et al. Shear-wave elastography of the liver and spleen identifies clinically significant portal hypertension: A prospective multicentre study. Liver International. 2017;**37**(3):396-405

[63] Fofiu R, Bende F, Popescu A, Sirli R, Lupusoru R, Ghiuchici AM, et al. Spleen

and liver stiffness for predicting high-risk Varices in patients with compensated liver cirrhosis. Ultrasound in Medicine & Biology. 2021;**47**(1):76-83

[64] Singh S, Eaton JE, Murad MH, Tanaka H, Iijima H, Talwalkar JA. Accuracy of spleen stiffness measurement in detection of esophageal varices in patients with chronic liver disease: Systematic review and meta-analysis. Clinical Gastroenterology and Hepatology. 2014;**12**(6):935-45e4

[65] Song J, Huang J, Huang H, Liu S, Luo Y. Performance of spleen stiffness measurement in prediction of clinical significant portal hypertension: A meta-analysis. Clinics and Research in Hepatology and Gastroenterology. 2018;**42**(3):216-226

[66] Wang QB, Zhu H, Liu HL, Zhang B. Performance of magnetic resonance elastography and diffusion-weighted imaging for the staging of hepatic fibrosis: A meta-analysis. Hepatology. 2012;**56**(1):239-247

[67] Singh S, Venkatesh SK, Wang Z, Miller FH, Motosugi U, Low RN, et al. Diagnostic performance of magnetic resonance elastography in staging liver fibrosis: A systematic review and meta-analysis of individual participant data. Clinical Gastroenterology and Hepatology. 2015;**13**(3):440-51e6

[68] Friedrich-Rust M, Poynard T, Castera L. Critical comparison of elastography methods to assess chronic liver disease. Nature Reviews Gastroenterology & Hepatology. 2016;**13**(7):402-411

[69] Wagner M, Hectors S, Bane O, Gordic S, Kennedy P, Besa C, et al. Noninvasive prediction of portal pressure with MR elastography and DCE-MRI of the liver and spleen: Preliminary results. Journal of Magnetic Resonance Imaging. 2018;**48**(4):1091-1103

[70] Jhang ZE, Wu KL, Chen CB, Chen YL, Lin PY, Chou CT. Diagnostic value of spleen stiffness by magnetic resonance elastography for prediction of esophageal varices in cirrhotic patients. Abdominal Radiology (NY). 2021;**46**(2):526-533

[71] Abe H, Midorikawa Y, Matsumoto N, Moriyama M, Shibutani K, Okada M, et al. Prediction of esophageal varices by liver and spleen MR elastography. European Radiology. 2019;**29**(12):6611-6619

[72] Hoffman DH, Ayoola A, Nickel D, Han F, Chandarana H, Babb J, et al. MR elastography, T1 and T2 relaxometry of liver: Role in noninvasive assessment of liver function and portal hypertension. Abdominal Radiology (NY). 2020;**45**(9):2680-2687

[73] Singh R, Wilson MP, Katlariwala P, Murad MH, McInnes MDF, Low G. Accuracy of liver and spleen stiffness on magnetic resonance elastography for detecting portal hypertension: A systematic review and meta-analysis. European Journal of Gastroenterology & Hepatology. 2021;**32**(2):237-245

Chapter 8

The Place of Elastography for Liver Tumors Assessment

Ana-Maria Ghiuchici and Mirela Dănilă

Abstract

Elastography is an ultrasound (US) based method widely used in the field of hepatology, particularly for liver stiffness assessment in patients with chronic liver disease. Elastography brings valuable information regarding tissue stiffness and could be considered a virtual biopsy. In the last years, the incidence of focal liver lesions (FLLs) has increased due to frequent detection during a routine abdominal US. The differential diagnosis of FLLs can be challenging, and it is important in terms of treatment options and prognosis. Currently, most FLLs require for diagnosis workup imaging methods with contrast (radiation exposure, potentially nephrotoxic contrast agents) and/or biopsy that are considered invasive procedures and could be contraindicated in particular cases. Avoidance of these invasive methods could be the main reason to perform elastography for FLLs evaluation as they are commonly first detected on US examination. Several studies showed that elastography could bring additional information regarding the stiffness of FLLs in order to predict their nature.

Keywords: strain elastography, shear-wave elastography, focal liver lesions, hepatocellular carcinoma, tissue stiffness

1. Introduction

In clinical practice, standard abdominal US is probably the most widely used imaging technique for liver examination due to the advantages of this method: non-invasive, availability, safe, low-cost. FLLs are often detected incidentally during routine US examinations [1–3]. The characterization and differential diagnosis of these lesions constitute a daily challenge for the practitioner. The continuous development of US tools (i.e., Color-Doppler; Tissue Harmonic Imaging; Contrast-Enhanced Ultrasound - CEUS, elastography) improved FLL characterization [4] and offered a new perspective for the clinician that led to a more complete evaluation of diffuse and focal liver disease.

US elastography is being widely used for liver stiffness assessment as a non-invasive marker of fibrosis useful for the management of patients with diffuse liver disease. Other clinical applications for liver elastography include diagnosing clinically significant portal hypertension and predicting high-risk varices, characterization of FLLs, and the prognosis of the clinical outcomes for chronic liver disease [5–9].

FLLs have different stiffness as the result of different histological structures. They can be classified as benign or malignant. The most frequent solid benign FLLs are hepatic hemangioma (HH), focal nodular hyperplasia (FNH), and hepatocellular adenoma (HA) [10]. Malignant FLLs can be primary liver tumors (hepatocellular carcinoma, HCC; cholangiocarcinoma, CC) or secondary lesions (metastases).

After detecting an FLL on the abdominal US, we must determine whether the tumor is benign or malignant; this is important for future follow-up, therapeutic management, and prognosis. In many cases, a second-line imaging method with contrast (CT/MRI) and/or biopsy is needed for a definite diagnosis. The need to develop less invasive methods to diagnose and characterize FLLs arises from the limitations of these currently used techniques that involve radiation exposure, potentially nephrotoxic contrast agents, limited availability, expensive and invasive methods.

Elastography can be added to a standard US and CEUS examination of an FLL, providing information regarding tissue stiffness and could be considered a virtual biopsy [11]. Several studies reported the possible role of different elastographic techniques to characterize diverse types of FLLs. They focused on the accuracy in discriminating between benign and malignant primary or secondary (metastases) liver tumors. The ability of US elastography to diagnose FLLs, including HCC, is still undergoing validation [12, 13]. In this chapter, we outline the recent advances regarding US elastography to evaluate FLLs.

2. Elastography for the evaluation of focal liver lesions in clinical practice

Currently, liver cancer is the sixth most common cancer and the fourth cause of cancer-related death worldwide [14]. Therefore, the clinical interest to rule out malignancy of FLLs is to diagnose liver cancer early and to allow prompt therapeutic intervention that can improve the prognosis of these patients. Starting from the premise that neoplastic disease can change the tissue structure/composition, elastography could help assess elasticity differences and predict the nature of an FLL [15, 16].

Elastographic assessment of an FLL must be performed knowing the clinical context and history of the patient (liver disease, previous cancer, medication, comorbidities, infections) [17, 18]. It is also essential to evaluate the liver parenchyma for steatosis or fibrosis, knowing the fact that some tumors are more common in particular clinical settings (i.e., cirrhosis represents the common underlying condition for HCC development).

US elastography is a noninvasive, noncontrast, rapid, cost-effective, easy to perform a method that can complete a standard US examination due to numerous elastographic techniques that are now available in different US machines.

According to elastography guidelines [13, 19–21], elastography techniques can be classified as qualitative (Strain elastography, SE) or quantitative (Shear Wave Elastography, SWE). **Figure 1** shows the types of US-based elastography used in clinical practice. Both SE and SWE techniques can assess tissue stiffness but use different principles. Measurement of minimal displacements in the tissue caused by mechanical compression or an enforced acoustic impulse that acts as a wavefront represents the fundamental principle of US elastography techniques [21].

2.1 Strain elastography for FLLs evaluation

Strain imaging is a qualitative technique that allows the measurement of physical tissue displacement parallel to the normally applied stress. The applied force can be: (a) mechanically induced by either active displacement of tissue surface

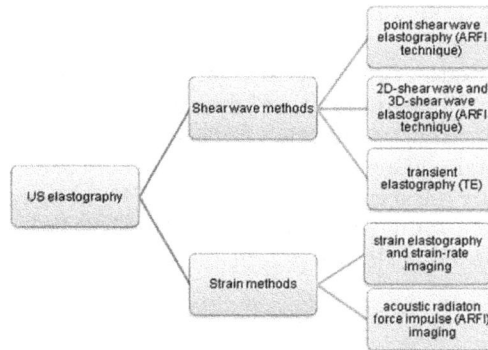

Figure 1.
Scheme of US-based elastography types in clinical practice.

(strain elastography, SE) or passive internal physiological induced (strain-rate imaging, SRI); (b) ultrasound induced by using acoustic radiation force impulse (ARFI) [21]. SE can provide information about the relative stiffness value between one tissue and another. This technique is limited by interobserver variability and can be challenging to apply in particular situations (i.e., patients with ascites; deep localization of the lesion). Although SE is the least used method for liver examination, studies show the utility of strain techniques in FLL evaluation by characterizing the lesion as either soft or hard.

In a recent study [22], benign FLL had a low strain ratio (mean ratio 1.08 ± 0.40) compared to malignant lesions with a high strain ratio (mean ratio 4.14 ± 1.25). The cut-off value for malignant lesions was 1.7 with a sensitivity of 100% and specificity of 93.10. The highest strain index was for CC (6.25 ± 0.44), followed by hepatoblastoma, HCC, and liver metastases [22].

The utility of semiquantitative strain elastography for FLL characterization was also evaluated in a previous study by Onur et al. [23] that obtained a different cut-off to discriminate between benign and malignant FLL. The cut-off value of the strain index for FLL differentiation was 1.28, with a sensitivity of 78% and a specificity of 65%. No difference in strain values between malignant FLLs was found.

A comprehensive evaluation of FLLs on qualitative and quantitative ARFI techniques was assessed in a study by Nagula et al. showing that malignant lesions were stiffer and larger, while benign lesions were softer and similar in size (P < 0.05) [24]. Also, using ARFI strain imaging, another study found that 83.8% malignant and 55% benign FLLs appeared stiffer as compared with the surrounding liver parenchyma having statistically significant differences (P < 0.05) [25].

The intra-operative (IO) application of SE was also studied [26–28]. In one study that compared the diagnostic accuracy of IO-SE to IO-CEUS for the differentiation between malignant and benign FLLs, the authors concluded that IO-CEUS is useful for localization and characterization of FLLs prior to surgical resection. In contrast, IO-SE provided correct characterization only for a limited number of lesions. The calculated sensitivity of the SE was 70.5%, specificity 60%, PPV 94%, NPV 18.75%, and accuracy 69% [28].

Because SE is a qualitative method, we can obtain the relative stiffness of a lesion compared with the surrounding liver parenchyma. The stiffness of the background liver can be variable depending on the degree of fibrosis and could be considered a limitation of SE for FLL examination. Another confounding factor could be that both benign and malignant lesions can be soft or hard compared to normal liver.

2.2 Shear wave elastography for FLLs evaluation

SWE assesses quantitative information regarding tissue stiffness by evaluating shear wave attenuation. These methods use dynamic ultrasound-induced force to generate shear waves by acoustic radiation force impulses [21]. Measuring the shear wave speed, we can obtain quantitative measurements of tissue elasticity. The stiffness value is provided by the shear wave velocity (SWV) in meters per second (m/sec) or by converting Young's modulus in kiloPascals (kPa) [21, 29]. The main three SWE techniques used in clinical practice are:

- Transient elastography (TE);

- Point shear wave elastography (pSWE);

- Two-dimensional shear wave elastography (2D-SWE).

TE is validated for liver fibrosis assessment [30]. However, it is not feasible for FLL stiffness evaluation because this method is used without direct B-mode US image guidance and cannot accurately where the lesion is localized.

2.2.1 Point shear wave elastography (pSWE): clinical applications for FLLs evaluation

Relied on ARFI technique, pSWE is available in different US machines and permits real-time non-invasive tissue stiffness assessment during US B-mode examination. Under US guidance, the operator can place the measurement box in any region of the hepatic parenchyma with no vasculature or in an FLL to a maximum depth of 8 cm from the skin plane, as shown in **Figure 2**. The SWV (m/sec) and depth (cm) of the region of interest (ROI) evaluated will be displayed.

Several meta-analysis focused on the performance of SWE in discriminating benign and malignant FLLs [31–33].

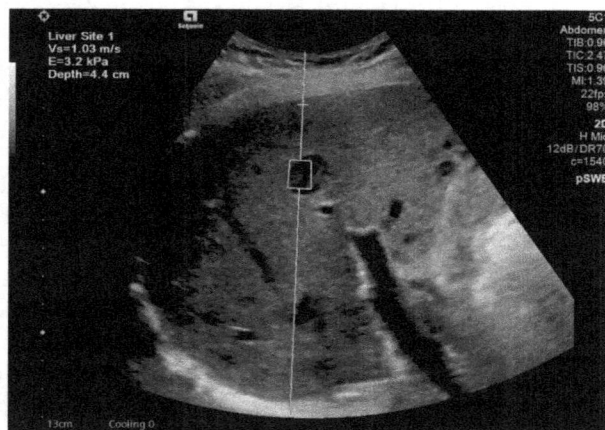

Figure 2.
pSWE measurement in metastasis using Siemens Acuson-Sequoia US system.

A meta-analysis performed by Jiao et al. [31] that included 9 prospective studies with a total of 1046 FLLs (malignant 679) showed a pooled sensitivity and specificity of 82.2% (95% CI: 73.4–88.5) and 80.2% (95% CI: 73.3–85.7), respectively. The positive likelihood ratio negative likelihood ratio and diagnostic odds ratio of SWE in differentiating malignant and benign liver lesions were 4.159 (95% CI: 2.899–5.966), 0.222 (95% CI: 0.140–0.352), and 18.749 (95% CI: 8.746–40.195), respectively. The area under the hierarchical summary receiver operating characteristic (HSROC) curve was 87% (95% CI: 84–90). The authors concluded that SWE complementary to the conventional US could be useful in FLL differentiation [31].

Another meta-analysis that included 8 studies with 590 lesions (228 benign and 362 malignant) showed that the cut-off value of SWV was different across studies, ranging from 1.5 to 2.7 m/sec. The sensitivity and specificity were 0.86 (95% CI 0.74–0.93) and 0.89 (95% CI 0.81–0.94). The HSROC curve was 0.94 (95% CI 0.91–0.96) [32].

Also, a recent meta-analysis of pSWE (12 studies) and 2D-SWE (3 studies) showed promising results for FLL evaluation [33]. The data included a total of 1894 FLLs from a large cohort (1728 patients). Comparing the methods, 2D-SWE had slightly higher sensitivity compared with pSWE (84% vs. 82%, $P < 0.01$) and no significant difference in the specificity for the two modalities ($P = 0.18$). SWE evaluation was useful for FLL differentiation with a mean sensibility of 0.72 (95% confidence interval [CI]: 0.59–0.83) and a mean specificity of 0.82 (95% CI: 0.43–0.97). The area under the operating curve (AUC) was 0.89 (95% CI: 0.86–0.91). The accuracy of the SWV ratio for the differentiation of benign and malignant FLLs was also assessed. The pooled sensitivity, specificity, PLR, and NLR, of the SWV ratio (FLL to surrounding liver parenchyma) for the differentiation of malignant and benign FLLs were 0.72 (95% CI: 0.59–0.83), 0.82 (95% CI: 0.43–0.97), 4.08 (95% CI: 0.88–18.89), and 0.33 (95% CI: 0.19–0.60), respectively. Using the Fagan plot demonstrated that SWE is fairly effective for FLL differentiation: 82% probability of malignant disease following a positive measurement, and the probability reduced to 18% when a negative measurement occurred [33].

Some published studies regarding FLL characterization using pSWE showed higher SWV in malignant tumors [34], and others showed similar SWV values in benign and malignant tumors [35–38]. The overlapping results can be explained by the level of fibrous tissue in an FLL and the level of vascularization [34].

The studies demonstrated that malignant FLLs are generally stiffer than benign lesions, reporting the following descending stiffness order: Liver metastases > HCC > FNH (focal nodular hyperplasia) > Hemangioma [17, 32, 34, 39]. In the setting of liver cirrhosis, HCC lesions may appear softer than the surrounding liver parenchyma and also softer than other malignant FLLs (metastases and cholangiocarcinoma) [40–42], with SWV values varying from 2.16 ± 0.75 m/s [43] to 3.07 ± 0.89 m/s in the Guo study [44]. SWE assessment of a lesion must be interpreted, considering the patient's clinical background [17, 33].

Table 1 shows the SWV mean values (m/sec) for different FLLS (HCC, Metastases, HH, FNH, and HA) and the cut-off values (m/sec) for discriminating between malignant and benign lesions obtained by different studies using pSWE for FLL evaluation.

2.2.2 Two-dimensional shear wave elastography (2D-SWE): clinical applications for FLLs evaluation

2D-SWE is another quantitative elastographic technique used in clinical practice to discriminate between malignant and benign lesions in the prostate [46], thyroid [47, 48],

Study	HCC	Metastases	HH	FNH	HA	Cut-off value malignant vs benign; P value
Dong et al. [35]	2.63 (range 1.84–5.68)	2.78 (range 1.02–3.15)	1.5 (range 0.79–2.61)	1.35 (range 0.69–2.94)	—	2.06 p < 0.005
Zhang et al. [36]	2.59 ± 0.91	3.20 ± 0.62	1.33 ± 0.38	1.90 ± 0.45	—	2.16 p < 0.01
Yu et al. [37]	2.49 ± 1.07	2.73 ± 0.89	1.75 ± 0.80	2.18 ± 0.84	1.79 ± 0.14	2.72 p < 0.01
Heide et al. [38]	2.63 ± 1.09	2.88 ± 1.16	2.36 ± 0.77	3.11 ± 0.93	2.23 ± 0.97	- p = 0.23
Akdoğan et al. [40]	2.75 ± 0.53	3.59 ± 0.51	2.15 ± 0.73	3.22 ± 0.18	—	2.32 p > 0.05
Kim et al. [41]	2.66 ± 0.94	2.82 ± 0.96 3.70 ± 0.61	1.80 ± 0.57	—	—	2.73 p > 0.05
Gallotti et al. [42]	2.17 ± 0.85	2.87 ± 1.13	2.30 ± 0.95	2.75 ± 0.95	1.25 ± 0.37	- p < 0.05
Ghiuchici et al. [43]	2.16 ± 0.75	—	—	—	—	- p < 0.001
Guo et al. [44]	3.07 ± 0.89	2.74 ± 1.06	1.48 ± 0.70	2.30 ± 1.18	—	2.13 p < 0.001
Galati et al. [45]	2.47 ± 1.42	3.29 ± 1.23	1.34 ± 0.91	—	—	2.0 -

Table 1.
Shear wave velocity values (m/sec, range) for FLLs in different studies using pSWE. Cut-off values (m/sec) for discriminating malignant versus benign FLLs.

breast [49], and FLLs [50–54]. This method allows real-time visualization of a color quantitative elastogram superimposed on a B-mode image. **Figures 3** and **4** show examples of 2D-SWE FLL evaluation implemented on different US devices.

Grgurevic et al. [52] aimed in a recent study to describe the stiffness of the most common benign and malignant FLLs by means of RT-2D-SWE (real-time

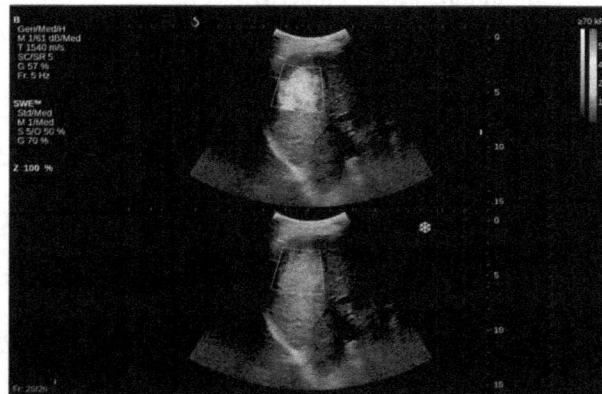

Figure 3.
2D-SWE elastogram in a large HCC using SSI–SuperSonic imagine, Aixplorer US system.

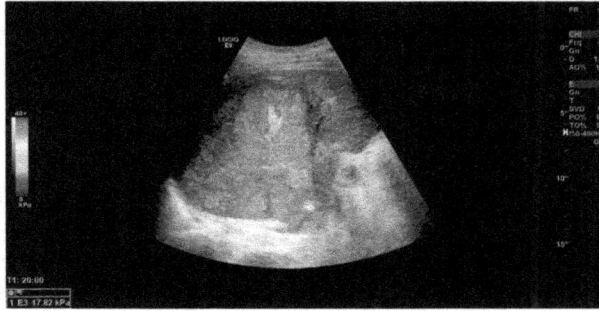

Figure 4.
2D-SWE.GE evaluation for a HCC using Logiq E9, GE Healthcare US system.

2-dimensional share-wave elastography), to analyze the ratio between the stiffness of FLL and surrounding liver parenchyma, and to determine the accuracy of RT-2D-SWE in differentiating benign and malignant FLLs. The authors developed a liver elastography malignancy prediction score (LEMP) for non-invasive characterization of FLLs that enabled correct differentiation of benign and malignant FLL in 96% of patients. This study concluded that RT-2D-SWE could be a reliable method for differentiating malignant from benign liver lesions with a comprehensive approach.

Two other 2D-SWE studies found no significant differences between malignant and benign FLL stiffness [51, 55]. Both studies showed that FNHs were significantly stiffer than HA. Regarding HCC nodules, studies showed 2D-SWE values that varied from19.6 kPa to 44.8 kPa (range 15.8 kPa–97 kPa) [51, 53]. This variability can be explained by many factors, including lesion dimensions and ROI positioning. Additionally, the background liver can influence the diagnostic capability of 2D-SWE [52, 54].

2.3 Limitations of elastography for FLL evaluation

Elastographic evaluation of FLLs has several limitations:

- Lesion position and size;

- Motion artifacts and patients features;

- Wide range of stiffness values in FLLs;

- The number of SWE measurements.

The location of the lesion can limit SWE evaluation; the maximum depth of SWE examination is limited to 8 cm from the skin [56]. The size of the lesion can lead to higher variability of elastographic values [43]. Patient-related limitations are connected to poor image acquisition due to poor intercostal window, obesity, and the patient's inability to hold respiration. Another confounding factor that must be mentioned is that the SWE values overlap between malignant and benign lesions, leading to diagnostic confusion. There is no consensus regarding the necessary number of elastographic measurements in FLLs [8, 18].

Nevertheless, elastography remains a powerful and essential diagnostic tool for FLL evaluation that can be added complementary to routine US examinations.

3. Conclusions

Elastography is a noninvasive, US-based, real-time imaging modality that can be a valuable tool in orienting the diagnosis and can be integrated into imaging protocols already involving the standard US to obtain a multiparametric approach. Although SWE has excellent potential in characterizing FLLs, further research is needed to evaluate the accuracy of these methods and set specific cut-off values.

Published studies have conflicting results, and no consensus has been so far established. This is the main reason that the WFUMB [13] and EFSUMB [21] guidelines do not recommend the use of elastography for differentiation between malignant and benign FLLs. Further multicentric studies with larger and homogenous cohorts are required for these techniques to be appropriately used routinely in a clinical setting.

Conflict of interest

The authors declare no conflict of interest.

Author details

Ana-Maria Ghiuchici[1,2] and Mirela Dănilă[1,2]*

1 Department of Gastroenterology and Hepatology, "Victor Babeş" University of Medicine and Pharmacy, Timişoara, Romania

2 Center of Advanced Research in Gastroenterology and Hepatology, "Victor Babeş" University of Medicine and Pharmacy, Timisoara, Romania

*Address all correspondence to: danila.mirela@umft.ro

IntechOpen

References

[1] Venkatesh SK, Chandan V, Roberts LR. Liver masses: A clinical, radiologic, and pathologic perspective. Clinical Gastroenterology and Hepatology. 2014;**12**(9):1414-1429. DOI: 10.1016/j. cgh.2013.09.017

[2] Dietrich CF, Sharma M, Gibson RN, Schreiber-Dietrich D, Jenssen C. Fortuitously discovered liver lesions. World Journal of Gastroenterology. 2013;**19**(21):3173-3188. DOI: 10.3748/wjg. v19.i21.3173

[3] Kaltenbach TE-M, Engler P, Kratzer W, Oeztuerk S, Seufferlein T, et al. Prevalence of benign focal liver lesions: Ultrasound investigation of 45,319 hospital patients. Abdominal Radiology. 2016;**41**(1):25-32. DOI: 10.1007/s00261-015-0605-7

[4] Sporea I, Sandulescu DL, Sirli R, Popescu A, Danila M, Sparchez Z, et al. Contrast-enhanced ultrasound for the characterization of malignant versus benign focal liver lesions in a prospective Multicenter experience - the SRUMB study. Journal of Gastrointestinal and Liver Diseases. 2019;**28**:191-196. DOI: 10.15403/jgld-180

[5] Fofiu R, Bende F, Popescu A, Şirli R, Lupuşoru R, Ghiuchici AM, et al. Spleen and liver stiffness for predicting high-risk varices in patients with compensated liver cirrhosis. Ultrasound in Medicine & Biology. 2021;**47**(1):76-83

[6] Gerber L, Fitting D, Srikantharajah K, Weiler N, Kyriakidou G, Bojunga J, et al. Evaluation of 2D- shear wave Elastography for characterisation of focal liver lesions. Journal of Gastrointestinal and Liver Diseases. 2017;**26**(3):283-290

[7] Ronot M, Di Renzo S, Gregoli B, Duran R, Castera L, Van Beers BE, et al. Characterization of fortuitously discovered focal liver lesions: Additional information provided by shearwave elastography. European Radiology. 2015;**25**(2):346-358. DOI: 10.1007/s00330-014-3370-z

[8] Lupsor-Platon M, Serban T, Silion AI, Tirpe A, Florea M. Hepatocellular carcinoma and non-alcoholic fatty liver disease: A step forward for better evaluation using ultrasound Elastography. Cancers. 2020;**12**(10):2778. DOI: 10.3390/cancers12102778

[9] Grgurevic I, Tjesic Drinkovic I, Pinzani M. Multiparametric ultrasound in liver diseases: An overview for the practising clinician. Postgraduate Medical Journal. 2019;**95**(1126):425-432. DOI: 10.1136/postgradmedj-2018-136111

[10] Oldhafer KJ, Habbel V, Horling K, Makridis G, Wagner KC. Benign Liver Tumors. Visceral Medicine. 2020;**36**(4):292-303. DOI: 10.1159/000509145

[11] Săftoiu A, Gilja OH, Sidhu PS, Dietrich CF, Cantisani V, Amy D, et al. The EFSUMB guidelines and recommendations for the clinical practice of Elastography in non-hepatic applications: Update 2018. Ultraschall in der Medizin. 2019;**40**:425-453. DOI: 10.1055/a-0838-9937

[12] Ferraioli G, Filice C, Castera L, Choi BI, Sporea I, Wilson SR, et al. WFUMB guidelines and recommendations for clinical use of ultrasound elastography: Part 3: Liver. Ultrasound in Medicine & Biology. 2015;**41**(5):1161-1179

[13] Ferraioli G, Wong VW, Castera L, Berzigotti A, Sporea I, Dietrich CF, et al. Liver ultrasound Elastography: An update to the world Federation for Ultrasound inMedicine and biology guidelines and recommendations. Ultrasound in Medicine & Biology. 2018;**44**(12):2419-2440. DOI: 10.1016/j.ultrasmedbio.2018.07.008

[14] Bray F, Ferlay J, Soerjomataram I, Siegel RL, Torre LA, Jemal A. Global cancer statistics 2018: GLOBOCAN estimates of incidence and mortality worldwide for 36 cancers in 185 countries. CA: A Cancer Journal for Clinicians. 2018;**68**:394-424. DOI: 10.3322/caac.21492

[15] Shiina T, Nightingale KR, Palmeri ML, Hall TJ, Bamber JC, Barr RG, et al. WFUMB guidelines and recommendations for clinical use of ultrasound elastography: Part 1: Basic principles and terminology. Ultrasound in Medicine & Biology. 2015;**41**(5):1126-1147. DOI: 10.1016/j.ultrasmedbio.2015.03.009

[16] Yeh WC, Li PC, Jeng YM, Hsu HC, Kuo PL, Li ML, et al. Elastic modulus measurements of human liver and correlation with pathology. Ultrasound in Medicine & Biology. 2002;**28**(4):467-474. DOI: 10.1016/s0301-5629(02)00489-1

[17] Berzigotti A, Ferraioli G, Bota S, Gilja OH, Dietrich CF. Novel ultrasound-based methods to assess liver disease: The game has just begun. Digestive and Liver Disease. 2018;**50**(2):107-112. DOI: 10.1016/j.dld.2017.11.019

[18] Martelletti C, Armandi A, Caviglia GP, Saracco GM, Pellicano R. Elastography for characterization of focal liver lesions: Current evidence and future perspectives. Minerva Gastroenterol. 2021;**67**(2):196-208. DOI: 10.23736/S2724-5985.20.02747-6

[19] Srinivasa Babu A, Wells ML, Teytelboym OM, Mackey JE, Miller FH, Yeh BM, et al. Elastography in chronic liver disease: Modalities, techniques, limitations, and future directions. Radiographics. 2016;**36**(7):1987-2006

[20] European Association for Study of Liver; Asociacion Latinoamericana para el Estudio del Higado. EASL-ALEH clinical practice guidelines: Non-invasive tests for evaluation of liver disease severity and prognosis. Journal of Hepatology. 2015;**63**(1):237-264. DOI: 10.1016/j.jhep.2015.04.006

[21] Dietrich CF, Bamber J, Berzigotti A, Bota S, Cantisani V, Castera L, et al. EFSUMBguidelinesandrecommendations on the clinical use of liver ultrasound Elastography, update 2017 (long version). Ultraschall in der Medizin. 2017;**38**(4):e16-e47. DOI: 10.1055/s-0043-103952

[22] Emara DM, El Shafei MM, El-Gendi A, Yousif AA. Is ultrasound elastography adding value in diagnosis of focal hepatic lesions? Our experience in a single-center study. Egyptian Journal of Radiology and Nuclear Medicine. 2019;**50**:103

[23] Onur MR, Poyraz AK, Ucak EE, Bozgeyik Z, Özercan IH, Ogur E. Semiquantitative strain elastography of liver masses. Journal of Ultrasound in Medicine. 2012;**31**(7):1061-1067. DOI: 10.7863/jum.2012.31.7.1061

[24] Nagolu H, Kattoju S, Natesan C, Krishnakumar M, Kumar S. Role of acoustic radiation force impulse Elastography in the characterization of focal solid hepatic lesions. Journal of Clinical Imaging Science. 2018;**8**:5

[25] Shuang-Ming T, Ping Z, Ying Q, Li-Rong C, Ping Z, Rui- ZL. Usefulness

of acoustic radiation force impulse imaging in the differential diagnosis of benign and malignant liver lesions. Academic Radiology. 2011;**18**(7):810-815

[26] Kato K, Sugimoto H, Kanazumi N, et al. Intra-operative application of real-time tissue elastography for the diagnosis of liver tumours. Liver International. 2008;**28**(9):1264-1271. DOI: 10.1111/j.1478-3231.2008.01701.x

[27] Inoue Y, Takahashi M, Arita J, Aoki T, Hasegawa K, Beck Y, et al. Intra-operative freehand real-time elastography for small focal liver lesions: "visual palpation" for non-palpable tumors. Surgery. 2010;**148**(5):1000-1011. DOI: 10.1016/j.surg.2010.02.009

[28] Jung EM, Batista P, da Silva N, Jung W, Farkas S, Stroszczynski C, et al. Is strain Elastography (IO-SE) sufficient for characterization of liver lesions before surgical resection--or is contrast enhanced ultrasound (CEUS) necessary? PLoS One. 2015;**10**(6):e0123737. DOI: 10.1371/journal.pone.0123737

[29] Sigrist RMS, Liau J, Kaffas AE, Chammas MC, Willmann JK. Ultrasound Elastography: Review of techniques and clinical applications. Theranostics. 2017;7(5):1303-1329. DOI: 10.7150/thno.18650

[30] European Association for the Study of the Liver. Electronic address: easloffice@easloffice.eu; Clinical Practice Guideline Panel; Chair:; EASL Governing Board representative:; Panel members. EASL clinical practice guidelines on non-invasive tests for evaluation of liver disease severity and prognosis - 2021 update. Journal of Hepatology. 2021;**75**(3):659-689. DOI: 10.1016/j.jhep.2021.05.025

[31] Jiao Y, Dong F, Wang H, Zhang L, Xu J, Zheng J, et al. Shear wave elastography imaging for detecting malignant lesions of the liver: A systematic review and pooled meta-analysis. Medical Ultrasonography. 2017;**19**(1):16-22. DOI: 10.11152/mu-925

[32] Ying L, Lin X, Xie ZL, Tang FY, Hu YP, Shi KQ. Clinical utility of acoustic radiation force impulse imaging for identification of malignant liver lesions: A meta-analysis. European Radiology. 2012;**22**(12):2798-2805. DOI: 10.1007/s00330-012-2540-0

[33] Hu X, Huang X, Chen H, Zhang T, Hou J, Song A, et al. Diagnostic effect of shear wave elastography imaging for differentiation of malignant liver lesions: A meta-analysis. BMC Gastroenterology. 2019;**19**(1):60. DOI: 10.1186/s12876-019-0976-2

[34] Wu JP, Shu R, Zhao YZ, Ma GL, Xue W, He QJ, et al. Comparison of contrast-enhanced ultrasonography with virtual touch tissue quantification in the evaluation of focal liver lesions. Journal of Clinical Ultrasound. 2016;**44**(6):347-353. DOI: 10.1002/jcu.22335

[35] Dong Y, Wang WP, Xu Y, Cao J, Mao F, Dietrich CF. Point shear wave speed measurement in differentiating benign and malignant focal liver lesions. Medical Ultrasonography. 2017;**19**(3):259-264. DOI: 10.11152/mu-1142

[36] Zhang P, Zhou P, Tian SM, Qian Y, Li JL, Li RZ. Diagnostic performance of contrast-enhanced sonography and acoustic radiation force impulse imaging in solid liver lesions. Journal of Ultrasound in Medicine. 2014;**33**(2):205-214. DOI: 10.7863/ultra.33.2.205

[37] Yu H, Wilson SR. Differentiation of benign from malignant liver masses with acoustic radiation force impulse technique. Ultrasound Quarterly.

2011;**27**(4):217-223. DOI: 10.1097/
RUQ.0b013e318239422e

[38] Heide R, Strobel D, Bernatik T, Goertz RS. Characterization of focal liver lesions (FLL) with acoustic radiation force impulse (ARFI) elastometry. Ultraschall in der Medizin. 2010;**31**(4):405-409. DOI: 10.1055/s-0029-1245565

[39] Hasab Allah M, Salama RM, Marie MS, Mandur AA, Omar H. Utility of point shear wave elastography in characterisation of focal liver lesions. Expert Review of Gastroenterology & Hepatology. 2018;**12**(2):201-207. DOI: 10.1080/17474124.2018.1415144

[40] Akdoğan E, Yılmaz FG. The role of acoustic radiation force impulse elastography in the differentiation of benign and malignant focal liver masses [published correction appears in Turk J Gastroenterol. 2018;29(6):722]. The Turkish Journal of Gastroenterology. 2018;**29**(4):456-463. DOI: 10.5152/tjg.2018.11710

[41] Kim JE, Lee JY, Bae KS, Han JK, Choi BI. Acoustic radiation force impulse elastography for focal hepatic tumors: Usefulness for differentiating hemangiomas from malignant tumors. Korean Journal of Radiology. 2013;**14**(5):743-753. DOI: 10.3348/kjr.2013.14.5.743

[42] Gallotti A, D'Onofrio M, Romanini L, Cantisani V, Pozzi Mucelli R. Acoustic radiation force impulse (ARFI) ultrasound imaging of solid focal liver lesions. European Journal of Radiology. 2012;**81**(3):451-455. DOI: 10.1016/j.ejrad.2010.12.071

[43] Ghiuchici AM, Sporea I, Dănilă M, Şirli R, Moga T, Bende F, et al. Is there a place for Elastography in the diagnosis of hepatocellular carcinoma? Journal of

Clinical Medicine. 2021;**10**(8):1710. DOI: 10.3390/jcm10081710

[44] Guo LH, Wang SJ, Xu HX, Sun LP, Zhang YF, Xu JM, et al. Differentiation of benign and malignant focal liver lesions: Value of virtual touch tissue quantification of acoustic radiation force impulse elastography. Medical Oncology. 2015;**32**(3):68. DOI: 10.1007/s12032-015-0543-9

[45] Galati G, De Vincentis A, Gallo P, Guidi A, Vespasiani-Gentilucci U, Picardi A. Diagnostic value of virtual touch quantification (VTQ®) for differentiation of hemangiomas from malignant focal liver lesions. Medical Ultrasonography. 2019;**21**(4):371-376. DOI: 10.11152/mu-2062

[46] Correas JM, Tissier AM, Khairoune A, Vassiliu V, Méjean A, Hélénon O, et al. Prostate cancer: Diagnostic performance of real-time shear-wave elastography. Radiology. 2015;**275**(1):280-289

[47] Zhang B, Ma X, Wu N, Liu L, Liu X, Zhang J, et al. Shear wave elastography for differentiation of benign and malignant thyroid nodules: A meta-analysis. Journal of Ultrasound in Medicine. 2013;**32**(12):2163-2169. DOI: 10.7863/ultra.32.12.2163

[48] Stoian D, Timar B, Craina M, Craciunescu M, Timar R, Schiller A. Elastography: A New Ultrasound Technique in Nodular Thyroid Pathology, Thyroid Cancer - Advances in Diagnosis and Therapy. Hojjat Ahmadzadehfar: IntechOpen; 2016. Available from: https://www.intechopen.com/chapters/51576

[49] Berg WA, Cosgrove DO, Doré CJ, Schäfer FK, Svensson WE, Hooley RJ, et al. Shear-wave elastography improves the specificity of breast US: The BE1

multinational study of 939 masses. Radiology. 2012;**262**(2):435-449

[50] Park HS, Kim YJ, Yu MH, Jung SI, Jeon HJ. Shear wave Elastography of focal liver lesion: Intraobserver reproducibility and elasticity characterization. Ultrasound Quarterly. 2015;**31**(4):262-271

[51] Ronot M, Di Renzo S, Gregoli B, Duran R, Castera L, Van Beers BE, et al. Characterization of fortuitously discovered focal liver lesions: Additional information provided by shearwave elastography. European Radiology. 2015;**25**(2):346-358. DOI: 10.1007/ s00330-014-3370-z

[52] Grgurevic I, Bokun T, Salkic NN, Brkljacic B, Vukelić-Markovic M, Stoos-Veic T, et al. Liver elastography malignancy prediction score for noninvasive characterization of focal liver lesions. Liver International. 2018;**38**(6):1055-1063. DOI: 10.1111/ liv.13611

[53] Gerber L, Fitting D, Srikantharajah K, Weiler N, Kyriakidou G, Bojunga J, et al. Evaluation of 2D- shear wave Elastography for characterisation of focal liver lesions. Journal of Gastrointestinal and Liver Diseases. 2017;**26**(3):283-290

[54] Hwang JA, Jeong WK, Song KD, Kang KA, Lim HK. 2-D shear wave Elastography for focal lesions in liver phantoms: Effects of background stiffness, depth and size of focal lesions on stiffness measurement. Ultrasound in Medicine & Biology. 2019;**45**(12):3261-3268. DOI: 10.1016/j. ultrasmedbio.2019.08.006

[55] Guibal A, Boularan C, Bruce M, Vallin M, Pilleul F, Walter T, et al. Evaluation of shearwave elastography for the characterisation of focal liver lesions on ultrasound. European Radiology. 2013;**23**(4):1138-1149. DOI: 10.1007/s00330-012-2692-y

[56] Frulio N, Laumonier H, Carteret T, Laurent C, Maire F, Balabaud C, et al. Evaluation of liver tumors using acoustic radiation force impulse elastography and correlation with histologic data. Journal of Ultrasound in Medicine. 2013;**32**(1):121-130. DOI: 10.7863/ jum.2013.32.1.121

Chapter 9

Endoscopic Ultrasound Elastography: New Advancement in Pancreatic Diseases

Bogdan Silviu Ungureanu and Adrian Saftoiu

Abstract

Elastography opened up new frontiers for pancreatic disease, as it may aid in tumor mass differentiation. Ultrasound strain elastography and ultrasound shear-wave elastography have been used so far by transabdominal transducers. New technological advancements have embedded elastography techniques in endoscopic ultrasound (EUS), thus enabling a better evaluation of patients with pancreatic tumors, chronic pancreatitis, autoimmune pancreatitis, gastrointestinal subepithelial lesions, and lymph node involvement. Moreover, EUS-E might help in guiding EUS-Fine Needle Aspiration or EUS-Fine Needle Biopsy when addressing solid pancreatic tumors, for proper tissue harvesting. Furthermore, artificial intelligence methods may bypass the human factor and lead to better diagnostic results.

Keywords: endoscopic ultrasound, elastography, pancreatic disease

1. Introduction

Elastography has surfaced in the early 1990s as a new noninvasive technique capable of offering new diagnostic opportunities for malignant diseases [1]. Initially, considered for superficial organs such as the breast [2, 3] or thyroid [4], elastography became to have an upward trend by covering most of the parenchymatous organs from the digestive system [5]. Over the years, new elastography techniques were integrated into ultrasound devices trying to create a foundational stage and to develop new standards by enhancing the spectrum of the available techniques [6]. However, the pancreas still stands as a challenge as it is hard to reach by elastography measurements.

When compared with other organs, the pancreas has by far a more limited number of studies. Due to its' retroperitoneal position, transabdominal ultrasound elastography may be rather difficult to be properly executed, and it may lead to an inaccurate or imprecise examination. The evolving field of evidence-based medicine has then focused on more precise imaging techniques used for the pancreas examination such as endoscopic ultrasound (EUS) [7]. This enhanced the spectrum of available techniques that might enable pancreatic disease diagnosis and lead to a pathbreaking development along with the endoscopic ultrasound fine-needle aspiration

(EUS-FNA) implementation as a standard and necessary method [8]. While EUS-FNA has laid the grounds for the current therapeutic techniques for pancreatic disease complications, it has also contributed to the elastography imaging, mainly by providing a pathological result, which is helped as the standard method for the elastography evaluation.

In the evolutionary steps of elastography, the first introduced method was strain elastography [9]. This technique measures the strain developed during external pressure, and its' results are considered inversely related, meaning that the tissue stiffness will be softer if the strain will be greater. The manual compression is acknowledged as a limitation in a pancreatic setting thus, it requires strain to be obtained from nearby structures. However, several limitations are encountered, as measurements may be obtained usually at the level of the pancreatic body, provided that no vascular elements are in the elastography region of interest.

Further on, other elastography techniques have tried to enlarge the current spectrum and to extend elastography to a more precise tool. Shear-wave elastography [10], which is based on a different principle, was then proposed to outcome the flaws of strain elastography. By generating shear waves from the transducer, pancreatic tissue is measured and its stiffness becomes more evident as the shear wave velocity is faster. This technique was recently introduced to a EUS setting and might strengthen the available data [11].

As part of ongoing technical developments, artificial intelligence methods have also been introduced in pancreatic elastography assessment [12]. Their potential is nonetheless beneficial, as they may avoid the human factor in some situations, thus covering new grounds in pancreatic elastography.

With this chapter, we try to explore the potential of elastography in different pancreatic diseases and try to answer some of the available questions about the future of elastography.

2. Endoscopic ultrasound elastography (EUS-E) techniques

Probably the major outcome of EUS-E is that it may reach structures that are rather hard to examine, such as the pancreas or adjacent lymph nodes. As mentioned above, there are two elastography techniques available on EUS systems that have been tested on pancreatic diseases: strain elastography and the recently introduced shear wave method [11].

2.1 Strain elastography

This technique was first considered a qualitative technique, with the elastography region of interest (ROI), which covered the ultrasound image showing a pattern of green and blue colors in correspondence to the tissue stiffness [12, 13]. Green areas were considered benign, whereas blue areas were related to a possible malignant tissue. Since this method requires the transducer to be placed near the examination tissue, it is recommended to cover up at least 50% of the targeted tissue. Also, since the compression will be performed with the echoendoscope, it is important not to produce too strong compressions, so that reproducible types of elastograms may be achieved. The targeted lesion should be in the center of the transducer so that the elastography image should cover it and avoid adjacent tissue as much as possible [14, 15].

Semiquantitative analysis was introduced by determining strain ratio [16, 17]. This concept allows the practitioner to select an ROI by highlighting a round-shaped area in the targeted tissue and a smaller ROI within the nearby normal tissue, which might be either the normal parenchyma or the gastrointestinal tract wall. Then, the strain ratio has resulted from the two selected areas, with a value displayed by the ultrasound software.

Another method is represented by the strain histogram, which is based on the hue histograms averaged over several compression cycles [18, 19]. The results are usually described by mean values and standard deviation, as well as other parameters characteristic to histograms (Kurtosis, skewness, etc.). This strain histogram will cover a scale of 256 colors, being now embedded in the software of most ultrasound systems.

2.2 Shear-wave elastography

Shear-wave elastography (SWE) also became recently available in the EUS setting [11]. While the concept of SWE is similar to strain elastography, it does not use a transducer to create pressure, but it creates an elasticity map by measuring shear wave parameters. Directed by the ultrasound beam, the tissue is targeted by a perpendicular "push-pulse," which generates shear waves. SWE is capable of providing direct stiffness measurements, which are translated either in kilopascal (kPa) or meter/second (m/s). This technique might be easier to use, as it may be performed much easier, and most of all since will directly provide quantitative values. However, it will require establishing cutoff values for every organ, which will be examined.

3. Clinical applications

Both strain and shear-wave elastography are available in the EUS setting for pancreatic disease [20, 21]. One of the major differences between these techniques is that when strain elastography is used only relative values are obtained as this is only a semiquantitative method, whereas shear-wave elastography produces absolute values, which may be more relevant. Thus, color pattern assessment with strain ratio and strain histogram analysis, as well as definite values for shear wave elastography may aid for pancreatic disease assessment and may represent an adjuvant method to confirm the diagnosis.

3.1 Pancreatic masses

There is always room for techniques improvement when discussing pancreatic tumors. Even though EUS-FNB is now considered the main method to confirm the diagnosis of a pancreatic tumor [22], elastography might aid in providing a larger panel when imaging examinations are performed.

Solid pancreatic lesions were classified by qualitative elastography into four different patterns presumably with their correspondent, normal tissue—green pattern, malignant tumor—mostly blue with small green areas and red lines, inflammatory mass—green with yellow and red lines or neuroendocrine tumor—homogeneous blue pattern [23]. When performing this procedure, it is important to avoid a smaller ROI, as the measurements will show a relative elasticity difference. Thus, the ROI should be large enough to include the tumor as well as normal adjacent tissue, and this is easily achievable in a clinical setting with a ratio of 50% for lesions and 50% for nearby tissues [24].

Along with the first study in 2006 [25], EUS was introduced as an optimistic technique that might be at least as useful as it was introduced in breast cancer. Moreover, due to the pancreatic adenocarcinoma characteristics as a tumor with high desmoplastic reaction, when performing EUS-E, the tumors should be much stiffer than the surrounding tissue [26]. However, no reliable correlation was successful so far with tumor grading.

Further on, the use of quantitative EUS-E suggested more reliable results, even though there were no differences in accuracy between these two techniques [27]. Iglesias-Garcia et al [28] mentioned that the strain ratio method had a higher accuracy (97.7%) and specificity (92.2%) than the qualitative analysis and that a cutoff value of the strain ratio higher than 6.04 with a lower elasticity index than 0.05% might be sensitive enough the difference between malignant and benign pancreatic tumors. He also concluded that this technique might properly differentiate from inflammatory masses with a sensitivity of 100% and a specificity of 96% and neuroendocrine tumors (sensitivity 100% and specificity 88%).

Histogram analysis also showed some promising results (**Figures 1** and **2**). In our own study published in 2008 [29], we reported a 91.4% sensitivity, 87.9% specificity, 88.9% positive predictive value (PPV), and 90.6% negative predictive value (NPV) for the diagnosis of pancreatic malignancies, based on a cutoff of 175. Even more, better results were obtained by Schrader et al [30], who obtained 100% sensitivity and 100% specificity for pancreatic ductal adenocarcinoma (PDAC) detection; however, they did mention the controls were patients with a normal pancreas. This might not be relevant, since chronic pancreatic or other masses would be the main objective to be compared with.

Currently, there are seven meta-analyses (**Table 1**) [31–37] that include strain EUS-E for pancreatic cancer and showed a specificity of 92–98% and a specificity of 67–76%. However, two studies assessed small pancreatic tumors of less than 15 and 20 mm, respectively, and pointed out that EUS-E might be confident in suggesting that PDAC is a stiff tumor [38, 39]. Kataoka et al [38] analyzed 126 cases of small pancreatic lesions associated or not with main pancreatic duct dilation. They concluded that a stiffness ratio was definitely higher for pancreatic cancer 62:3 vs. 29:32, $P < 0.001$. Also, when comparing lesions with PC vs. without main pancreatic duct dilation, the sensitivity (94 vs 100%), specificity (23 vs 60%), and predictive value (60 vs 100%) were different suggesting that a small lesion might be excluded from being pancreatic cancer without main pancreatic duct dilation with high confidence and concordance.

As this technique may be used as an adjuvant tool for pancreatic masses diagnosis, it may be included in a panel of procedures to enhance the diagnosis process. Combining EUS-E with contrast-enhanced endoscopic ultrasound (CEUS), it could help patients with a negative FNA, if a PDAC is strongly suspected. For EUS-FNA negative cases, we compared PDAC patients with chronic pancreatitis and suggested that a hypovascular, hard tumor might suggest a PDAC with 75.8% sensitivity, 85.2% specificity, 83.3% PPV, and 96.2% NPV [40].

A different approach was tested by Yamada et al [41], which tried to assess vascular invasion of PDAC using EUS-E. They defined vascular invasions as seen in EUS by their exerting pressure characteristics. They considered that if two tissues with different stiffness are in close contact, but not fixed, their border will move when compression is made, which will translate in EUS-E as a softer tissue with adjacent artifacts with red, yellow, and green. On the other hand, if their border moves at a time, they will not have any artifacts there, thus they might have a vascular invasion. EUS-E showed a high diagnostic ability with a sensitivity of 0.917 a specificity of 0.900, and

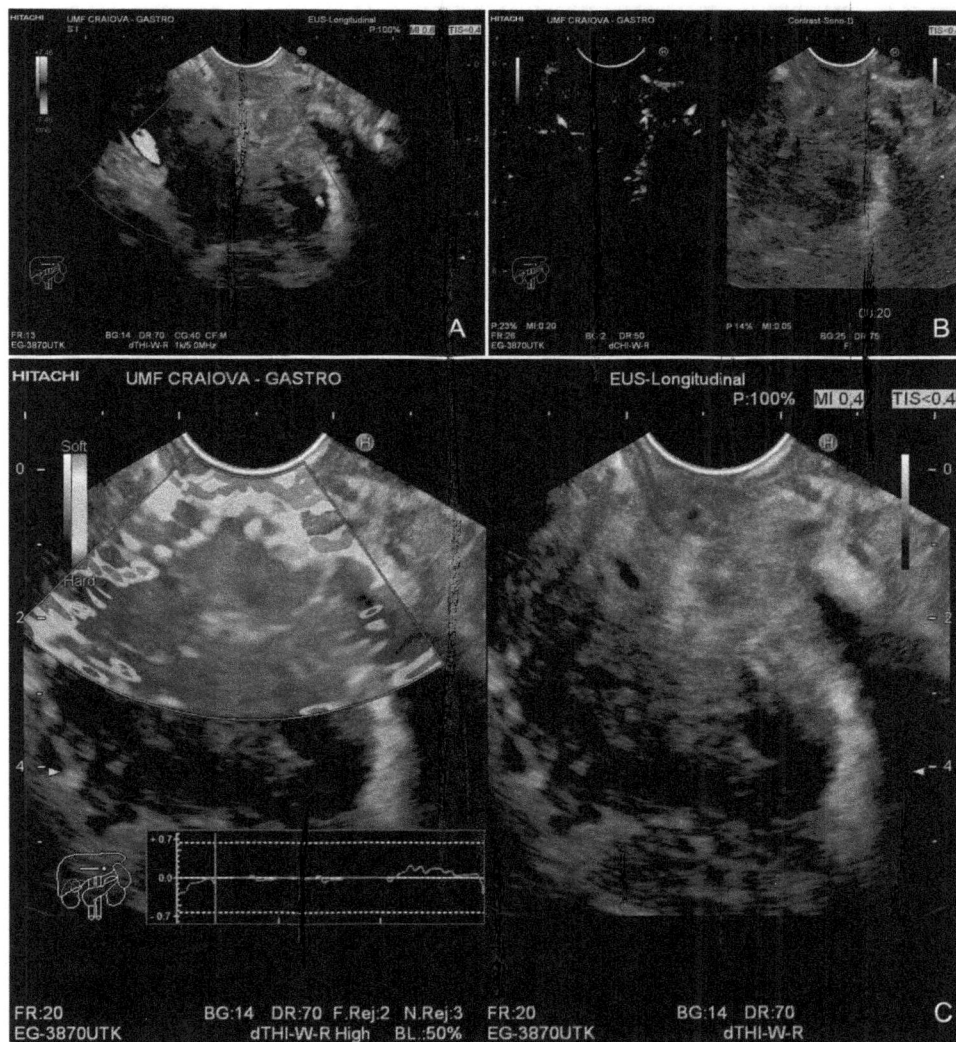

Figure 1.
Multimodal EUS imaging of a solid pancreatic tumor, pancreatic adenocarcinoma. A EUS – Doppler imaging. B Contrast-enhanced ultrasound imaging. C. EUS-E imaging with strain histogram.

an accuracy of 0.906, and after the interobserver agreement, they obtained higher k-coefficients than the B mode k −0.542 vs. $k = 0.625$, suggesting a possible method to assess vascular invasion. However, they used six different ultrasound settings, and this may hamper their results.

In a research setting, Mazzawi et al [42] published two cases where they tested EUS-E after radiofrequency ablation. Based on the fact that after ablation is difficult to distinguish residual from a recurrent tumor or fibrotic tissue, while the mass is only visible at CT/MR as decreased or unchanged by RFA, they USED EUS-E to figure out if there is any tumor tissue left. First, EUS-E was performed before the RFA procedure showing blue colored mass suggesting a hard tissue. Second, after RFA, the CT scan showed an increase in tumor diameter without any other characterization. While performing EUS-E, a mixture of blue and green areas was seen, suggesting central

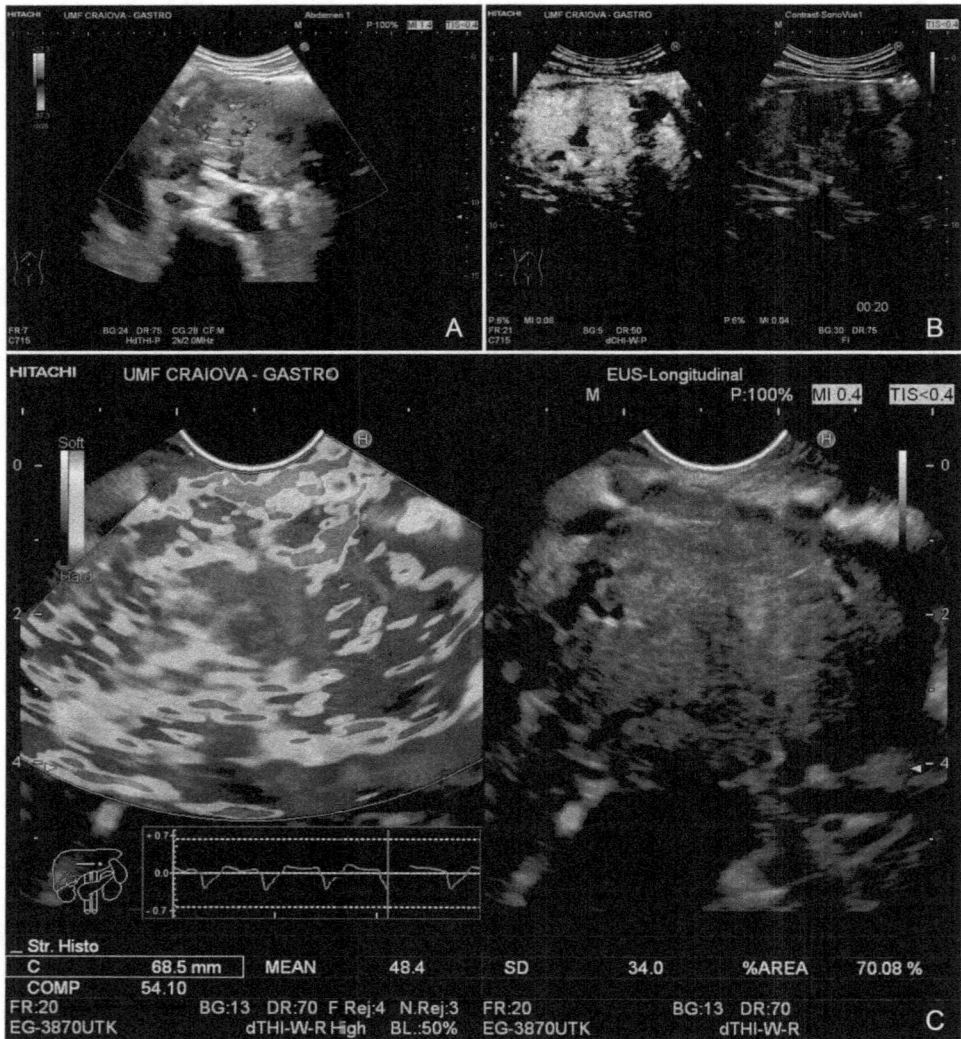

Figure 2.
Multimodal imaging of a solid pancreatic tumor, neuroendocrine tumor. A. EUS – Doppler imaging. B Contrast-enhanced ultrasound imaging. C. EUS-E imaging with strain histogram.

anechoic areas indicating necrosis and another hypoechoic region of the tumor mass. Thus, they suggest that since RFA could be performed sequentially, EUS-E might help in determining which region should be reassessed on future procedures.

The second technique available for EUS-E in a pancreatic setting, the shear-wave measurement, has only one study published so far on pancreatic masses with inconclusive results [43]. Shear wave velocity is measured, and faster propagation will be related to greater tissue elasticity. Ohno et al [43] compared EUS-SWM and EUS-E for 64 consecutive cases with solid pancreatic lesions and pointed out that the velocity of the shear wave when comparing pancreatic cancer to mass-forming pancreatitis was not statistically significant (p 0.5687), while the mean strain value was lower for pancreatic cancer 45.4 vs. 74.5; p 0.0007. They used an Arietta 850 (Hitachi Medical Systems Europe, Zug, Switzerland) device, which unfortunately may not visualize

Year	Author	Number of patients	Sensitivity (%)	Specificity (%)
2012	Pei et al. [31]	1042	95	69
2013	Mei et al. [32]	1044	95	67
2013	Ying et al. [33]	893	98	69
2013	Li et al. [34]	781	99	76
2013	Hu et al. [35]	752	97	76
2013	Xu et al. [36]	752	99	74
2017	Lu et al. [37]	1537	97	67

Table 1.
Available meta-analyses that focus in EUS-E strain assessment on pancreatic cancer.

the propagation status of shear waves in the ROI. Moreover, as they mention, many artifacts may be encountered due to various reasons, such as tissue motion, nearby blood vessels, distortion, or precompression artifacts, as well as breathing, because the procedures are usually performed under conscious sedation. Thus, their conclusion was that this set of EUS-SWM is not feasible for pancreatic solid masses assessment and that EUS-E with strain ratios and histogram still remain the main adjuvant method to be considered.

3.2 Chronic pancreatitis

Currently, EUS-E is considered for pancreatic fibrosis assessment (as well as stiffness) by both strain and shear-wave elastography [44]. Even though transabdominal US-E has been reported at first [45, 46], EUS-E is the preferred method, due to its capability to better visualize the pancreas, regardless of the patient's body size. However, the technique still requires a highly experienced endoscopist (**Figure 3**).

Itoh et al [47] used quantitative analysis to diagnose pancreatic fibrosis using EUS-E of surgically resected specimens. They included 58 patients who underwent EUS-EG of the distal pancreas before performing a pancreatectomy of pancreatic tumor based on the concept that if a tumor is present in the pancreatic head, fibrosis might be present in the tail due to obstructive pancreatitis. When compared with histology, they maintained the same image as the EUS-E pattern by providing a median of 2.0 sections. They quantified four parameters of tissue elasticity (mean, standard deviation, skewness, and kurtosis) and obtained a significant correlation between all of them and the grade of pancreatic fibrosis. They concluded that with fibrosis progression, the skewness and kurtosis increased, whereas the standard deviation and mean decreased.

While this concept might be the ideal one, it is difficult to be introduced without comparing it to surgical specimens. On the other hand, EUS by itself is not standardized and has a low reproducibility in diagnosing chronic pancreatitis. Thus, by performing a histogram analysis, these drawbacks might be overcome. Kuwahara et al [48] published in 2017 their experience on using EUS on 96 patients. They performed EUS-E on the head of the pancreas and compared the mean values with no substantial difference (68.8 vs. 71.3); however, the interobserver reliability of chronic pancreatitis was substantial with a k value of 0.648 and a consistency ratio of 73%. They also mention that EUS characteristics with hyperechoic foci with shadowing and lobularity and honeycomb appearance, as well as the Rosemont Criteria, were correlated with

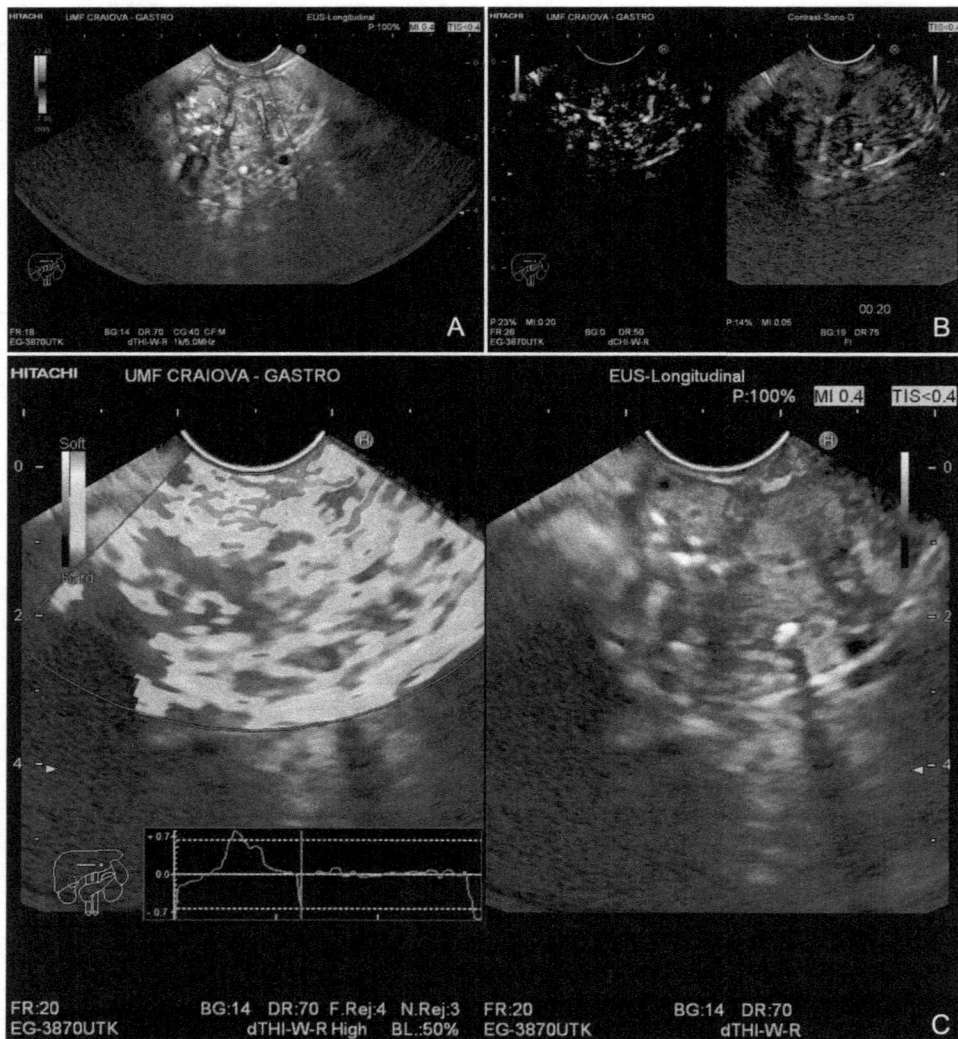

Figure 3.
Multimodal imaging of chronic pancreatitis A. EUS – Doppler imaging. B. Contrast-enhanced ultrasound imaging. C. EUS-E imaging with strain histogram.

EUS-E. In conclusion, they suggest that EUS-E is an objective method for the diagnosis of chronic pancreatitis and should be considered when performing EUS.

The elastography spectrum was enhanced with the shear wave devices implemented on EUS systems. Nonetheless, chronic pancreatitis benefited from this breakthrough, and recent studies have already been published. The first reports of EUS shear wave elastography [43, 49] compared the resulting values with the Rosemont classification and EUS criteria with positive results and suggested that shear wave values may assess the fibrotic changes, which occur in chronic pancreatitis. They obtained a high sensitivity of 100%, specificity 94%, and an AUROC (Area Under the Receiver Operating Characteristics) of 0.97, which highlights the EUS-SWM diagnostic capability and that also may surpass other imaging techniques. The exocrine and endocrine functions were also discussed if they might be correlated with

EUS-SWM since in chronic pancreatitis, they are both altered [50]. The EUS-SWM sensitivity, specificity, and AUROC obtained for diagnosing chronic pancreatitis were 83%, 100%, and 0.92. When discussing exocrine dysfunction with pancreatic function diagnostic tests, the AUROC was 0.78 with a cutoff value of 1.96, whereas for the endocrine dysfunction associated with diabetes mellitus, it was 0.63 with a cutoff value of 2.34.

EUS-E is a promising asset for chronic pancreatitis; however, there is a need for more studies since some limitations are still encountered. While the proper way to validate its use is represented by histology as a reference, in chronic pancreatitis this might be rather difficult, thus another setting should be proposed. Also, the use of shear waves seems to provide better data, as they estimate the stiffness of the tissue.

3.3 Autoimmune pancreatitis

Exploring new diagnostic paths, EUS-E might be a valid tool for AP assessment. The first cases were reported by Dietrich et al [51] after suspicion of chronic pancreatitis but had a final diagnosis of AIP after EUS. The stiffness that covers the entire pancreas is characteristic for AIP, which enables to easily distinguish AIP and pancreatic adenocarcinoma. Only one study tested EUS-E with strain ratio on AIP. The authors tried to show a positive relationship after steroid treatment in AIP by examining the patient before and 2 weeks after therapy. The patients showed a decrease in the strain ratio from (8.04 ± 2.29 to 3.44 ± 1.97 ($P < 0.0001$). This might promote EUS-E as a response to the therapy, which might be useful for clinicians.

Additionally, there is also a study published on SWE that compared patients with AIP with controls, yielding different values of share wave velocity (2.57 m/s vs. 1.89 m/s) ($P = 0.0185$). The study also tested the response to steroid therapy, and Vs significantly decreased from 3.32 to 2.46 m/s ($n = 6$) (P 0.0234), which highlights the technique's capability in AIP [49, 51, 52].

3.4 Pancreatic fistulas

EUS-E has also been tested in the particular setting of pancreatic fistula following pancreaticoduodenectomy [53]. This is a possible complication that may occur and can have dramatic consequences. Mean elasticity was measured and proved to be significantly higher in patients with pancreatic fistula as compared with the ones without ($p < 0.001$). The AUROC for EUS-E to determine pancreatic fistula was higher than the operator who appreciated the tissue by hand; however, no statistical significance was present ($p = 0.132$).

4. Conclusions

EUS-E is a complementary tool for pancreatic disease assessment with a continuous endeavor to aid as a proper diagnosis method. While this method may not replace EUS tissue acquisition, it may be used as an additional method to help the decision-making process.

While strain EUS-E was the first technique used, with various results, the recent EUS-SWM in a pancreatic setting still requires more investigations. With only a few studies, and perhaps more to come in the next years, perhaps SWM will overcome the flaws of strain EUS-E and will be used more for pancreatic disease assessment.

Moreover, new software developments, such as artificial intelligence tools could also be an alternative, by enabling a more rapid diagnostic based on image analysis.

In conclusion, EUS-E might require more attention, because of its potential, and in combination with other methods, such as CEUS, may maximize the efforts for pancreatic disease management.

Acknowledgements

This chapter was supported by the Executive Unit for the Financing of Higher Education, Research, Development and Innovation (UEFISCDI) of the Ministry of National Education (project "PREdictive Machine Learning Algorithm for the Dynamic Evaluation of Pancreatic Cancer during Therapy Multimodal Therapy"— PREDYCT, code PN-III-P4-ID-PCE2020-0884 within PNCDI III).

Conflict of interest

The authors declare no conflict of interest.

Author details

Bogdan Silviu Ungureanu* and Adrian Saftoiu
Research Center of Gastroenterology and Hepatology Craiova, University of Medicine and Pharmacy of Craiova, Craiova, Romania

*Address all correspondence to: boboungureanu@gmail.com

IntechOpen

References

[1] Ophir J, Céspedes I, Ponnekanti H, Yazdi Y, Li X. Elastography: A quantitative method for imaging the elasticity of biological tissues. Ultrasonic Imaging. 1991;**13**(2):111-134. DOI: 10.1177/016173469101300201

[2] Gheonea IA, Stoica Z, Bondari S. Differential diagnosis of breast lesions using ultrasound elastography. Indian Journal of Radiology Imaging. 2011;**21**(4):301-305. DOI: 10.4103/0971-3026.90697

[3] Garra BS, Cespedes EI, Ophir J, Spratt SR, Zuurbier RA, Magnant CM, et al. Elastography of breast lesions: Initial clinical results. Radiology. 1997;**202**(1):79-86. DOI: 10.1148/radiology.202.1.8988195

[4] Sandrin L, Fourquet B, Hasquenoph JM, Yon S, Fournier C, Mal F, et al. Transient elastography: A new noninvasive method for assessment of hepatic fibrosis. Ultrasound in Medicine & Biology. 2003;**29**(12):1705-1713. DOI: 10.1016/j.ultrasmedbio.2003.07.001

[5] Moon HJ, Sung JM, Kim EK, Yoon JH, Youk JH, Kwak JY. Diagnostic performance of gray-scale US and elastography in solid thyroid nodules. Radiology. 2012;**262**(3):1002-1013. DOI: 10.1148/radiol.11110839

[6] Sigrist RMS, Liau J, Kaffas AE, Chammas MC, Willmann JK. Ultrasound elastography: Review of techniques and clinical applications. Theranostics. 2017;**7**(5):1303-1329. DOI: 10.7150/thno.18650

[7] Xu MM, Sethi A. Imaging of the pancreas. Gastroenterology Clinics of North America. 2016;**45**(1):101-116. DOI: 10.1016/j.gtc.2015.10.010

[8] Cazacu IM, Luzuriaga Chavez AA, Saftoiu A, Vilmann P, Bhutani MS. A quarter century of EUS-FNA: Progress, milestones, and future directions. Endoscopic Ultrasound. 2018;**7**(3): 141-160. DOI: 10.4103/eus.eus_19_18

[9] Lee TH, Cha SW, Cho YD. EUS elastography: Advances in diagnostic EUS of the pancreas. Korean Journal of Radiology. 2012;**13**(Suppl. 1):S12-S16. DOI: 10.3348/kjr.2012.13.S1.S12

[10] Kawada N, Tanaka S. Elastography for the pancreas: Current status and future perspective. World Journal of Gastroenterology. 2016;**22**(14):3712-3724. DOI: 10.3748/wjg.v22.i14.3712

[11] Yamamiya A, Irisawa A, Hoshi K, Yamabe A, Izawa N, Nagashima K, et al. Recent advances in endosonography-elastography: Literature review. Journal of Clinical Medicine. 2021;**10**(16)

[12] Săftoiu A, Vilmann P, Gorunescu F, Janssen J, Hocke M, Larsen M, et al. Efficacy of an artificial neural network-based approach to endoscopic ultrasound elastography in diagnosis of focal pancreatic masses. Clinical Gastroenterology and Hepatology. 2012;**10**(1):84-90.e1. DOI: 10.1016/j.cgh.2011.09.014

[13] Itokawa F, Itoi T, Sofuni A, Kurihara T, Tsuchiya T, Ishii K, et al. EUS elastography combined with the strain ratio of tissue elasticity for diagnosis of solid pancreatic masses. Journal of Gastroenterology. 2011;**46**(6):843-853. DOI: 10.1007/s00535-011-0399-5

[14] Kim SY, Cho JH, Kim YJ, Kim EJ, Park JY, Jeon TJ, et al. Diagnostic efficacy of quantitative endoscopic ultrasound elastography for differentiating

pancreatic disease. Journal of Gastroenterology and Hepatology. 2017;**32**(5):1115-1122. DOI: 10.1111/jgh.13649

[15] Havre RF, Ødegaard S, Gilja OH, Nesje LB. Characterization of solid focal pancreatic lesions using endoscopic ultrasonography with real-time elastography. Scandinavian Journal of Gastroenterology. 2014;**49**(6):742-751. DOI: 10.3109/00365521.2014.905627

[16] Carrara S, Di Leo M, Grizzi F, Correale L, Rahal D, Anderloni A, et al. EUS elastography (strain ratio) and fractal-based quantitative analysis for the diagnosis of solid pancreatic lesions. Gastrointestinal Endoscopy. 2018;**87**(6):1464-1473. DOI: 10.1016/j.gie.2017.12.031

[17] Okasha H, Elkholy S, El-Sayed R, Wifi MN, El-Nady M, El-Nabawi W, et al. Real time endoscopic ultrasound elastography and strain ratio in the diagnosis of solid pancreatic lesions. World Journal of Gastroenterology. 2017;**23**(32):5962-5968. DOI: 10.3748/wjg.v23.i32.5962

[18] Opačić D, Rustemović N, Kalauz M, Markoš P, Ostojić Z, Majerović M, et al. Endoscopic ultrasound elastography strain histograms in the evaluation of patients with pancreatic masses. World Journal of Gastroenterology. 2015;**21**(13):4014-4019. DOI: 10.3748/wjg.v21.i13.4014

[19] Costache MI, Cazacu IM, Dietrich CF, Petrone MC, Arcidiacono PG, Giovannini M, et al. Clinical impact of strain histogram EUS elastography and contrast-enhanced EUS for the differential diagnosis of focal pancreatic masses: A prospective multicentric study. Endosc Ultrasound. 2020;**9**(2):116-121. DOI: 10.4103/eus.eus_69_19

[20] Kuwahara T, Hara K, Mizuno N, Haba S, Okuno N. Present status of ultrasound elastography for the diagnosis of pancreatic tumors: Review of the literature. Journal of Medical Ultrasonics (2001). 2020;**47**(3):413-420. DOI: 10.1007/s10396-020-01026-6

[21] Cui XW, Chang JM, Kan QC, Chiorean L, Ignee A, Dietrich CF. Endoscopic ultrasound elastography: Current status and future perspectives. World Journal of Gastroenterology. 2015;**21**(47):13212-13224. DOI: 10.3748/wjg.v21.i47.13212

[22] Marques S, Bispo M, Rio-Tinto R, Fidalgo P, Devière J. The impact of recent advances in endoscopic ultrasound-guided tissue acquisition on the management of pancreatic cancer. GE Portuguese Journal of Gastroenterology. 2021;**28**(3):185-192. DOI: 10.1159/000510730

[23] Dietrich CF, Burmeister S, Hollerbach S, Arcidiacono PG, Braden B, Fusaroli P, et al. Do we need elastography for EUS? Endosc Ultrasound. 2020;**9**(5):284-290. DOI: 10.4103/eus.eus_25_20

[24] Dietrich CF, Barr RG, Farrokh A, Dighe M, Hocke M, Jenssen C, et al. Strain elastography: How to do it? Ultrasound International Open. 2017;**3**(4):E137-Ee49. DOI: 10.1055/s-0043-119412

[25] Giovannini M, Hookey LC, Bories E, Pesenti C, Monges G, Delpero JR. Endoscopic ultrasound elastography: The first step towards virtual biopsy? Preliminary results in 49 patients. Endoscopy. 2006;**38**(4):344-348. DOI: 10.1055/s-2006-925158

[26] Giovannini M, Thomas B, Erwan B, Christian P, Fabrice C, Benjamin E, et al. Endoscopic ultrasound elastography

for evaluation of lymph nodes and
pancreatic masses: A multicenter study.
World Journal of Gastroenterology.
2009;**15**(13):1587-1593. DOI: 10.3748/
wjg.15.1587

[27] Săftoiu A, Vilmann P. Differential
diagnosis of focal pancreatic masses
by semiquantitative EUS elastography:
Between strain ratios and strain
histograms. Gastrointestinal Endoscopy.
2013;**78**(1):188-189. DOI: 10.1016/j.
gie.2013.01.024

[28] Iglesias-Garcia J, Lindkvist B,
Lariño-Noia J, Abdulkader-Nallib I,
Dominguez-Muñoz JE. Differential
diagnosis of solid pancreatic masses:
Contrast-enhanced harmonic (CEH-
EUS), quantitative-elastography
(QE-EUS), or both? United European
Gastroenterology Journal. 2017;**5**(2):236-
246. DOI: 10.1177/2050640616640635

[29] Săftoiu A, Vilmann P, Gorunescu F,
Gheonea DI, Gorunescu M, Ciurea T,
et al. Neural network analysis of
dynamic sequences of EUS elastography
used for the differential diagnosis of
chronic pancreatitis and pancreatic
cancer. Gastrointestinal Endoscopy.
2008;**68**(6):1086-1094. DOI: 10.1016/j.
gie.2008.04.031

[30] Schrader H, Wiese M,
Ellrichmann M, Belyaev O, Uhl W,
Tannapfel A, et al. Diagnostic value
of quantitative EUS elastography
for malignant pancreatic tumors:
Relationship with pancreatic
fibrosis. Ultraschall in der
Medizin. 2012;**33**(7):E196-e201.
DOI: 10.1055/s-0031-1273256

[31] Mei M, Ni J, Liu D, Jin P, Sun L.
EUS elastography for diagnosis of
solid pancreatic masses: A meta-
analysis. Gastrointestinal Endoscopy.
2013;**77**(4):578-589. DOI: 10.1016/j.
gie.2012.09.035

[32] Ying L, Lin X, Xie ZL, Hu YP,
Tang KF, Shi KQ. Clinical utility of
endoscopic ultrasound elastography for
identification of malignant pancreatic
masses: A meta-analysis. Journal of
Gastroenterology and Hepatology.
2013;**28**(9):1434-1443. DOI: 10.1111/
jgh.12292

[33] Li X, Xu W, Shi J, Lin Y, Zeng X.
Endoscopic ultrasound elastography
for differentiating between pancreatic
adenocarcinoma and inflammatory
masses: A meta-analysis. World Journal
of Gastroenterology. 2013;**19**(37):6284-
6291. DOI: 10.3748/wjg.v19.i37.6284

[34] Hu DM, Gong TT, Zhu Q.
Endoscopic ultrasound elastography
for differential diagnosis of pancreatic
masses: A meta-analysis. Digestive
Diseases and Sciences. 2013;**58**(4):
1125-1131. DOI: 10.1007/s10620-
012-2428-5

[35] Xu W, Shi J, Li X, Zeng X, Lin Y.
Endoscopic ultrasound elastography for
differentiation of benign and malignant
pancreatic masses: A systemic review
and meta-analysis. European Journal
of Gastroenterology & Hepatology.
2013;**25**(2):218-224. DOI: 10.1097/
MEG.0b013e32835a7f7c

[36] Lu Y, Chen L, Li C, Chen H,
Chen J. Diagnostic utility of endoscopic
ultrasonography-elastography in the
evaluation of solid pancreatic masses:
A meta-analysis and systematic
review. Medical Ultrasonography.
2017;**19**(2):150-158. DOI: 10.11152/
mu-987

[37] Hewitt MJ, McPhail MJ, Possamai L,
Dhar A, Vlavianos P, Monahan KJ.
EUS-guided FNA for diagnosis of
solid pancreatic neoplasms: A meta-
analysis. Gastrointestinal Endoscopy.
2012;**75**(2):319-331. DOI: 10.1016/j.
gie.2011.08.049

[38] Kataoka K, Ishikawa T, Ohno E, Iida T, Suzuki H, Uetsuki K, et al. Endoscopic ultrasound elastography for small solid pancreatic lesions with or without main pancreatic duct dilatation. Pancreatology. 2021;**21**(2):451-458. DOI: 10.1016/j.pan.2020.12.012

[39] Ignee A, Jenssen C, Arcidiacono PG, Hocke M, Möller K, Saftoiu A, et al. Endoscopic ultrasound elastography of small solid pancreatic lesions: A multicenter study. Endoscopy. 2018;**50**(11):1071-1079. DOI: 10.1055/a-0588-4941

[40] Iordache S, Costache MI, Popescu CF, Streba CT, Cazacu S, Săftoiu A. Clinical impact of EUS elastography followed by contrast-enhanced EUS in patients with focal pancreatic masses and negative EUS-guided FNA. Medical Ultrasonography. 2016;**18**(1):18-24. DOI: 10.11152/mu.2013.2066.181.ich

[41] Yamada K, Kawashima H, Ohno E, Ishikawa T, Tanaka H, Nakamura M, et al. Diagnosis of vascular invasion in pancreatic ductal adenocarcinoma using endoscopic ultrasound elastography. BMC Gastroenterology. 2020;**20**(1):81. DOI: 10.1186/s12876-020-01223-9

[42] Mazzawi T, Chaiyapo A, Kongkam P, Ridtitid W, Rerknimitr R. Elastography of pancreatic ductal adenocarcinoma following EUS-guided radiofrequency ablation (with video). Arabian Journal of Gastroenterology. 2020;**21**(2):128-131. DOI: 10.1016/j.ajg.2020.04.014

[43] Ohno E, Kawashima H, Ishikawa T, Iida T, Suzuki H, Uetsuki K, et al. Diagnostic performance of endoscopic ultrasonography-guided elastography for solid pancreatic lesions: Shear-wave measurements versus strain elastography with histogram analysis. Digestive Endoscopy. 2021;**33**(4):629-638. DOI: 10.1111/den.13791

[44] Yamashita Y, Kitano M. Benefits and limitations of each type of endoscopic ultrasonography elastography technology for diagnosis of pancreatic diseases. Digestive Endoscopy. 2021;**33**(4):554-556. DOI: 10.1111/den.13870

[45] Kuwahara T, Hirooka Y, Kawashima H, Ohno E, Ishikawa T, Yamamura T, et al. Usefulness of shear wave elastography as a quantitative diagnosis of chronic pancreatitis. Journal of Gastroenterology and Hepatology. 2018;**33**(3):756-761. DOI: 10.1111/jgh.13926

[46] Kuwahara T, Hirooka Y, Kawashima H, Ohno E, Sugimoto H, Hayashi D, et al. Quantitative evaluation of pancreatic tumor fibrosis using shear wave elastography. Pancreatology. 2016;**16**(6):1063-1068. DOI: 10.1016/j.pan.2016.09.012

[47] Itoh Y, Itoh A, Kawashima H, Ohno E, Nakamura Y, Hiramatsu T, et al. Quantitative analysis of diagnosing pancreatic fibrosis using EUS-elastography (comparison with surgical specimens). Journal of Gastroenterology. 2014;**49**(7):1183-1192. DOI: 10.1007/s00535-013-0880-4

[48] Kuwahara T, Hirooka Y, Kawashima H, Ohno E, Ishikawa T, Kawai M, et al. Quantitative diagnosis of chronic pancreatitis using EUS elastography. Journal of Gastroenterology. 2017;**52**(7):868-874. DOI: 10.1007/s00535-016-1296-8

[49] Ohno E, Hirooka Y, Kawashima H, Ishikawa T, Tanaka H, Sakai D, et al. Feasibility and usefulness of endoscopic ultrasonography-guided shear-wave measurement for assessment of autoimmune pancreatitis activity: A prospective exploratory study. Journal of Medical Ultrasonics (2001). 2019;**46**(4):425-433. DOI: 10.1007/s10396-019-00944-4

[50] Yamashita Y, Tanioka K, Kawaji Y, Tamura T, Nuta J, Hatamaru K, et al. Endoscopic ultrasonography shear wave as a predictive factor of endocrine/exocrine dysfunction in chronic pancreatitis. Journal of Gastroenterology and Hepatology. 2021;**36**(2):391-396. DOI: 10.1111/jgh.15137

[51] Dietrich CF, Hirche TO, Ott M, Ignee A. Real-time tissue elastography in the diagnosis of autoimmune pancreatitis. Endoscopy. 2009;**41**(8):718-720. DOI: 10.1055/s-0029-1214866

[52] Ishikawa T, Kawashima H, Ohno E, Mizutani Y, Fujishiro M. Imaging diagnosis of autoimmune pancreatitis using endoscopic ultrasonography. Journal of Medical Ultrasonics (2001). 2021;**48**(4):543-553. DOI: 10.1007/s10396-021-01143-w

[53] Kuwahara T, Hirooka Y, Kawashima H, Ohno E, Yokoyama Y, Fujii T, et al. Usefulness of endoscopic ultrasonography-elastography as a predictive tool for the occurrence of pancreatic fistula after pancreatoduodenectomy. Journal of Hepato-Biliary-Pancreatic Sciences. 2017;**24**(12):649-656. DOI: 10.1002/jhbp.514

Chapter 10

Renal Elastography for the Assessment of Chronic Kidney Disease

Flaviu Bob

Abstract

For the assessment of chronic kidney disease, point shear wave elastography (pSWE) and shear wave speed imaging (2D-SWE) are suitable, but the use of elastography in the assessment of the kidneys is more difficult compared to the use in other organs, because of the complex architecture of the kidneys, characterized by a high anisotropy and also by the limited size of the renal parenchyma, where the measurements are performed. Despite the difficulties of renal elastography, the reproducibility of the method is good. Kidney shear wave speed values are influenced mainly by age and gender, while in chronic kidney disease, renal stiffness is sometimes decreased in more advanced disease and is not influenced mainly by the progression of fibrosis. There are studies proving that a decreased renal blood flow is associated with a decrease in kidney shear wave speed, the fact that could explain why patients with CKD tend to have lower kidney stiffness. Elastography is a real-time imaging method that could be useful in the assessment of the kidneys, but more extensive studies and even some improvements of the processing algorithms of raw data of elastography machines seem to be needed to implement the use in clinical practice.

Keywords: chronic kidney disease, kidney shear wave speed, renal stiffness, point shear wave elastography, shear wave speed imaging

1. Introduction

Chronic kidney disease (CKD), a progressive disease, with high morbidity and mortality, therefore associated with increased health costs, is becoming a public health problem because of the increasing incidence and prevalence. For the diagnosis of CKD, biochemical markers are used—glomerular filtration rate, estimated from the level of serum creatinine and urinary albumin/creatinine ratio. For the assessment of the progression of CKD histology can often be helpful, and different new biomarkers are emerging as important tools as well [1].

The use of imagistic methods in the early diagnosis, or to assess the progression of CKD is very limited. Conventional ultrasound is helpful in diagnosing cystic kidney diseases, which represent a small proportion of the causes of CKD. Regarding the most frequent etiologies of CKD (diabetes mellitus, arterial hypertension, glomerular diseases, or chronic tubulointerstitial diseases) information provided by ultrasound is of limited help. Using conventional ultrasound we can quantify the renal size and parenchymal thickness, both decreasing in advanced stages of CKD, when due to the progression of fibrosis, the echogenicity of the renal cortex is increasing [2].

The increased echogenicity, observed by the investigator is however not quantifiable using conventional ultrasound, being therefore subjective. An ultrasound-based method that has proven its utility in the assessment of fibrosis in different other organs (liver in both, diffuse [3, 4] or focal lesions [5], spleen [6, 7], thyroid [8, 9] or prostate [10]), by measuring the stiffness of the tissue is elastography.

2. Renal elastography- method

Elastography is a method used to quantify the elasticity of tissues. Elasticity is an intrinsic property of tissue, that permits after initial stress, the deformation with a subsequent return to the normal shape [11].

2.1 The types of elastography

Different methods, corresponding to different technologies can be used to measure tissue elasticity:

1. Strain elastography (SE) is a qualitative method, the strain images being obtained from the tissue displacement, due to pressure applied by the transducer. SE is mentioned in experimental studies performed in renal transplant recipients when the assessed kidney is superficial [12].

2. Shear wave elastography

This is a quantitative method, that in contrast to SE does not use the transducer pressure, but high-intensity pulses that generate shear waves in the different tissues. The tissue shear wave speed (SWS) is expressed in m/s and is correlating with tissue stiffness expressed by Young's modulus (kPa). Performing this method in a stiffer tissue leads to a higher SWS.

   a. Transient elastography (TE) or Fibroscan is known from liver stiffness assessment. Shear waves in TE are generated by controlled external vibration, however, the fact that the obtained image is not superimposed on an ultrasound image, makes it difficult to use in renal assessment. The conclusions of the few published studies using TE in kidneys, underline the fact that the results can be affected by the heterogeneous kidney morphology [13–15].

   b. Acoustic radiation force impulse (ARFI), in contrast to TE, uses the same transducer to generate shear waves and to image their propagation. The system is integrated into an ultrasound machine, and the ultrasound image is used to guide the site of elastography measurements. As a principle, in ARFI, shear waves are generated inside the organ due to focused acoustic radiation force pushing pulses. After generation the shear waves propagate through the soft tissue, their speed represents the SWS and are progressively attenuated due to their absorption in the soft tissue [16]. There are two different types of ARFI, corresponding to the different methods of obtaining and reporting information:

- Point shear wave elastography (pSWE): The result is an average value inside a region of interest (ROI) and the systems/machines that use pSWE are: Virtual touch quantification (VTQ) (Siemens S2000, S3000) (**Figure 1**), elastography point quantification (ElastPQ) (Phillips Affiniti) (**Figure 2**).

- Shear wave speed imaging (2D-SWE). Instead of an average value, the ROI appears as a color-coded map mosaic inside which the measurement is performed. The systems that use this method are: 2D SWE.SSI technique (Aixplorer) (**Figure 3**) and 2D SWE.GE (General Electric) (**Figure 4**).

Only the two ARFI-based shear wave elastography methods (pSWE and 2D-SWE) seem to be suitable for the assessment of renal diseases.

2.2 Method description

Both mentioned renal elastography methods (pSWE and 2D-SWE) are ultrasound-based. The image obtained is a normal ultrasound image, and superimposed on it there is the region of interest (ROI), inside which the kidney shear wave speed is measured (**Figures 1–4**). The result is displayed on the screen and is expressed either in m/s or in kPa.

The preparation of the patient should be the one used for a conventional ultrasound examination, but because the results obtained with elastography are quantifiable, the position of the examined subject should be standardized. Renal elastography should be thus performed with the patient in lateral decubitus, asked to stop breathing for a moment, to minimize breathing motion (**Figure 5**). Because the elastography method is ultrasound-based, the obtained B-mode US image should have a good quality, to obtain a reliable elastography measurement. Thus, before starting elastography acquisition, the correct scan of the kidneys should be obtained, using the best acoustic window.

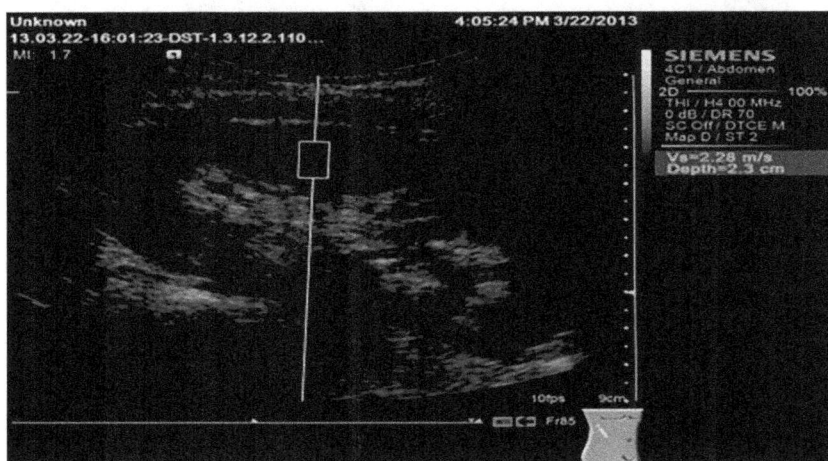

Figure 1.
Kidney SWS (expressed in m/s) measured with a pSWE method: Virtual TouchTM tissue quantification (VTQ), software version 2.0, on a Siemens Acuson S2000TM ultrasound system (Siemens AG, Erlangen, Germany) with a 4CI transducer.

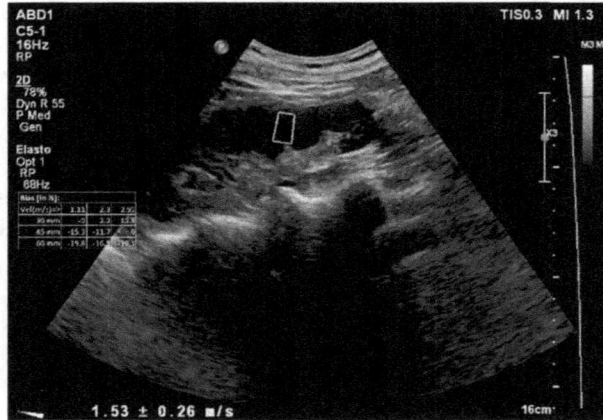

Figure 2.
Kidney SWS (expressed in m/s) measured with a pSWE method: Elatography point quantification system (ElastPQ) on a Phillips Affiniti ultrasound system with a 4CI transducer.

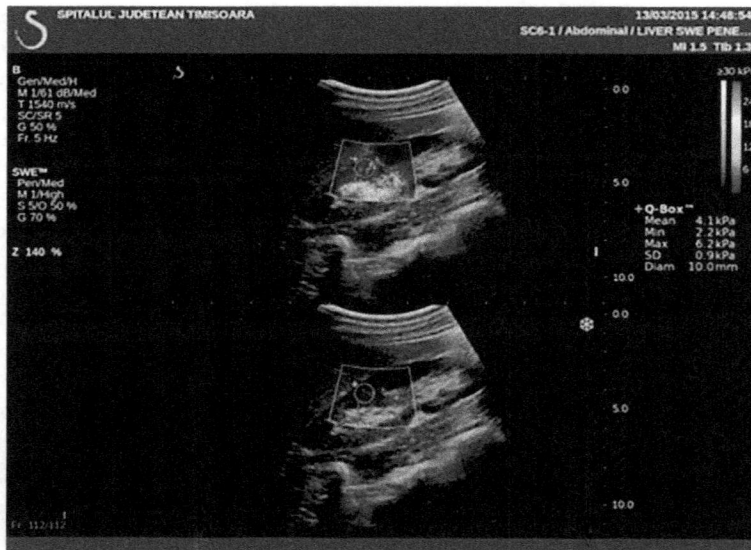

Figure 3.
Kidney stiffness (expressed in kPa) measured with a 2D-SWE method: 2D-SWE.SSI technique on a SuperSonic imagine Aixplorer® ShearWave™ Elastography machine with a SuperCurved™ SC6-1 transducer.

The need for a good standardization of this method comes from the complex architecture of the kidney, which is composed of cortex, medulla, central fat, vasculature, collecting system, and a capsule [17]. This complex structure leads to a high degree of anisotropy, especially at the level of the medulla, composed of tubules that are aligned perpendicular to the renal capsule [17]. Anisotropy is present at the level of the renal cortex as well and is due to the spherical glomeruli and proximal and distal tubules which have a convoluted shape [18].

The consequence of anisotropy of the renal structure is represented by the influence on the kidney stiffness measured using elastography [19]. The results are influenced

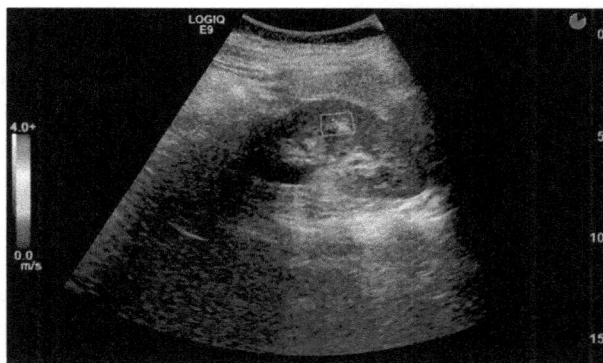

Figure 4.
Kidney SWS measured with a 2D SWE.GE technique using a Logiq E9- General Electric ultrasound system.

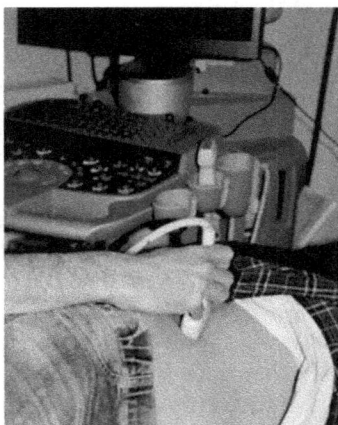

Figure 5.
For elastography, the patient should be examined in lateral decubitus, to obtain the best acoustic window.

by the relationship between the direction of the ultrasound main axis and the renal pyramid axis. Thus, if the ROI is put in the mid-portion of the renal parenchyma the two axes are parallel, while if the ROI is at the level of the renal poles the two axes are perpendicular and the obtained SWS is different [20]. To have a standardized approach and because the placement of the ROI in the poles is sometimes difficult, the most common way to place the ROI is in the mid-portion of the renal parenchyma.

Anisotropy of the renal tissue can however be beneficial and used as a diagnostic tool. Standardizing the variation of SWS in the kidney can be used to obtain an anisotropic ratio, that could represent a diagnostic and monitoring marker in CKD [21].

When performing renal elastography, another important issue is the one regarding the positioning of the ROI, because theoretically the measurements should be performed in the renal cortex. It is known that the stiffness of the cortex is higher compared to the stiffness of the medulla [22]. In practice, however, because of the fixed dimension of the ROI, of 1 cm, it is difficult to differentiate between cortex and medulla, and therefore, the measurements will be performed in the renal parenchyma, which contains both cortex and medulla. This difficulty resulting from the dimension of the ROI is further increased in patients with advanced CKD, that have thin parenchyma (sometimes below 1 cm), and elastography results could be biased.

The limited size of the renal parenchyma (compared to the size of the ROI), even in normal kidneys, leads to the necessity of positioning the ROI just beneath the renal capsule. The vicinity of the renal capsule can lead to the appearance of some common ultrasound artifacts that occurs when a sound pulse reverberates back and forth between two strong parallel reflectors, and that leads to increased measured values. These reverberation artifacts are the reason for the recommendation in liver elastography, for example, to put the ROI 1.5–2 cm beneath the capsule to avoid these artifacts, a recommendation that is impossible to use in renal elastography [23].

Despite the above-mentioned difficulties in performing renal elastography, if the approach of the kidneys is standardized, it has been proven that the method has good inter-observer reproducibility, and thus has the potential to be used in clinical practice [24, 25].

3. Renal elastography- normal values

In practice and considering the results of the majority of published studies the kidney shear wave speed value should be reported as the median value of five valid measurements, although it has been proven that even three valid measurements are enough [26].

It is difficult to establish the normal values of kidney shear wave speed because even if the measurement is performed at the same cortical level, the reported results are different depending on the different elastography systems used. For pSWE, the normal values range between 2.15 and 2.54 m/s (for the VTQ system) and between 1.23 and 1.54 m/s (for the ElastPQ system) [27]. For 2DSWE-GE, normal values range between 1.71 and 1.79 m/s [28].

An important limitation of elastography is the fact that the different methods that are available, and that have been mentioned previously, are coming from different providers and no correlation tables are available to compare results obtained with different transducers from different manufacturers.

Kidney shear wave speed seems to be influenced by age, with a decrease of renal stiffness in older subjects, and also by gender, with men showing lower values compared to women [29, 30].

The results obtained when performing renal elastography are influenced also by the depth of the kidneys. Kidney shear wave speed is decreasing with increasing organ depth [29, 31, 32]. The assessment becomes difficult in very deep kidneys because the maximum depth of the ROI is 8 cm.

But very superficial kidneys can be difficult to assess as well, because the results are potentially biased due to the different compression of the transducer, being thus operator dependent. It has been proven in a study published by Correas et al., that cortex stiffness is increasing with the increased transducer compression [22]. This problem could influence especially measurements performed in superficial kidneys when the different non-quantifiable transducer force applied, could intervene, leading to different SWSs.

4. The assessment of chronic kidney disease

The most promising use of elastography in the hands of a nephrologist should be for the assessment of CKD, to diagnose and quantify the progression, as it has been mentioned in the introduction of this chapter.

There are several studies that are showing that kidney SWS values are significantly increased in patients with CKD compared to normal controls, pointing out that kidneys are stiffer because of chronic disease [33–37]. These observations are, however, not confirmed in every published study. Other authors have shown that renal stiffness is significantly lower in patients with CKD [24, 38, 39]. A statistically significant relationship between kidney shear wave speed values and renal function, expressed by estimated glomerular filtration rate (eGFR), has been shown as well, with lower kidney SWS associated with lower eGFR [40–42].

Despite the decrease of kidney SWS with the decrease of eGFR, mentioned in some studies, it was not possible to use elastography to differentiate between the different stages of CKD, because no significant differences could be found between the SWS levels in the different CKD stages [28, 43].

In a meta-analysis comprising seven studies including 639 patients with CKD and 640 normal controls, it has been shown that kidney SWS is decreased in patients with CKD, and there is a decrease of kidney SWS with the progression of CKD (decrease of eGFR). However, the included studies showed an increased heterogeneity [44].

To implement the use of renal elastography in the current practice, for the diagnosis of CKD for example, the finding of cut-off values would be important. However, the attempts published so far are presenting cut-off values for the diagnosis of more advanced stages of CKD, and not for incipient CKD.

Thus, diabetic kidney disease with an eGFR of below 60 ml/min could be predicted using the VTQ system (pSWE) with a sensitivity of 67.4% and a specificity of 67.8%, if kidney SWS was less than 2.32 m/s [45]. Better sensitivity (89.2%) and specificity (76.9%) have been obtained with 2D SWE GE, which predicted CKD if SWS was 1.47 m/s or below [28].

When combining elastography with clinical parameters, such as albuminuria or diabetes duration, and using a logistic regression model, the accuracy of diagnosing even early stages of diabetic kidney disease could be significantly improved, in contrast to the independent use of the different methods [36, 46].

5. Fibrosis and elastography

From the studies using liver elastography, we know that fibrosis, which occurs due to the progression of liver disease, leads to an increase in liver stiffness. Because the histological background of chronic kidney disease is renal fibrosis, and especially tubulointerstitial fibrosis, it can be hypothesized that similar changes occur in the kidneys, and therefore, the progression of kidney disease should lead to an increase of SWS. However, as mentioned in the previous chapter, the studies published so far, that compare elastography performed in patients with CKD and normal controls, have shown that not always CKD is associated with an increase in renal stiffness.

Therefore, it would be useful to take a look at those studies that compare histological changes with results obtained using elastography, and to see if there is a relationship between fibrosis and kidney SWS, and to find an explanation to the observation mentioned in some studies that kidney SWS is decreasing in advanced stages of CKD.

The first studies that compare elastography with histological parameters have been performed in renal transplant recipients. Those studies using transient elastography (TE) show a positive correlation between renal stiffness and fibrosis [13–15, 47], but as already mentioned the use of Fibroscan in the assessment of the kidneys is especially biased by the renal structure. In the studies using pSWE or 2D

SWE in transplanted patients, there was a lack of correlation between fibrosis and renal stiffness [48–51].

In native kidneys, there are studies using different elastography systems (VTQ, ElastPQ) that show, as expected, that severe histological changes, both glomerular and tubulointerstitial, are associated with a statistically significant increase in kidney SWS [33, 52]. Moreover, in a study performed using the 2D-SWE – SSI elastography method, it has been shown that the degree of glomerulosclerosis and tubulointersti-tial fibrosis is associated with higher levels of kidney stiffness and that patients with lower kidney SWS showed a better response to corticotherapy [53]. This observation could be explained by the fact that corticotherapy is not effective on fibrosis, but on active glomerular lesions, which probably do not influence renal stiffness.

However not all published studies sustain the mentioned conclusions regarding the relationship between kidney elastography and histological changes, and thus in some studies, no correlations at all have been found between histology and elastography. This is the case of a small study performed in 45 patients with CKD in which no statistically significant correlation of kidney SWS with the studied histological parameters (glomerulosclerosis index, tubular atrophy, interstitial fibrosis) has been found [54]. In another study that has been performed in kidneys used for transplant from living donors, elastography and renal biopsies have been performed before nephrectomy. Although the kidneys with more pronounced interstitial fibrosis had a lower SWS, none of the correlations between histology and elastography was statistically significant [31].

Even more surprising are those studies that show an association of a decreased renal stiffness with fibrosis, for example, that severe histological impairment in CKD is associated with significantly reduced kidney SWS [41], or even that the presence of tubulointerstitial fibrosis or arteriolar hyalinosis leads to significantly decreased values of SWS [55].

Combining elastography with conventional ultrasound features (renal length, parenchymal thickness, resistance index) can improve the predictive value and offer better diagnostic performance in the evaluation of pathological changes in CKD., as it has been shown in a study performed in patients with IgA nephropathy, that had a significantly lower kidney SWS in more severe diseases [56].

One explanation for the different pattern of results and the different relationship between renal stiffness and elastography provided by the different studies could be the fact that histological changes in renal diseases are heterogenous, showing a non-uniform involvement of the compartments of the renal tissue (glomerular, vascular, or tubulointerstitial). However, another explanation could be the fact, that maybe other factors, besides histological changes (renal fibrosis) are involved in influencing renal stiffness.

6. Urinary pressure or renal blood flow

Besides fibrosis, the stiffness of the renal tissue could be theoretically influenced by urinary pressure, which could be increased in case of urinary obstruction, but again the results of the published studies that are addressing this topic are not consistent. As expected, kidney SWS was increased in children with different degrees of hydrone-phrosis compared to normal controls, as it has been shown in a study performed on 51 children [57]. But, however, in another study performed on 88 children with vesico-ureteric reflux, SWS decreased with the increasing grades of the reflux [58], while a third smaller study (37 children) was not able to discriminate between obstructive and unobstructive hydronephrosis using shear wave elastography [59].

Another factor, besides the structure of the renal tissue and urinary obstruction, that could influence renal tissue stiffness could be renal blood flow. The background for this hypothesis is represented by the fact that the vascularization of the kidney is increased, with 20% of the cardiac outflow running into the kidneys [60, 61].

The relationship between renal blood flow and elastography has been hinted at by experimental data using an *ex vivo* kidney that has been cannulated and in which an increased renal pressure has been obtained by introducing saline into the kidney. The result was an increase in renal stiffness measured using 2D-SWE (Aixplorer) [62]. When performing elastography in experimental animal kidneys, the ligation of the renal artery, with the subsequent reduction of renal blood flow, leads to a decrease of SWS. The ligation of the renal vein, however, leads to an increase of renal SWS [63, 64].

A similar situation to the latter one mentioned above has been reported in a patient with renal vein thrombosis, which led to an increased value of kidney shear wave speed compared to the contralateral kidney [65].

There are also clinical studies that are sustaining the renal blood flow hypothesis. Asano et al. show in a study performed in over 300 CKD patients that increased arterial stiffness, measured through pulse wave velocity (PWV), is associated with a low kidney SWS [60]. These results have been confirmed in another study performed in patients with diabetic kidney disease, that showed a negative, statistically significant correlation of kidney SWS not only with PWV but with the aortic augmentation index as well [66]. This means that in patients in whom there is a progression of arteriosclerosis in the large vessels (high PWV and aortic augmentation index), which leads to a decreased renal blood flow, the kidney SWS is subsequently low.

There are also indirect proofs of the validity of the hypothesis of an existing relationship between renal blood flow and renal stiffness. In patients with gestational hypertension, characterized by renal hypoperfusion, it has been shown that high blood pressure was associated with a low renal elasticity [67].

A study performed in renal transplant recipients showed that interstitial fibrosis/tubular atrophy has no influence on kidney SWS, but adaptive glomerular hyperfiltration leads to an increase in kidney SWS. This observation is in favor of the hypothesis that renal hemodynamics influences renal stiffness [50].

Considering the supposed relationship between renal blood flow and elastography findings, it has been proposed to use pre-procedural elastography to predict the risk of bleeding after renal biopsy, but the results show a low sensitivity, with high specificity for the method [68].

A new experimental elastography-based method that could explain the described results and relationships is two-dimensional time-harmonic ultrasound elastography. When using this method, the patient is placed on a vibration bed that produces continuous vibrations and thus the 2D-SWE elastography covers the entire kidney and is not limited to a superficial ROI [69]. Performing this enhanced elastography Grossman et al. showed that renal SWS decreased significantly in CKD stage 1 (patients with glomerulonephritis) compared to normal controls. Moreover, there was a statistically significant negative correlation with the resistive index, the fact that could underline that renal blood flow is influencing renal stiffness [70].

The decrease of renal blood flow could have a higher influence on renal stiffness, compared to fibrosis, leading to the decrease of kidney SWS. The progression of renal fibrosis, which should increase renal stiffness, is on the other hand associated with a

	Study	Elastography method	Patient population (number, type of subjects)	Histology	SWS in CKD[*]
1	Arndt et al. [13]	TE	57 transplant patients (20 with renal biopsy)	yes	increase
2	Syversveen et al. [48]	VTQ	30 transplant patients	yes	no relationship
3	Stock et al. [51]	VTQ	18 transplant patients	yes	moderate positive
4	Grenier et al. [49]	SSI	43 transplant patients	yes	no relationship
5	Sommerer et al. [14]	TE	164 transplant patients	yes	increase
6	Guo et al. [30]	VTQ	64 CKD patients/327 healthy subjects	no	decrease
7	Lukenda et al. [15]	TE	52 (23 with renal biopsy)	yes	increase
8	Hu et al. [41]	VTQ	163 CKD patients/32 healthy subjects	yes	decrease
9	Yu et al. [34]	VTQ	120 diabetic patients/30 healthy subjects	no	increase
10	Asano et al. [60]	VTQ	309 CKD patients/14 healthy subjects	no	decrease
11	Wang et al. [54]	VTQ	45 CKD patients	yes	no relationship
12	Cui et al. [33]	VTQ	76 CKD patients	yes	increase
13	Nakao et al. [47]	TE	35 transplant patients (27 with renal biopsy)	yes	increase
14	Lee et al. [50]	VTQ	73 transplant patients	yes	no correlation
15	Bob et al. [42]	VTQ	46 CKD patients/58 healthy subjects	no	decrease
16	Samir et al. [36]	2D SWE-SSI	25 CKD patients/20 healthy subjects	no	increase
17	Alan et al. [40]	VTQ	76 coronary artery disease patients/79 healthy subjects	no	decrease
18	Bob et al. [45]	VTQ	80 diabetic kidney disease patients/84 healthy subjects	no	decrease
19	Bilgici et al. [38]	VTQ	30 CKD patients/38 healthy subjects - pediatric patients	no	decrease
20	Bob et al. [55]	VTQ	20 CKD patients	yes	moderate decrease
21	Sasaki et al. [43]	VTQ	187 CKD patients	no	no relationship
22	Yang et al. [35]	VTQ	90 idiopatic nephrotic syndrome CKD patients/30 healthy subjects	no	increase
23	Grosu et al. [39]	E ast PQ	102 CKD patients/22 healthy subjects	no	decrease

	Study	Elastography method	Patient population (number, type of subjects)	Histology	SWS in CKD*
24	Liu et al. [46]	Elast PQ	69 diabetic kidney disease patients/40 diabetic controls	no	increase
25	Hu et al. [56]	VTQ	146 IgA nephropathy patients/39 healthy volunteers	yes	decrease
26	Grosu et al. [28]	2D SWE- GE	42 CKD patients/50 healthy subjects	no	decrease
27	Sumbul et al. [37]	Elast PQ	125 diabetic, prediabetic patients and controls	no	increase
28	Yang et al. [53]	2D-SWE- SSI	120 idiopathic nephrotic syndrome - CKD patients	yes	increase
29	Lee et al. [31]	VTQ	73 (biopsies of kidney donors before transplant)	yes	no (tendency of SWS to **decrease** with advanced renal changes)
30	Leong et al. [52]	ElastPQ	75 CKD patients	yes	increase

The terms "increase" or "decrease" are representing a statistically significant change of SWV in CKD compared to healthy subjects, or in more severe CKD compared to less advanced stages.

Table 1.
Main published studies on renal elastography.

decrease in intrarenal blood flow, leading to opposite effects on renal SWS. This could explain why renal fibrosis is not associated with an increase in renal stiffness in some of the cited studies (**Table 1**) [41, 55, 56].

7. Conclusions and future perspectives of renal elastography

Shear wave elastography could be an ideal imaging modality to assess CKD because it combines all the well-known advantages of ultrasound examination, which is noninvasive, performed in real time, and does not imply high costs with the possibility to deliver quantifiable results. However, because of the complexity of the kidney architecture and its tissue properties, it seems that the results obtained using renal SWE are affected by numerous confounding elements, a fact that affects the reliability of the method and limits its application to clinical trials [71]. Therefore, it is very important to try to find those methods that could improve the use of SWE (**Figure 6**).

It has already been shown that combining SWE with other US methods (B-mode ultrasound and color Doppler) increases the prognostic value. The combination of the different ultrasound-based methods could be a step toward the use of multiparametric ultrasound imaging in the assessment of the kidney.

Another step forward could be the use of artificial intelligence. In a study performed in 208 CKD patients machine learning techniques have been used to combine multiple ultrasound characteristics of SWE, B-mode, and color Doppler flow imaging to assess the prognostic value of SWE for kidney tubulointerstitial fibrosis grades among the studied CKD patients. SWE ultrasound fitting machine learning improved

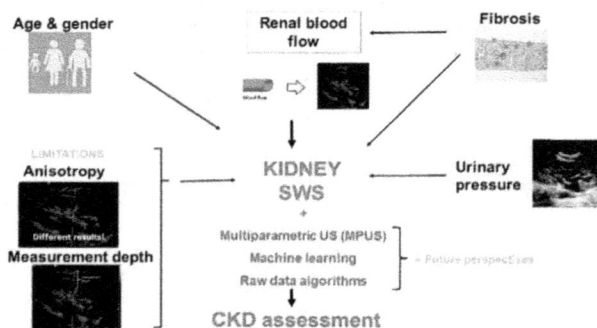

Figure 6.
Factors that influence kidney shear wave speed (SWS).

the diagnostic performances and also explained the lack of a linear correlation between kidney stiffness and CKD stages [72].

An improvement of the use of renal elastography could emerge from the analysis of raw data of the different systems used. Such an analysis has recently been published by Richard Barr using raw data of different three machines (Siemens, Phillips, and Aixplorer), and the conclusion was that an improvement of processing algorithms could lead to more accurate renal stiffness data from an elastographic system [73]. It is possible that assessing raw data with a new algorithm can overcome the existing limitations of the method, and make kidney elastography a feasible method [17].

Considering all the presented aspects, at the moment, no evidence-based recommendations can be offered for the use of SWE in the assessment of the kidneys [27]. Therefore, more extensive studies are needed to find the place and indication of renal elastography in clinical practice.

Acknowledgements

The personal research cited and the elastography images inserted in this chapter have been performed with the support of the Center of Elastography of the University of Medicine and Pharmacy "Victor Babes" Timisoara, Romania.

Conflict of interest

The author declares no conflict of interest.

Appendices and Nomenclature

2D SWE	shear wave speed imaging
CKD	chronic kidney disease
eGFR	estimated glomerular filtration rate
ElastPQ	elastography point quantification
pSWE	point shear wave elastography

PWV	pulse wave velocity
ROI	region of interest
SWE	shear wave elastography
SWS	shear wave speed
VTQ	virtual touch quantification

Author details

Flaviu Bob[1,2]

1 Nephrology Clinic, Department of Internal Medicine 2, "Victor Babes" University of Medicine and Pharmacy, Timisoara, Romania

2 Centre for Molecular Research in Nephrology and Vascular Disease, Faculty of Medicine, "Victor Babes," University of Medicine and Pharmacy, Timisoara, Romania

*Address all correspondence to: flaviu_bob@yahoo.com

IntechOpen

References

[1] Turner N, Lameire N, Goldsmith D, et al. Oxford Textbook of Clinical Nephrology. 4th ed. Oxford, UK: Oxford University Press; 2016

[2] Skorecki K, Chertow GM, Taal MW, Alan SL, Luyckx V. Brenner & Rector's the kidney. In: Marsden PA, editor. Philadelphia, PA, USA: Elsevier; 2016

[3] Bota S, Herkner H, Sporea I, et al. Meta-analysis: ARFI elastography versus transient elastography for the evaluation of liver fibrosis. Liver International. 2013;**33**(8):1138-1147

[4] Nierhoff J, Chávez Ortiz AA, Herrmann E, Zeuzem S, Friedrich-Rust M. The efficiency of acoustic radiation force impulse imaging for the staging of liver fibrosis: A meta-analysis. European Radiology. 2013;**23**(11):3040-3053

[5] Ying L, Lin X, Xie ZL, Tang FY, Hu YP, Shi KQ. Clinical utility of acoustic radiation force impulse imaging for identification of malignant liver lesions: A meta-analysis. European Radiology. 2012;**22**:2798-2805

[6] Bota S, Sporea I, Sirli R, Focsa M, Popescu A, Danila M, et al. Can ARFI elastography predict the presence of significant esophageal varices in newly diagnosed cirrhotic patients? Annals of Hepatology. 2012;**11**:519-525

[7] Takuma Y, Nouso K, Morimoto Y, Tomokuni J, Sahara A, Toshikuni N, et al. Measurement of spleen stiffness by acoustic radiation force impulse imaging identifies cirrhotic patients with esophageal varices. Gastroenterology. 2013;**144**:92-101.e2

[8] Zhang B, Ma X, Wu N, Liu L, Liu X, Zhang J, et al. Shear wave elastography for differentiation of benign and malignant thyroid nodules: A meta-analysis. Journal of Ultrasound in Medicine. 2013;**32**:2163-2169

[9] Hou XJ, Sun AX, Zhou XL, Ji Q, Wang HB, Wei H, et al. The application of virtual touch tissue quantification (VTQ) in diagnosis of thyroid lesions: A preliminary study. European Journal of Radiology. 2013;**82**:797-801

[10] Zhai L, Madden J, Foo WC, Mouraviev V, Polascik TJ, Palmeri ML, et al. Characterizing stiffness of human prostates using acoustic radiation force. Ultrasonic Imaging. 2010;**32**:201-213

[11] Dietrich CF, Bamber J, Berzigotti A, Bota S, Cantisani V, Castera L, et al. EFSUMB guidelines and recommendations on the clinical use of liver ultrasound Elastography, update 2017 (long version). Ultraschall in der Medizin-European Journal of Ultrasound. 2017;**38**(4):e16-e47. English. DOI: 10.1055/s-0043-103952 Erratum in: Ultraschall Med. 2017 Aug;38(4):e48. PMID: 28407655.

[12] Qi R, Yang C, Zhu T. Advances of contrast-enhanced ultrasonography and Elastography in kidney transplantation: From microscopic to microcosmic. Ultrasound in Medicine & Biology. 2021;**47**(2):177-184. DOI: 10.1016/j.ultrasmedbio. 2020.07.025

[13] Arndt R, Schmidt S, Loddenkemper C, Grünbaum M, Zidek W, et al. Noninvasive evaluation of renal allograft fibrosis by transient elastography-a pilot study. Transplant International. 2010; **23**:871-877

[14] Sommerer C, Scharf M, Seitz C, Millonig G, Seitz HK, et al. Assessment of renal allograft fibrosis by transient

elastography. Transplant International. 2013;**26**:545-551

[15] Lukenda V, Mikolasevic I, Racki S, Jelic I, Stimac D, Orlic L. Transient elastography: A new noninvasive diagnostic tool for assessment of chronic allograft nephropathy. International Urology and Nephrology. 2014;**46**(7):1435-1440

[16] Shiina T, Nightingale KR, Palmeri ML, Hall TJ, Bamber JC, Barr RG, et al. WFUMB guidelines and recommendations for clinical use of ultrasound elastography: Part 1: Basic principles and terminology. Ultrasound in Medicine & Biology. 2015;**41**(5):1126-1147. DOI: 10.1016/j.ultrasmedbio.2015.03.009

[17] Ferraioli G, Barr RG, Farrokh A, Radzina M, Cui XW, Dong Y, et al. How to perform shear wave elastography. Part II. Medical Ultrasonography. 2021;**0**:1-15. DOI: 10.11152/mu-3342

[18] Madsen K. NSTC: Anatomy of the kidney. In: B B, editor. The Kidney. Philadelphia: Sanders Elsevier; 2008. pp. 25-90

[19] Leong SS, Wong JHD, Md Shah MN, Vijayananthan A, Jalalonmuhali M, Mohd Sharif NH, et al. Stiffness and anisotropy effect on shear wave Elastography: A phantom and in vivo renal study. Ultrasound in Medicine & Biology. 2020;**46**(1):34-45. DOI: 10.1016/j.ultrasmedbio.2019.08.011

[20] Grenier N, Gennisson JL, Cornelis F, Le Bras Y, Couzi L. Renal ultrasound elastography. Diagnostic and Interventional Imaging. 2013;**94**:545-550

[21] Wang L. New insights on the role of anisotropy in renal ultrasonic elastography: From trash to treasure. Medical Hypotheses. 2020;**143**:110146. DOI: 10.1016/j.mehy.2020.110146

[22] Correas JM, Anglicheau D, Joly D, Gennisson JL, Tanter M, Hélénon O. Ultrasound-based imaging methods of the kidney-recent developments. Kidney International. 2016;**90**(6):1199-1210

[23] Bruce M, Kolokythas O, Ferraioli G, Filice C, O'Donnell M. Limitations and artifacts in shear-wave elastography of the liver. Biomedical Engineering Letters. 2017;**7**(2):81-89

[24] Bob F, Bota S, Sporea I, Sirli R, Petrica L, Schiller A. Kidney shear wave speed values in subjects with and without renal pathology and inter-operator reproducibility of acoustic radiation force impulse Elastography (ARFI) - preliminary results. PLoS One. 2014;**9**(11):e113761

[25] Hwang J, Kim HW, Kim PH, Suh CH, Yoon HM. Technical performance of acoustic radiation force impulse imaging for measuring renal parenchymal stiffness: A systematic review and meta-analysis. Journal of Ultrasound in Medicine. 2021;**40**(12):2639-2653. DOI: 10.1002/jum.15654

[26] Bob F, Bota S, Sporea I, Gradinaru-Tascau O, Popescu M, Popescu A, Schiller A. How many measurements are needed for kidney stiffness assessment by acoustic radiation force impulse (ARFI) elastography? 26th Congress of the European Federation of Societies for Ultrasound in Medicine and Biology (EFSUMB) EUROSON; May 26-28 2014; Tel Aviv, Israel, Congress Program and Abstracts CD, Israel Society for Diagnostic Ultrasound in Medicine, 2014, Tel Aviv, Israel

[27] Saftoiu A, Gilja OH, Sidhu PS, Dietrich CF, Cantisani V, Amy D, et al. The EFSUMB guidelines and recommendations for the clinical practice of Elastography in non-hepatic applications: Update 2018. Ultraschall

in der Medizin-European Journal of Ultrasound. 2019;**40**(4):425-453. DOI: 10.1055/a-0838-9937

[28] Grosu I, Bob F, Sporea I, Popescu A, Sirli R, Schiller A. Two-Dimensional Shear-Wave Elastography for Kidney Stiffness Assessment. Ultrasound Q. 2019 Jun 4;**37**(2):144-148. DOI: 10.1097/RUQ.0000000000000461. PMID: 31166295

[29] Bota S, Bob F, Sporea I, Sirli R, Popescu A. Factors that influence kidney shear wave speed assessed by acoustic radiation force impulse Elastography in patients without kidney pathology. Ultrasound in Medicine & Biology. 2015;**41**(1):1-6

[30] Guo LH, Xu HX, Fu HJ, Peng A, Zhang YF, et al. Acoustic radiation force impulse imaging for noninvasive evaluation of renal parenchyma elasticity: Preliminary findings. PLoS One. 2013;**8**:e68925

[31] Lee A, Joo DJ, Han WK, Jeong HJ, Oh MJ, Kim YS, et al. Renal tissue elasticity by acoustic radiation force impulse: A prospective study of healthy kidney donors. Medicine (Baltimore). 2021;**100**(3):e23561. DOI: 10.1097/MD.0000000000023561

[32] Zhao H, Song P, Urban MW, Kinnick RR, Yin M, Greenleaf JF, et al. Bias observed in time-offlight shear wave speed measurements using radiation force of a focused ultrasoundbeam. Ultrasound in Medicine & Biology. 2011;**370**:1884-1892

[33] Cui G, Yang Z, Zhang W, et al. Evaluation of acoustic radiation force impulse imaging for the clinicopathological typing of renal fibrosis. Experimental and Therapeutic Medicine. 2014;**7**(1):233-235. DOI: 10.3892/etm.2013.1377

[34] Yu N, Zhang Y, Xu Y. Value of virtual touch tissue quantification in stages of diabetic kidney disease. Journal of Ultrasound in Medicine. 2014;**33**(5):787-792

[35] Yang X, Yu N, Yu J, Wang H, Li X. Virtual touch tissue quantification for assessing renal pathology in idiopathic nephrotic syndrome. Ultrasound in Medicine & Biology. 2018;**44**(7):1318-1326. DOI: 10.1016/j.ultrasmedbio.2018.02.012

[36] Samir AE, Allegretti AS, Zhu Q, Dhyani M, Anvari A, Sullivan DA, et al. Shear wave elastography in chronic kidney disease: A pilot experience in native kidneys. BMC Nephrology. 2015;**16**:119

[37] Sumbul HE, Koc AS, Gülümsek E. Renal cortical stiffness is markedly increased in pre-diabetes mellitus and associated with albuminuria. Singapore Medical Journal. 2020;**61**(8):435-442. DOI: 10.11622/smedj.2019052

[38] Bilgici MC, Bekci T, Genc G, Tekcan D, Tomak L. Acoustic radiation force impulse quantification in the evaluation of renal parenchyma elasticity in Pediatric patients with chronic kidney disease: Preliminary results. Journal of Ultrasound in Medicine. 2017;**36**(8):1555-1561. DOI: 10.7863/ultra.16.08033

[39] Grosu I, Bob F, Sporea I, Popescu A, Şirli R, Schiller A. Correlation of point shear wave velocity and kidney function in chronic kidney disease. Journal of Ultrasound in Medicine. 2018;**37**(11):2613-2620. DOI: 10.1002/jum.14621

[40] Alan B, Göya C, Aktan A, Alan S. Renal acoustic radiation force impulse elastography in the evaluation of coronary artery disease. Acta

Radiologica. 2017;**58**(2):156-163. DOI:
10.1177/0284185116638569

[41] Hu Q, Wang XY, He HG, Wei HM,
Kang LK, Qin GC. Acoustic radiation
force impulse imaging for non-invasive
assessment of renal histopathology
in chronic kidney disease. PLoS One.
2014;**9**(12):e115051

[42] Bob F, Bota S, Sporea I, Sirli R,
Popescu A, Schiller A. Relationship
between the estimated glomerular
filtration rate and kidney shear wave
speed values assessed by acoustic
radiation force impulse elastography:
A pilot study. Journal of Ultrasound in
Medicine. 2015;**34**(4):649-654. DOI:
10.7863/ultra.34.4.649.ISSN 0278-4297

[43] Sasaki Y, Hirooka Y,
Kawashima H, Ishikawa T, Takeshita K,
Goto H. Measurements of renal shear
wave velocities in chronic kidney
disease patients. Acta Radiologica.
2018;**59**(7):884-890. DOI:
10.1177/0284185117734417

[44] Bob F, Grosu I, Sporea I, Popescu A,
Sirli R, Schiller A. Kidney shear wave
speed is lower in patients with chronic
kidney disease compared to normal
controls—A meta-analysis. 30th
Congress of the European Federation of
Societies for Ultrasound in Medicine and
Biology (EFSUMB) EUROSON. Poznan,
Poland; 6-9 September 2018. (Online
abstract book, Poznan, Poland)

[45] Bob F, Grosu I, Sporea I, Bota S,
Popescu A, Sima A, et al. Ultrasound-
based shear wave Elastography in the
assessment of patients with diabetic
kidney disease. Ultrasound in Medicine
& Biology. 2017;**43**(10):2159-2166. DOI:
10.1016/j.ultrasmedbio.2017.04.019

[46] Liu QY, Duan Q, Fu XH, Fu LQ,
Xia HW, Wan YL. Value of elastography
point quantification in improving the

diagnostic accuracy of early diabetic
kidney disease. World Journal of Clinical
Cases. 2019;**7**(23):3945-3956. DOI:
10.12998/wjcc.v7.i23.3945

[47] Nakao T, Ushigome H, Nakamura T,
Harada S, Koshino K, Suzuki T, et al.
Evaluation of renal allograft fibrosis
by transient elastography (fibro
scan). Transplantation Proceedings.
2015;**47**(3):640-643

[48] Syversveen T, Brabrand K,
Midtvedt K, Strøm EH, Hartmann A, et
al. Assessment of renal allograft fibrosis
by acoustic radiation force impulse
quantification--a pilot study. Transplant
International. 2011;**24**:100-105

[49] Grenier N, Poulain S,
Lepreux S, Gennisson JL, Dallaudière B,
et al. Quantitative elastography of renal
transplants using supersonic shear
imaging: A pilot study. European
Radiology. 2012;**22**:2138-2146

[50] Lee J, Oh YT, Joo DJ, Ma BG,
Lee AL, Lee JG, et al. Acoustic Radiation
Force Impulse Measurement in Renal
Transplantation: A Prospective,
Longitudinal Study With Protocol
Biopsies. Medicine (Baltimore). 2015
Sep;**94**(39):e1590. DOI: 10.1097/
MD.0000000000001590

[51] Stock KF, Klein BS, Cong MT,
Regenbogen C, Kemmner S, et al. ARFI-
based tissue elasticity quantification and
kidney graft dysfunction: First clinical
experiences. Clinical Hemorheology and
Microcirculation. 2011;**49**:527-535

[52] Leong SS, Wong JHD, Md Shah MN,
Vijayananthan A, Jalalonmuhali M,
Chow TK, et al. Shear wave elastography
accurately detects chronic changes
in renal histopathology. Nephrology
(Carlton, Vic.). 2021;**26**(1):38-45.
DOI: 10.1111/nep.13805

[53] Yang X, Hou FL, Zhao C, Jiang CY, Li XM, Yu N. The role of real-time shear wave elastography in the diagnosis of idiopathic nephrotic syndrome and evaluation of the curative effect. Abdominal Radiology (NY). 2020;**45**(8):2508-2517. DOI: 10.1007/s00261-020-02460-3

[54] Wang L, Xia P, Lv K, et al. Assessment of renal tissue elasticity by acoustic radiation force impulse quantification with histopathological correlation: Preliminary experience in chronic kidney disease. European Radiology. 2014;**24**(7):1694-1699

[55] Bob F, Grosu I, Sporea I, Bota S, Popescu A, Sirli R, et al. Is there a correlation between kidney shear wave velocity measured with VTQ and histological parameters in patients with chronic glomerulonephritis? A pilot study. Medical Ultrasonography. 2018;**1**(1):27-31. DOI: 10.11152/mu-1117

[56] Hu Q, Zhang WJ, Lin ZQ, Wang XY, Zheng HY, Wei HM, et al. Combined acoustic radiation force impulse and conventional ultrasound in the quantitative assessment of immunoglobulin a nephropathy. Ultrasound in Medicine & Biology. 2019;**45**(9):2309-2316. DOI: 10.1016/j.ultrasmedbio. 2019. 05.013

[57] Sohn B, Kim MJ, Han SW, Im YJ, Lee MJ. Shear wave velocity measurements using acoustic radiation force impulse in young children with normal kidneys versus hydronephrotic kidneys. Ultrasonography. 2014;**33**(2):116-121

[58] Göya C, Hamidi C, Ece A, Okur MH, Taşdemir B, Çetinçakmak MG, et al. Acoustic radiation force impulse (ARFI) elastography for detection of renal damage in children. Pediatric Radiology. 2015;**45**(1):55-61

[59] Dillman JR, Smith EA, Davenport MS, DiPietro MA, Sanchez R, Kraft KH, et al. Can shear-wave Elastography be used to discriminate obstructive Hydronephrosis from nonobstructive Hydronephrosis in children? Radiology. 2015;**277**(1):259-267

[60] Asano K, Ogata A, Tanaka K, et al. Acoustic radiation force impulse elastography of the kidneys: Is shear wave velocity affected by tissue fibrosis or renal blood flow? Journal of Ultrasound in Medicine. 2014;**33**(5):793-801

[61] Grenier N, Gennisson JL, Cornelis F, Le Bras Y, Couzi L. Renal ultrasound elastography. Diagnostic and Interventional Imaging. 2013;**94**:545-550

[62] Locke S. The Effect of Interstitial Pressure on Tumour Stiffness. [Thesis: Master of Science]. Graduate Department of Medical Biophysics. Toronto, Canada: University of Toronto; 2014. Available from: https://tspace.library.utoronto.ca>bitstream

[63] Gennisson JL, Grenier N, Combe C, Tanter M. Supersonic shear wave elastography of in vivo pig kidney: Influence of blood pressure, urinary pressure and tissue anisotropy. Ultrasound in Medicine & Biology. 2012;**38**(9):1559-1567

[64] Liu X, Li N, Xu T, Sun F, Li R, Gao Q, et al. Effect of renal perfusion and structural heterogeneity on shear wave elastography of the kidney: An in vivo and ex vivo study. BMC Nephrology. 2017;**18**(1):265. DOI: 10.1186/s12882-017-0679-2

[65] Grosu I, Bob F, Sporea I et al. Assessment of renal vein thrombosis using renal acoustic radiation force impulse (ARFI) imaging in a systemic lupus erythematosus (SLE) patient: A case report. [abstract] Medical Ultrasonography, The 17th National

Conference of the Romanian Society of Ultrasound in Medicine and Biology. Timisoara, Romania: Congress abstract book; 2014

[66] Bob F, Grosu I, Sporea I, Timar R, Lighezan D, Popescu A, et al. Is kidney stiffness measured using Elastography influenced mainly by vascular factors in patients with diabetic kidney disease? Ultrasonic Imaging. 2018;**40**(5):300-309. DOI: 10.1177/0161734618779789

[67] Wang Y, Feng Y, Yang X, Zhang L, Zhang T, Wang W. Clinical values of studying kidney elasticity with virtual touch quantification in gestational hypertension patients. Medical Science Monitor. 2016;**22**:403-407. DOI: 10.12659/msm.895567

[68] Çildağ MB, Gök M, Abdullayev O. Pre-procedural shear wave elastography on prediction of hemorrhage after percutaneous real-time ultrasound-guided renal biopsy. La Radiologia Medica. 2020;**125**(8):784-789. DOI: 10.1007/s11547-020-01176-0

[69] Marticorena Garcia SR, Grossmann M, Lang ST, Nguyen Trong M, Schultz M, Guo J, et al. Full-field-of-view time-harmonic Elastography of the native kidney. Ultrasound in Medicine & Biology. 2018;**44**(5):949-954. DOI: 10.1016/j.ultrasmedbio.2018.01.007

[70] Grossmann M, Tzschätzsch H, Lang ST, Guo J, Bruns A, Dürr M, et al. US time-harmonic Elastography for the early detection of glomerulonephritis. Radiology. 2019;**292**(3):676-684. DOI: 10.1148/radiol.2019182574

[71] Lim WTH, Ooi EH, Foo JJ, Ng KH, Wong JHD, Leong SS. Shear wave Elastography: A review on the confounding factors and their potential mitigation in detecting chronic kidney disease. Ultrasound in Medicine &

Biology. 2021;**47**(8):2033-2047. DOI: 10.1016/j.ultrasmedbio.2021.03.030

[72] Zhu M, Ma L, Yang W, Tang L, Li H, Zheng M, Mou S. Elastography ultrasound with machine learning improves the diagnostic performance of traditional ultrasound in predicting kidney fibrosis. Journal of the Formosan Medical Association. 2021 Aug 24:S0929-6646(21)00387-9. DOI: 10.1016/j.jfma.2021.08.011

[73] Barr RG. Can accurate shear wave velocities Be obtained in kidneys? Journal of Ultrasound in Medicine. 2020;**39**(6):1097-1105. DOI: 10.1002/jum.15190

Section 2

Non-Abdominal Application of Elastography

Chapter 11

Breast Elastography

Dominique Amy

Abstract

Breast elastography has become a key complementary technique. A modality in the framework of breast pathology, complementary of B-mode imaging and colour doppler analysis. Breast ultrasound has provided morphological grayscale images and functional flow analysis of the soft breast tissues. Elastography now brings new physio-pathological information through the assessment of tissue elasticity. There are two different modalities: Real Time Elastography (RTE) and Shear Waves (SWE) ultrafast Imaging. Both techniques require a minimum adhesion to the skill rules for acquisition and interpretation so as to limit the operator dependant dimension and diagnostic errors. Elastography thus becomes perfectly reproducible with good accuracy in the different scores of the RTE or SWE classification. The aim of elastography in cancer screening is to achieve reliable lesion characterisation and better therapy monitoring/management.

Keywords: Strain Real Time Elastography (RTE), Shear wave Elastography (SWE), lesion identification, Lymph node analysis, prognostic + lesion aggressiveness, oncologic management

1. Introduction

No one denies anymore the use of ultrasound which is now part and parcel of the different techniques used in medical imagery for the diagnosis of mammary pathologies. The complementarity of these techniques (mammography, MR and ultrasound) is perfectly accepted, as each of them suffers from a certain number of shortcomings. The development of elastography has deeply improved the management of the monitoring of mammary lesions thanks to a better identification of the anomalies of the breast, a more accurate measuring of the lesions, a guiding of the biopsies of the lesions and of the lymph nodes, an approach to probably benign lesions, a management of those which are highly likely to be suspicious and a better planning of the surgical and therapeutic interventions. It is important to limit to the utmost the number of breast biopsies, when one bears in mind that between 40% and 50% of these biopsies concern benign lesions which, as a rule, do not require these punctures.

Echography (B-mode imagery-colour Doppler) can claim an excellent over 90% sensitivity, with a very good negative predictive value (NPV) (around 90%). But its specificity and its positive predictive value (PPV) are less accurate, by 40–60% according to various publications.

IntechOpen

It is essential, when choosing an echography machine to select one with a good elastography attachment, as well as to have a minimum training to practice elastography so as to curb as much as possible the operator-dependent dimension of the examination, optimise the criteria of interpretation and finally ensure a good reproducibility of the results obtained.

It appears that the use of elastography has clearly contributed to limit the technical shortcomings of conventional echography. In order to achieve this, it is absolutely essential to abide by a minimum number of technical rules (like the correct positioning of the probe which must be horizontal and strictly perpendicular to the skin, as well as a good positioning of the patient in relation to the anatomical zones of the breast to be explored, and lastly a mastering of the micro-sismo-echography technique or vibrating technique or parkinson like vibrations (for Real Time Elastography Strain).

Though falling short of perfection, two important studies were commissioned in 2013 by EFSUMB (European Federation of the Societies of Ultrasound in Medicine and Biology): *Guidelines and Recommendations on the Clinical Use of Ultrasound Elastography* [1] and in 2015 by WFUMB (World Federation of Ultrasound in Medicine and Biology): *Guidelines and Recommendations for the Clinical Use of Ultrasound Elastography* [2]. Since these two dates, technical evolution as well as very numerous publications bear witness to very important improvements and a better approach to clinical applications for elastography.

2. Two elastography techniques

Two different sorts of medical equipment can make use of elastography:

1. Nuclear Magnetic Resonance (MR)

2. Ultrasound Echography (US). This latter technique is the only one currently used in daily practice;

US elastography is of two different types:

Real Time Elastography Strain (RTES) using an external constraint
Shear Wave Elastography (SWE) using an internal constraint.

For both techniques, the results of the 'estimation of tissue stiffness' are either qualitative or quantitative.

2.1 RTES: (SE)

This technique uses an external constraint induced to the tissue which is generated by the physician himself by positioning the probe in contact with the skin. The probe allows him to apply repetitive minimal compression/vibration to the breast tissue, the compression wave being propagated at the speed of 1500 m/s. The software of the echography machine allows the analysis of the relative movements of the different tissues thanks to the stress/strain ratio distribution providing an image of relative tissue stiffness, classified with the Tsukuba coloured criteria of stiffness of the lesion itself and of the surrounding tissues (classification in keeping with the BI-RADS radiological classification) with five scores [3]:

Score 1—No difference between the different tissues
Scores 2 and 3: Increasing proportion of the stiffer zone
Score 4: typical permanent internal stiffness of the lesion itself
Score 5: stiffness extends beyond the margins of the lesion to the background
(**Figures 1** and **2**).

The real cut-off point between benign and malignant corresponds to the score 3–4 boundary.

The use of the (ROI) region of interest on the most reproducible frame (selected with cine-loop) can be placed to cover the lesion and its adjacent tissue (as softly as possible, ideally just under the skin) to allow calculation of the fat/lesion ratio.

These data increase the diagnostic confidence in the differentiation between benign and malignant diseases without adding significantly to the length of the examination.

The sensitivity is over 90%, the specificity 88% when adding US elastography in multicentric series of several thousands of breast lesions with a good accuracy and reproducibility [4].

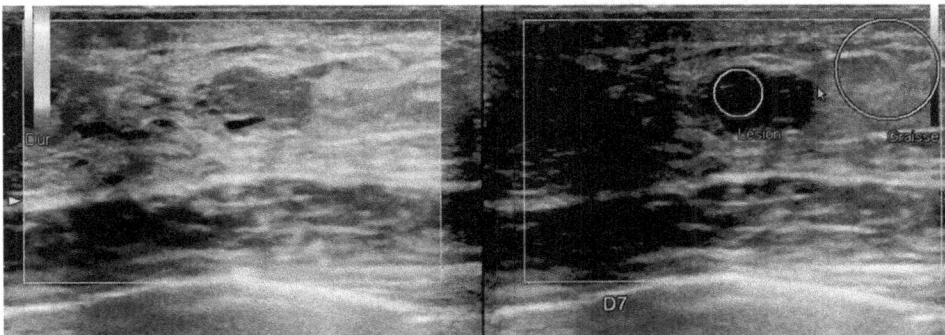

Figure 1.
Strain elastography: benign fibro-adenoma: fat to lesion ratio = 1.65.

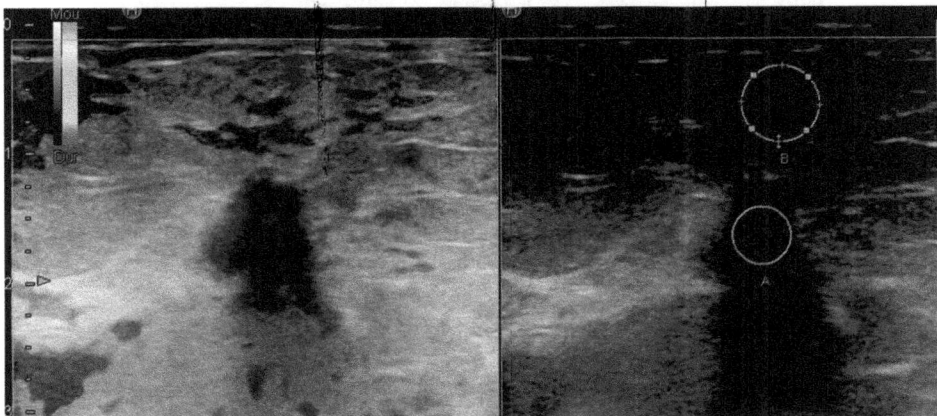

Figure 2.
Strain elastography: malignant lesion with a fat/lesion ratio = 17.47.

2.2 SWE

A third dimension, that is a piece of histo-pathological information obtained through the assessment of time elasticity is achieved by the Shear Wave Elastography technique (SWE), the first two dimensions being morphological grey scale images on the one hand and functional flow imaging of soft tissue on the other.

The waves travel in these tissues at 1–10 m/s with Shear Waves.

Focused ultrasound beams are automatically generated at supersonic speed by the probe and received back for analysis. The analysis of the propagation of ultrasound wave trains in the tissue structures is the trademark of SWE.

A mind-boggling calculation capacity is needed to capture shear waves and measure their propagation speed at the frame rate of up to 20,000 images per second.

Shear waves propagate faster in hard tissue than in soft one. The shear wave speed can be converted in colour (optionally in grey scale) or in kilo Pascal (kPa).

A specific region of interest (ROI) of different stiffer parts of the lesion or of adjacent tissue gives precise information on the variations in stiffness. This measurement in kilo-Pascal is a characteristic of the SWE technique. It allows extremely precise results.

Fat elasticity varies from 3 to 9 kPa; glandular stroma elasticity from 11 to 50 kPa. The average figure for the elasticity of malignant lesions is higher than 100 kPa and can even reach over 150–200 kPa (in 13 published studies).

All the lesions with a figure higher than 50/60 kPa are to be biopsied, thanks to an impressive improvement in the sensitivity and the negative predictive value up to 100% according to EVANS. The specificity as well as the positive predictive value are also significantly improved with a better evaluation of the 3–4 BI-RADS

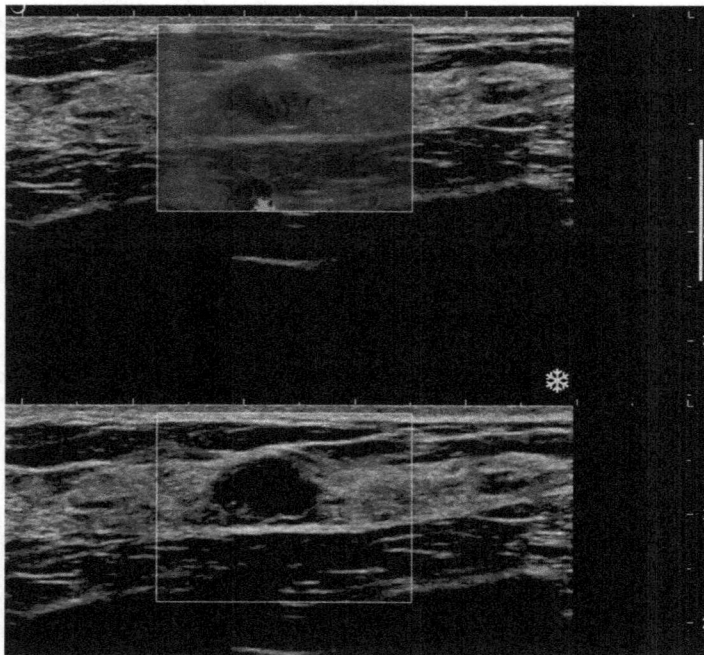

Figure 3.
SWElastography: benign lesion without colour modification +28 kPa.

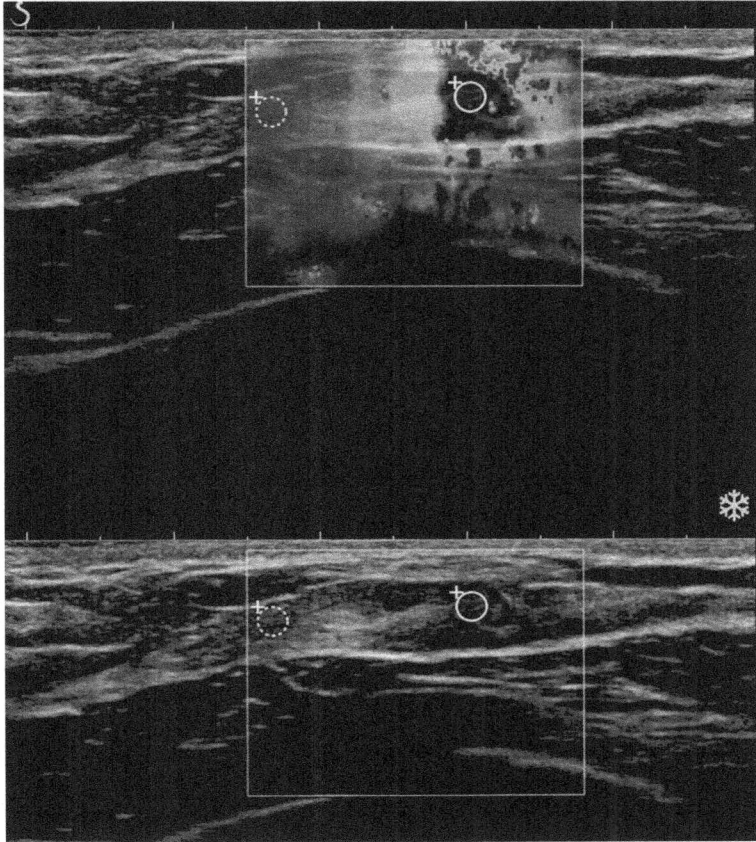

Figure 4.
SWE with a sub-cutaneous malignant invasive carcinoma = 284 kPa.

cases which can thus be reclassified upward or downward as the case may be, which leads to a considerable reduction in the number of unnecessary biopsies (**Figures 3** and **4**) [5].

3. Limitations and artefact

1. Some cysts have heterogenous contents which are difficult to analyse.

2. The viscous contents of these atypical cysts require light pre-compression for a better analysis (**Figures 5** and **10**);

3. The very superficial location of a lesion next to the skin, or on the contrary against a rib in a breast without fatty cover may cause difficulties by making it impossible to position the ROIs or achieve the fat to lesion ratios.

4. There exist 'soft' cancers of the cancer in situ type, colloid or mucoid cancers, diffuse ones (no mass cancers). On the other hand, mucinous cancers have been described by some as 'hard', between 95 and 270 kPa.

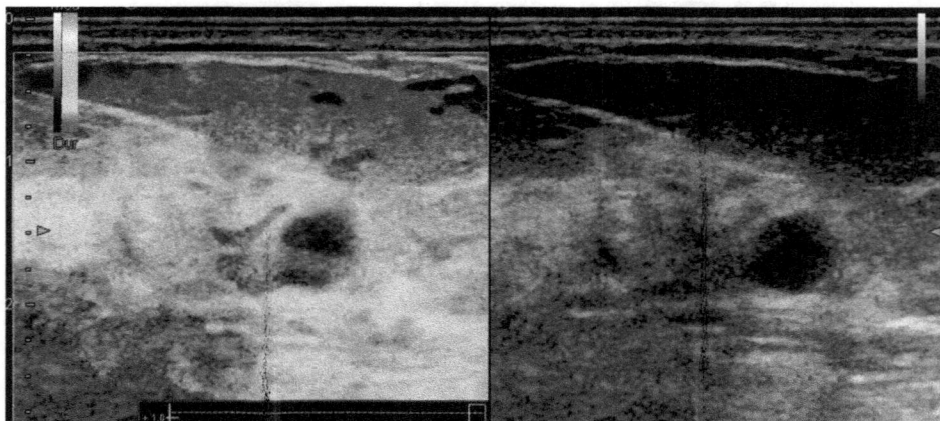

Figure 5.
Typical strain elastography of liquid structure: BGR sign (blue/green/red).

5. Lastly some old, very fibrous fibroadenomas may seem 'hard' but are without any hypervascularisation, and without very suspicious ultrasound signs. A perfect mastery of the technique of positioning the 'elasticity boxes' is essential for their correct analysis.

4. Contribution of elastography to the diagnosis of breast cancer

4.1 The coupling of conventional echography

The coupling of conventional echography (which underestimates the size of the lesions) with Strain or SWE elastography has resulted in a significant improvement in the measurement of the size and extent of the lesions (calculation of the longest axis, the perimeter and the extent). The histological sections and the SWE measurements were identical (give or take 2 mm) according to some authors. In its calculations, elastography integrates changes in extra cellular matrix, inflammation and stroma remodelling (myofibroblasts and collagen) in invasive cancers (**Figure 12**).

4.2 Echo-guided punctures

Echo-guided punctures are made easier in areas displaying maximum modification in elasticity. The centre of the tumour is not always the area with the highest density in cancerous cells (central necrosis) which are to be found in larger numbers at the periphery of the tumour (**Figure 6**).

Patients having a second reading echography after an MR showing subtle or difficult to interpret images have benefitted from a better biopsy carried out under echo-elastography (29% improvement of the sensitivity). Decrease in the number of false positives and 40–50% reduction of biopsies concerning benign lesions for which puncturing is not needed, thanks to an improvement in the sensitivity of mammary echography (**Figure 7**).

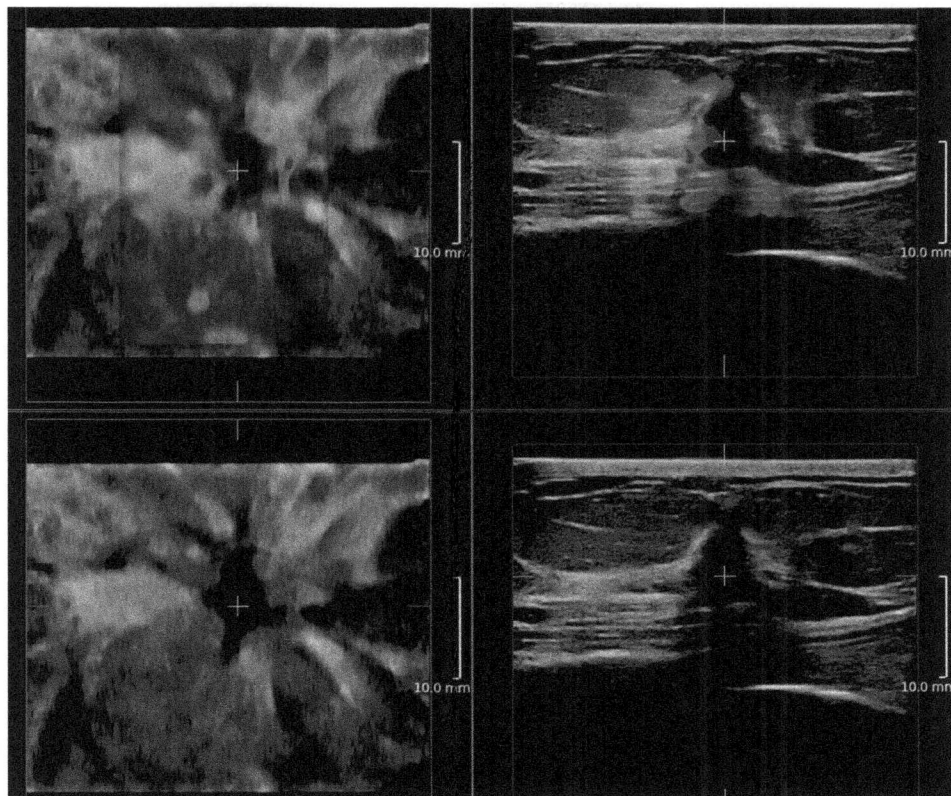

Figure 6.
SWE 2D with coronal section of a carcinoma.

4.3 Better identification of the pathological lymph nodes

he analysis of the lymph nodes through echography and elastography requires a good deal of experience and a thorough exploration of all the zones of the breast where these nodes are to be found (axillary, para-sternal intra-mammary, intra-pectoral, supra-clavicular, mediastinal, contralateral axillary and internal mammary zones)

Most lymph nodes (75%) are to be found in the axillary zone.

90% of the lymph nodes larger than 5 mm can be identified [6].

The modifications of the lymph nodes can be inflammatory, related to a systemic disease, to granulomatosis, or lastly to a metastasis of melanoma, lymphoma or breast cancer. There is a subtle classification of the metastatic criteria of the lymph nodes which are often difficult to identify Axillary metastatic nodes are to be found in half the number of breast cancers.

Lymph node elastography has a 42% sensitivity. There is a significant number of false positives. The correct positioning of the elasticity box is essential in the case of small lymph node structures.

In the case of metastatic lymph nodes, elasticity is around 20–25 kPa.

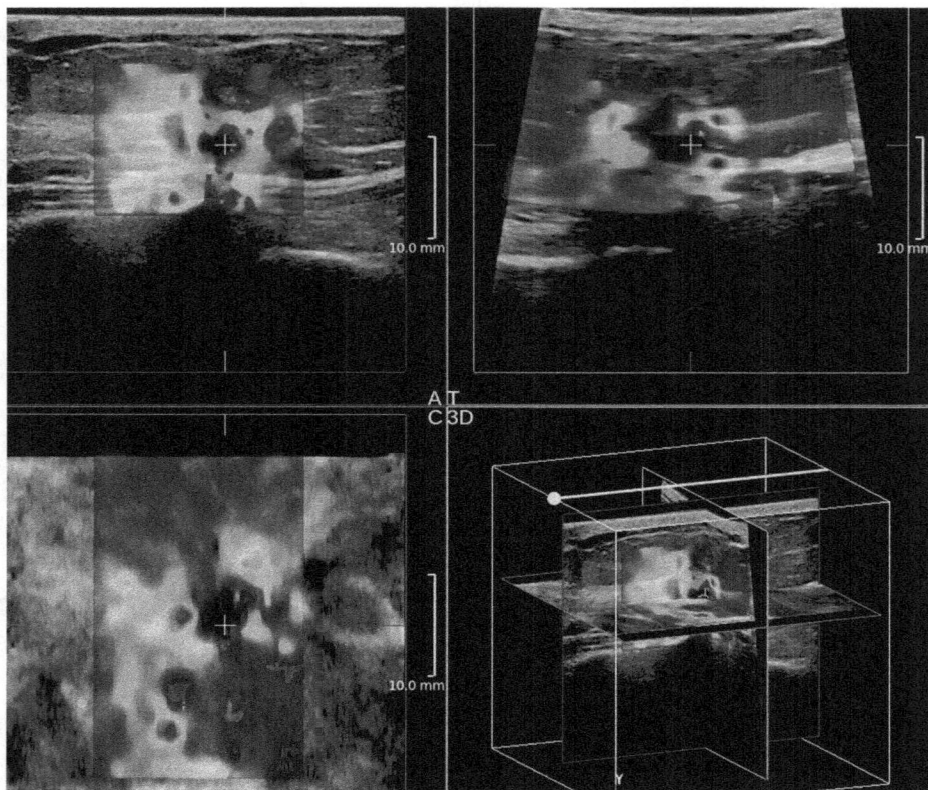

Figure 7.
SWE + 3D malignant tumour =110 kPa.

A perfectly round lymph node without hyperechoic hilum is highly suspicious. To analyse it, it is important to make use of a Doppler examination.

A lymph node less than 2 mm large bears micro-metastases which will have but little influence on the evolution of the disease.

Lymph nodes larger than 3 mm or more bear macro-metastases which will modify significantly the general evolution of the patient.

90% of the metastatic nodes over 5 mm are thus analysed for an accurate pre-operative stage, with a significant saving of time, diagnostic accuracy and cost effectiveness.

The identification of the sentinel node is important if it can be carried out.

The taking of sample cells through fine needle aspiration or core biopsy makes it possible to assert there is an invasion of the lymph nodes, thus avoiding unnecessary complete axillary lympho-node dissection.

4.4 Better analysis of the zones of micro-calcifications detected through mammography

The vast majority of micro-calcifications are badly identified in echography. Elastography may allow a study of the zones targeted through the radiological examination as containing micro-calcifications. Ultrasound evidences the zones of intra-ductal or lobular epithelial proliferation (**Figure 8**).

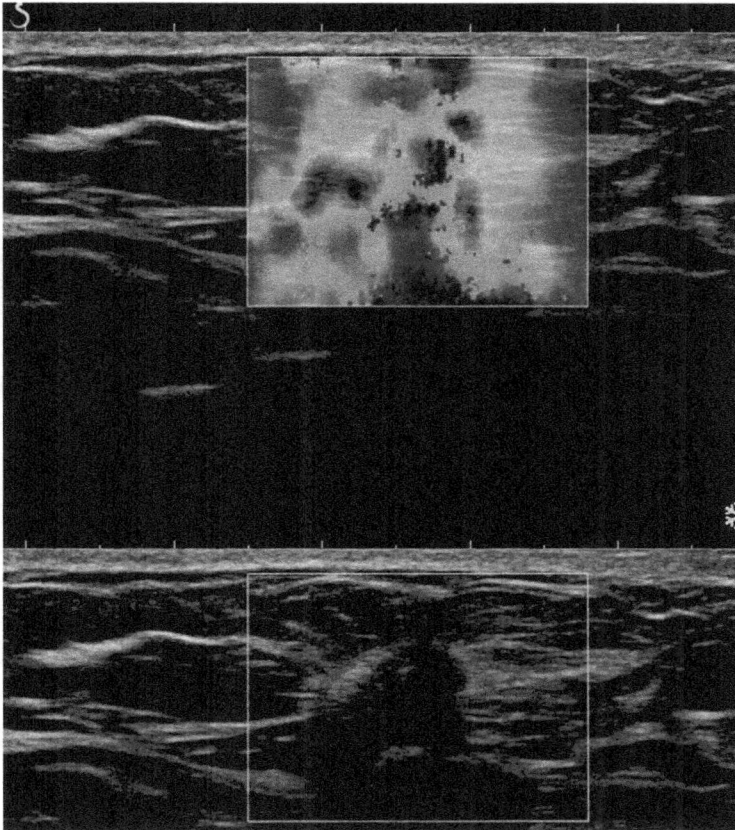

Figure 8.
SWE non evident 2D malignant lesion =148 kPa.

Colour Doppler (ultra fast, angio-plus Doppler) coupled with 3D imagery allows a reconstruction of lobar anatomy with its possible pathological modifications, but it is obvious that it is impossible to distinguish simple epithelial proliferation from florid hyperplasia, from a case of CIS in situ or from a millimetric invasive cancer at its very beginning.

Echography coupled with elastography enables one to select a risk zone (to be monitored or punctured) with or without micro-calcifications (**Figures 9–11**).

4.5 Prognostic study of a lesion and its aggressiveness

In 2011 and 2014, Evans was one of the pioneers in the description of the relationships between the size of the lesions, the increase in elasticity and the aggressiveness of the tumour, the contamination of the lymph nodes, the lympho-vascular invasion and the histological grade of the cancer [7–10].

The hardest cancers are more invasive with a median value of 180 kPa and the highest histological grade. Median elasticity values of 126 kPa correspond to ductal cancers in situ. Benign lesions have a median score of 45 kPa. Lipomas have a score of 14 kPa, with 97% sensitivity and 88% specificity. These data can thus be considered as predictive (**Figures 8 and 12**).

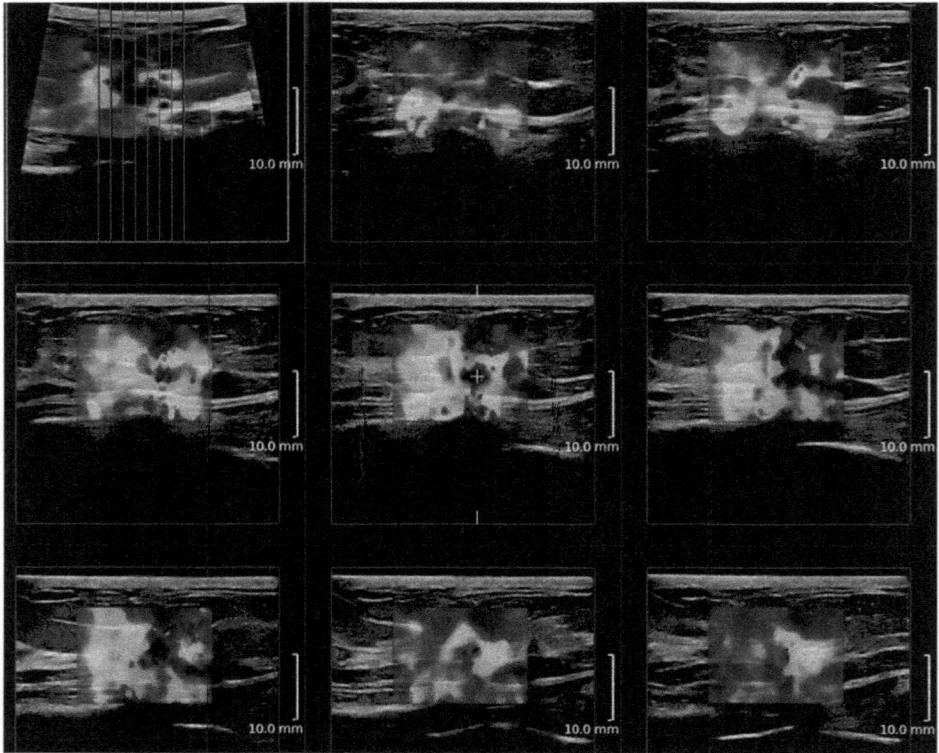

Figure 9.
SWE multi-slides technic of a malignant lesion = 123 kPa.

4.6 Oncologic management and monitoring in the course of neoadjuvant chemotherapy

There is a significant link between the pre-operative elasticity values and the evolution of elasticity during the treatment, and this allows us to assess its efficiency. The decrease in elasticity and heterogenicity of the tumour corresponds to a good response to the treatment. Therapeutic monitoring is thus improved.

These results have proved to be more relevant than those achieved by dynamic MR with a contrasting agent, even though MR is considered as a golden rule in the monitoring of pre-operative therapy.

5. Practical information for the use of mammary elastography

5.1 Colour map code

The Hitachi company, a pioneer of strain elastography (SE) have expressed the modifications in the elasticity of mammary tissues through a colorimetric chart known as the 'Tsukuba score'. Reds and yellows correspond to very supple tissues, green has a slightly higher elasticity score and blue a much increased gradient in elasticity; last of all, a deep blue zone surrounded with a pale blue halo is the sign of a lesion which is very likely to be malignant [4].

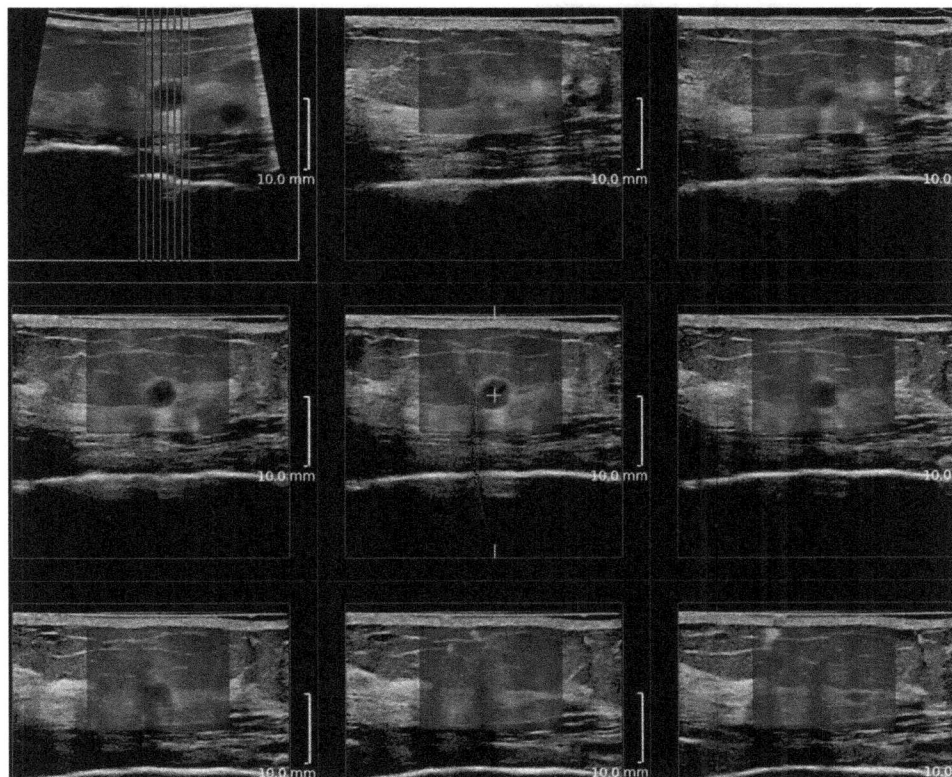

Figure 10.
SWE multi plane benign cyst = 20 kPa.

Another pioneer in Shear Wave Elastography (SWE), the Supersonic image group have chosen the opposite colour coding, red for a hard, probably malignant lesion, blue for low score, supple elasticity which is therefore benign. This latter, more 'European' colorimetric representation (red = danger) can very easily be reversed electronically through a simple modification in the software, and this applies to both SE and SWE techniques. This colour inversion is not a major difficulty for the user who, most of the time, does not use the two techniques simultaneously; he must simply make sure he follows some basic, standard rules (e.g. no hyper-pressure with the probe which must be strictly perpendicular to the skin, etc.) which he will have had fully described in the course of his training.

The use of a dual mode (mode B image joined to the elastography image in colour) enables a perfect synchronisation in the analysis of the lesion, either in SE or in SWE. The colour mode indicates very rapidly the suspicious (or non suspicious) character of an anomaly detected through echography [11].

As the appreciation of colours may vary from one user to another, the builders of these machines have turned towards more precise and measurable quantitative data.

The 'fat to lesion ratio' makes it possible to measure the variations in elasticity between the hardest tissues and the supplest fatty tissue with great precision.

The use of ROI (region of interest) or of the Q Box has to be well handled: one ROI/Q Box is positioned on the suspicious coloured lesion, the other is placed on the supplest possible tissue, generally the subcutaneous fatty tissue.

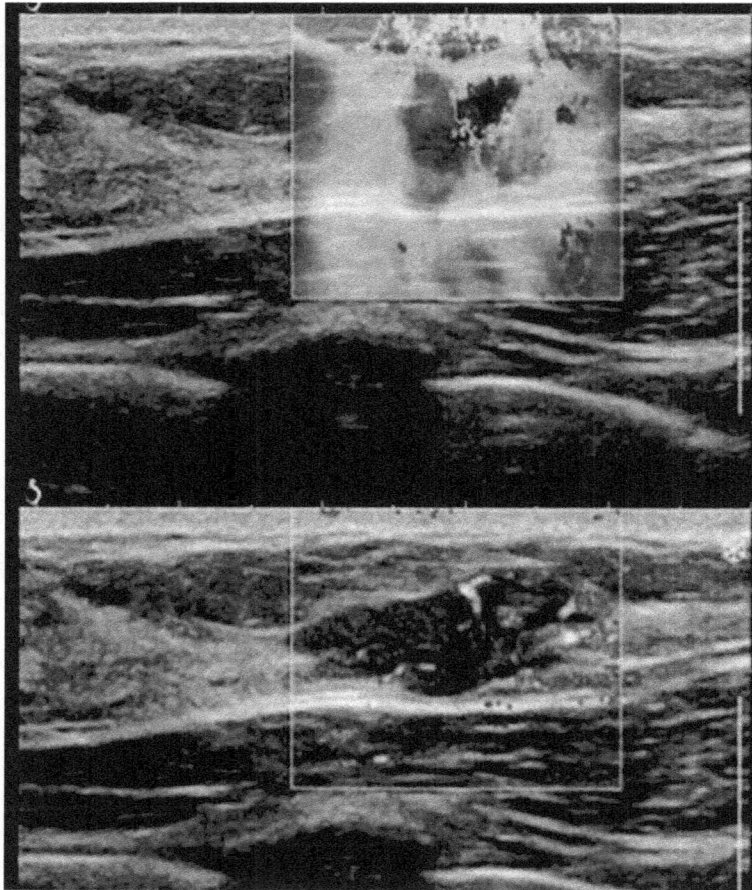

Figure 11.
Ultrafast doppler + SWE of a carcinoma =160 kPa.

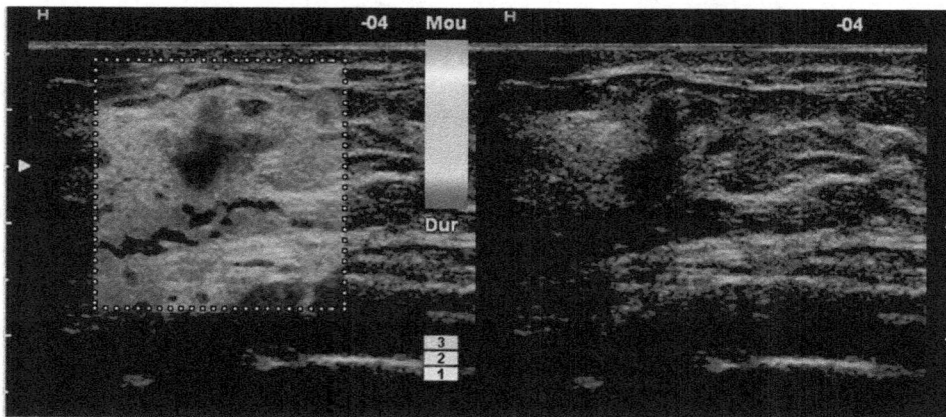

Figure 12.
Srain elastography of a non-evident 2D lesion with a F/L ratio = 15.21.

In SE, the ratio is graded from 1 to 10 (or more) with a 'cut off point' between 3 and 4 (lesion likely to be benign, or likely to be suspicious). In SWE the mean and standard deviations are provided in kPa (KiloPascal), ratio and averages derive from the quantitative measurements.

Evans has determined the threshold of 50 kPa for Birads 3 or below lesions which are benign as a rule. According to him, scores over 50/60 kPa correspond to Birads 4/5 lesions which are to be biopsied, scores higher than 100 kPa or more are a certainty of malignancy.

The most interesting case is that of the lesions graded Birads 3, when one keeps in mind that 2% in this category correspond to malignant lesions and that, furthermore, there exist 'soft' cancers (mucoid, colloid, in situ or no mass cancers). Mucinous cancers considered as 'soft' tumours reach high scores in SWE (from 95 to over 200 kPa). Quite obviously, one must take into account complementary factors such as the age of the patient, the size of the breast, the distance between the skin and the lesion, the fibrous or involuted character of the breast, all of which take their share in the Birads 3/4 scoring.

5.2 Regrading of these 3/4 Birads lesions = upgrade/downgrade:

Elastography allows to reduce the number of unnecessary biopsies through a better specificity and PPV (Positive Predictive Value). It guides the decision not to biopsy a Birads 4a lesion with a negative reassuring elastography and to suggest instead an echography follow-up 6 months later, or on the contrary, to biopsy a Birads 3 lesion with a suspicious elastography response. Such a way of dealing was presented by the Korean Society of Ultrasound (KSUM) in 2014 [12].

In the case of a negative Birads 3 lesion, the follow-up will be the same as for a Birads 2 lesion.

a. Negative Birads 4a = Birads 3

b. Positive Birads3 = Biopsy

c. Negative Birads 4a = Birads 2

5.3 Follow-up of treatment efficiency in a proven cancer

If mode B echography alone underestimates the size of the cancer, with the contribution of elastography, it produces a perfect assessment of the histological size of the lesion.

The prediction of the response to the neoadjuvant chemotherapy treatment has been studied by different groups who confirm that there is a relationship between the score of pre-operative elasticity and the response to the treatment.

The maximum score in elasticity of the tumour is related to its histological severity:

Invasive cancer elasticity score = between 140 and 180 kPa.
Ductal cancer in situ = between 70 and 180 kPa.
Benign lesion medium elasticity score = 45 kPa.
Lipoma = 15 kPa.

The 180 kPa is predictive of nodular metastasis. If information on the size of the tumour, the lymph node and vascular invasion and the histological grade of the cancer is added, capital information is obtained on the prognosis of the evolution of the cancer.

Modification of stiffness (up or down) seems to be a very relevant parameter to access treatment efficacy.

5.4 Assessment of echo graphically revealed micro-calcifications

Two conditions are to be faced: either micro-calcifications with an obvious focal lesion, or micro-calcifications without echo graphically visible lesions. A very small number only of these micro-calcifications can be detected through mode B echography. They are the indirect signs of an intra-ductal or intra-lobular disruption. In comparison to mammography, echography offers the added bonus to visualise directly the epithelial structure of the epithelial proliferation or hyperplasia type. Their development may correspond to a physiological character, an inflammation or a tumoral process. And it is only the bringing together of mode B echography, ultra fast Doppler, elastography and possibly 3D analysis, that allows to distinguish a probably benign lesion from a well-defined or a diffuse lesion, but it remains difficult, if not impossible, to distinguish between the successive stages in epithelial modifications: physiologic proliferation, florid hyperplasia, border line or cancer in situ in its earliest stages. The role of echography is to allow a selection of the patients at risks (with a thickening of epithelial structures) for whom follow-ups or further investigations must be considered.

5.5 Role of elastography in mammary pathology

The diagnosis of breast lesions and the way in which they are dealt with has progressed dramatically thanks to the use of new technologies in breast imaging. Among these techniques, ultrasound elastography has become an essential, unavoidable tool. It combines rapidity of execution, diagnostic reliability and remarkable reproducibility. It allows to put forward dubious cases and patients at risk who have to have regular check-ups. And it also allows a reduction in the high number of ultrasound false positives, a regular follow-up of probably benign lesions and a monitoring of the efficiency of neoadjuvant treatments [13].

At this stage, however, the study of lymph nodes invasion remains difficult and the understanding of the relationship between the maximum elasticity score of a tumour and its immuno-histological phenotype is not conclusive. Let us hope that future progress in echography will soon enable us to fill in these gaps.

6. Conclusion

The coupling of 3D Breast Echography + Angio-plus-Ultra-fast Colour Doppler with elastography has allowed significant improvements in evidencing the location of the breast lesions, their qualification and the management of pre-operative neoadjuvant chemotherapy. A better collaboration with the team who is in charge of the patient (surgeon, oncologist, doctor, radiotherapist, nurse etc....) can thus be achieved to the patient's greatest benefit.

In qualifying the grade of the tumour, the presence of metastases in the lymph nodes and in offering a prognosis linked to the aggressiveness of the tumour, the radiologist allows a significant saving of time for the therapeutic approach of the patient and a better targeted, more personalised therapy.

The evaluation of therapeutic care strategies is better adapted than a standard protocol. There are close relations between the modification of elasticity, the size of the tumour, the metastatic invasion of the lymph nodes, the more or less aggressive nature of the cancer and the choice of the suitable neoadjuvant chemotherapy.

The decrease in recall rate as well as in unnecessary punctures (40–50%) amounts to serious cost effectiveness.

Inter or intra-operator perfect reproducibility, fair possibility to repeat the examinations in over 85% of the cases and lastly outstanding sensitivity and specificity explain why the echography-elastography coupling has achieved a significant beneficial impact on breast imaging. Future developments are still to improve the diagnosis and follow up of breast cancer [10, 14–62].

Author details

Dominique Amy
Breast Center, Aix-en-Provence, France

*Address all correspondence to: domamy@wanadoo.fr

IntechOpen

References

[1] Cosgrove D et al. EFSUMB guideline and recommendations on the clinical use of ultrasound elastograpy. Ultraschall in der Medizin. 2013;**34**:238-253

[2] Barr RG, Nakashima K, Amy D, Cosgrove D, Farrokh A, Schafer F, et al. WFUMB guidelines and recommendations for clinical use of ultrasound elastography; Part 2. Breast. Ultrasound in Medicine & Biology. 2015;**41**(5):1148-1160. DOI: 10.1016/j.ultrasmedbio.2015.03.008. Epub 2015 Mar 18

[3] Itoh A, Ueno E, Tohno E, Kamma H, Takahashi H, Shiina T, et al. Breast disease: Clinical application of US elastography for diagnosis. Radiology. 2006;**239**:341-350

[4] Ueno E, Tohno E, Morishima I, Umemoto T, Waki K. A preliminary prospective study to compare the diagnostic performance of assist strain ratio versus manual strain ratio. Journal of Medical Ultrasonics. 2015;**42**(4):521-531

[5] Evans A, Whelehan P, Thomson K, Brauer K, Jordan L, Purdie C, et al. Differentiating benign from malignant solid breast masses: Value of shear wave elastography according to lesion stiffness combined with greyscale ultrasound according to BI-RADS classification. British Journal of Cancer. 2012;**107**(2):224-229

[6] Fournier D. Lymph node staging with US (and FNA). In: Amy D, editor. Lobar Approach to Breast Ultrasound. Springer International Publishing AG Part of Springer Nature; 2018

[7] Chang JM, Park IA, Lee SH, Kim WH, Bae MS, Koo HR, et al. Stiffness of tumours measured by shear-wave elastography correlated with subtypes of breast cancer. European Radiology. 2013;**23**(9):2450-2458

[8] Evans A, Whelehan P, Thomson K, McLean D, Brauer K, Purdie C, et al. Invasive breast cancer: Relationship between shear-wave elastographic findings and histologic prognostic factors. Radiology. 2012;**263**(3):673-677

[9] Ganau S, Andreu FJ, Escribano F, Martín A, Tortajada L, Villajos M, et al. Shear-wave elastography and immunohistochemical profiles in invasive breast cancer: Evaluation of maximum and mean elasticity values. European Journal of Radiology. 2015;**84**(4):617-622

[10] Lee SH, Moon WK, Cho N, Chang JM, Moon HG, Han W, et al. Shear-wave elastographic features of breast cancers: Comparison with mechanical elasticity and histopathologic characteristics. Investigative Radiology. 2014;**49**(3):147-155

[11] Amy D, Bercoff J, Bibby E. Breast elastography. In: Amy D, editor. Lobar Approach to Breast Ultrasound. Springer International Publishing AG Part of Springer Nature; 2018

[12] Lee SH, Chang JM, Cho N, Koo HR, Yi A, Kim SJ, et al. Practice guideline for the performance of breast ultrasound elastography. Ultrasonography. 2014;**33**(1):3-10

[13] Cosgrove DO, Berg WA, Doré CJ, Skyba DM, Henry JP, Gay J, et al. Shear wave elastography for breast masses is highly reproducible. European Radiology. 2012;**22**(5):1023-1032

[14] Abdullah N, Mesurolle B, El-Khoury M, Kao E. Breast imaging reporting and data system lexicon for US: Interobserver agreement for assessment of breast masses. Radiology. 2009;**252**(3):665-672

[15] Alvarez S, Anorbe E, Alcorta P, Lopez F, Alonso I, Cortes J. Role of sonography in the diagnosis of axillary lymph node metastases in breast cancer: A systematic review. American Journal of Roentgenology. 2006;**186**:1342-1348

[16] Athanasiou A, Tardivon A, Tanter M, Sigal-Zafrani B, Bercoff J, Deffieux T, et al. Breast lesions: Quantitative elastography with supersonic shear imaging--preliminary results. Radiology. 2010;**256**(1):297-303

[17] Athanasiou A, Latorre-Ossa H, Criton A, Tardivon A, Gennisson JL, Tanter M. Feasibility of Imaging and treatment monitoring of breast lesions with three-dimensional shear wave elastography. Ultraschall in der Medizin. 2017;**38**:51-59

[18] Au FW, Ghai S, Moshonov H, Kahn H, Brennan C, Dua H, et al. Diagnostic performance of quantitative shear wave elastography in the evaluation of solid breast masses: Determination of the most discriminatory parameter. AJR. American Journal of Roentgenology. 2014;**203**(3):W328-W336

[19] Au FW, Ghai S, Lu FI, Moshonov H, Crystal P. Quantitative shear wave elastography: Correlation with prognostic histologic features and immuno histo chemical biomarkersof breast cancer. Academic Radiology. 2015;**22**(3):269-277

[20] Awad FM. Role of supersonic shear wave imaging quantitative elastography (SSI) in differentiating benign and malignant solid breast masses. The Egyptian Journal of Radiology and Nuclear Medicine. 2013;**44**:681-685

[21] Barr RG, Zhang Z, Cormack JB, Mendelson EB, Berg WA. Probably benign lesions at screening breast US in a population with elevated risk: Prevalence and rate of malignancy in the ACRIN 6666 trial. Radiology. 2013;**269**(3):701-712

[22] Barr RG, Zhang Z. Effects of precompression on elasticity imaging of the breast: Development of a clinically useful semiquantitative method of precompression assessment. Journal of Ultrasound in Medicine. 2012;**31**(6):895-902

[23] Berg WA, Cosgrove DO, Doré CJ, Schäfer FK, Svensson WE, Hooley RJ, et al. Shear-wave elastography improves the specificity of breast US: TheBE1 multinational study of 939 masses. Radiology. 2012;**262**(2):435-449

[24] Berg WA, Mendelson EB, Cosgrove DO, Doré CJ, Gay J, Henry JP, et al. Quantitative maximum shear-wave stiffness of breast masses as a predictor of histopathologic severity. AJR. American Journal of Roentgenology. 2015;**205**(2):448-455

[25] Boisserie-Lacroix M, MacGrogan G, Debled M, Ferron S, Asad-Syed M, Brouste V, et al. Radiological features of triple-negative breast cancers (73 cases). Diagnostic and Interventional Imaging. 2012;**93**(3):183-190

[26] Brkljaçiç B, Divjak E, Tomasoviç-Lonçariç Ç, Tešiç V, Ivanac G. Shear-wave sonoelastographic features of invasive lobular breast cancers. Croatian Medical Journal. 2016;**57**:42-50

[27] Çebi Olgun D, Korkmazer B, Kılıç F, Dikici AS, Velidedeoglu M, Aydogan F,

et al. Use of shear wave elastography to differentiate benign and malignant breast lesions. Diagnostic and Interventional Radiology. 2014;**20**(3):239-244

[28] Chang JM, Moon WK, Cho N, Yi A, Koo HR, Han W, et al. Clinical application of shear wave elastography (SWE) in the diagnosis of benign and malignant breast diseases. Breast Cancer Research and Treatment. 2011;**129**(1):89-97

[29] Chang JM, Won JK, Lee KB, Park IA, Yi A, Moon WK. Comparison of shear-wave and strain ultrasound elastography in the differentiation of benign and malignant breast lesions. AJR. American Journal of Roentgenology. 2013;**201**(2):W347-W356

[30] Corsetti V, Houssami N, Ferrari A, Ghirardi M, Bellarosa S, Angelini O, et al. Breast screening with ultrasound in women with mammography-negative dense breasts: Evidence on incremental cancer detection and false positives, and associated cost. European Journal of Cancer. 2008;**44**(4):539-544

[31] Dobruch-Sobczak K, Nowicki A. Role of shear wave sonoelastography in differentiation between focal breast lesions. Ultrasound in Medicine & Biology. 2015;**41**(2):366-374

[32] Drukteinis JS, Mooney BF, Flowers CI, Gatenby RA. Beyond mammography: New frontiers in breast cancer screening. The American Journal of Medicine. 2013;**126**(6):472-479

[33] Džoiç Dominkoviç M, Ivanac G, Kelava T, Brkljaçiç B. Elastographic features of triple negative breast cancers. European Radiology. 2016;**26**(4):1090-1097

[34] Elverici E, Zengin B, Nurdan Barca A, Didem Yilmaz P, Alimli A,

Araz L. Interobserver and Intraobserver agreement of sonographic BIRADS lexicon in the assessment of breast masses. Iranian Journal of Radiology. 2013;**10**(3):122-127

[35] Esen G, Gurses B, Yilmaz MH, Ilvan S, Ulus S, Celik V, et al. Gray scale and power Doppler US in the preoperative evaluation of axillary metastases in breast cancer patients with no palpable lymph nodes. European Radiology. 2005;**15**:1215-1223

[36] Evans A, Armstrong S, Whelehan P, Thomson K, Rauchhaus P, Purdie C, et al. Can shear-wave elastography predict response to neoadjuvant chemotherapy in women with invasive breast cancer? British Journal of Cancer. 2013;**109**(11):2798-2802

[37] Evans A, Whelehan P, Thomson K, McLean D, Brauer K, Purdie C, et al. Quantitative shear wave ultrasound elastography: Initial experience in solid breast masses. Breast Cancer Research. 2010;**12**(6):R104

[38] Evans A, Rauchhaus P, Whelehan P, Thomson K, Purdie CA, Jordan LB, et al. Does shear wave ultrasound independently predict axillary lymph node metastasis in women with invasive breast cancer? Breast Cancer Research and Treatment. 2014;**143**(1):153-157

[39] Feldmann A, Langlois C, Dewailly M, Martinez EF, Boulanger L, Kerdraon O, et al. Shear wave elastography (SWE): An analysis of breast lesion characterization in 83 breast lesions. Ultrasound in Medicine & Biology. 2015;**41**(10):2594-2604

[40] Gweon HM, Youk JH, Son EJ, Kim JA. Clinical application of qualitative assessment for breast masses in shear-wave elastography. European Journal of Radiology. 2013;**82**(11):e680-e685

[41] Kim MY, Choi N, Yang JH, Yoo YB, Park KS. False positive or negative results of shear-wave elastography in differentiating benign from malignant breast masses: Analysis of clinical and ultrasonographic characteristics. Acta Radiologica. 2015;**56**(10):1155-1162

[42] Kim H, Youk JH, Gweon HM, Kim JA, Son EJ. Diagnostic performance of qualitative shear-wave elastography according to different color map opacities for breast masses. European Journal of Radiology. 2013;**82**(8):e326-e331

[43] Ko KH, Jung HK, Kim SJ, Kim H, Yoon JH. Potential role of shear-wave ultrasound elastography for the differential diagnosis of breast non-mass lesions: Preliminary report. European Radiology. 2014;**24**(2):305-311

[44] Lee SH, Cho N, Chang JM, Koo HR, Kim JY, Kim WH, et al. Two-view versus single-view shear-wave elastography: Comparison of observer performance in differentiating benign from malignant breast masses. Radiology. 2014;**270**(2):344-353

[45] Lee SH, Chang JM, Kim WH, Bae MS, Seo M, Koo HR, et al. Added value of shear-wave elastography for evaluation of breast masses detected with screening US imaging. Radiology. 2014;**273**(1):61-69

[46] Lee EJ, Jung HK, Ko KH, Lee JT, Yoon JH. Diagnostic performances of shearwave elastography: Which parameter to use in differential diagnosis of solid breastmasses? European Radiology. 2013;**23**(7):1803-1160

[47] Mendelson EB, Böhm-Vélez M, Berg WA, et al. ACR BI-RADS® Ultrasound. In: ACR BI-RADS® Atlas, Breast Imaging Reporting and Data System. Reston, VA: American College of Radiology; 2015

[48] Moorman AM, Bourez RL, de Leeuw DM, Kouwenhoven EA. Pre-operative ultrasonographic evaluation of axillary Lymph nodes in breast cancer patients: For which group still of additional value and in which group cause for special attention? Ultrasound in Medicine and Biology. 2015;**41**(11):2842-2848. DOI: 10.1016/j.ultrasmedbio.2015.06.013

[49] Mori M, Tsunoda H, Kawauchi N, Kikuchi M, Honda S, Suzuki K, et al. Elastographic evaluation of mucinous carcinoma of the breast. Breast Cancer. 2012;**19**(1):60-63

[50] Mullen R, Thompson JM, Moussa O, Vinnicombe S, Evans A. Shear-wave+elastography contributes to accurate tumour size estimation when assessing small breast cancers. Clinical Radiology. 2014;**69**(12):1259-1263

[51] Ohuchi N, Suzuki A, Sobue T, Kawai M, Yamamoto S, Zheng YF, et al. Sensitivity and specificity of mammography and adjunctive ultrasonography to screen for breast cancer in the Japan Strategic Anti-cancer Randomized Trial (J-START): A randomised controlled trial. Lancet. 201623;**387**(10016):341-8.11

[52] Park CS, Lee JH, Yim HW, Kang BJ, Kim HS, Jung JI, et al. Observer agreement using the ACR breast imaging reporting and data system (BI-RADS)-ultrasound, first edition (2003). Korean Journal of Radiology. 2007;**8**(5):397-402

[53] Plecha DM, Pham RM, Klein N, Coffey A, Sattar A, Marshall H. Addition of shear-wave elastography during second-look MR imaging-directed breast US: Effect onlesion detection and biopsy targeting. Radiology. 2014;**272**(3):657-664

[54] Rzymski P, Skórzewska A, Skibinska-Zielinska M, Opala T. Factors

influencingbreast elasticity measured by the ultrasound shear wave elastography—Preliminary results. Archives of Medical Science. 2011;**7**(1):127-133

[55] Schwab F, Redling K, Siebert M, Schötzau A, Schoenenberger CA, Zanetti-Dällenbach R. Inter- and intra-observer agreement in ultrasound BI-RADS classification and real-time elastography Tsukuba score assessment of breast lesions. Ultrasound in Medicine and Biology. 2016;**42**(11):2622-2629

[56] Tozaki M, Fukuma E. Pattern classification of ShearWave™ elastography images for differential diagnosis between benign and malignant solid breast masses. Acta Radiologica. 2011;**52**(10):1069-1075

[57] Yoon JH, Jung HK, Lee JT, Ko KH. Shear-wave elastography in the diagnosis of solid breast masses: What leads to false-negative or false-positive results? European Radiology. 2013;**23**(9):2432-2440

[58] Youk JH, Son EJ, Gweon HM, Kim H, Park YJ, Kim JA. Comparison of strain and shear wave elastography for the differentiation of benign from malignant breast lesions, combined with B-mode ultrasonography: Qualitative and quantitative assessments. Ultrasound in Medicine & Biology. 2014;**40**(10):2336-2344

[59] Youk JH, Gweon HM, Son EJ, Chung J, Kim JA, Kim EK. Three-dimensional shear-wave elastography for differentiating benign and malignant breast lesions: Comparison with two-dimensional shear-wave elastography. European Radiology. 2013;**23**(6):1519-1527

[60] Youk JH, Gweon HM, Son EJ, Han KH, Kim JA. Diagnostic value of commercially available shear-wave elastography for breast cancers: Integration into BI-RADS classification with sub categories of category 4. European Radiology. 2013;**23**(10):2695-2704

[61] Youk JH, Gweon HM, Son EJ, Kim JA, Jeong J. Shear-wave elastography of invasive breast cancer: Correlation between quantitative mean elasticity value andimmunohistochemical profile. Breast Cancer Research and Treatment. 2013;**138**(1):119-126

[62] Zhou J, Zhan W, Chang C, Zhang X, Jia Y, Dong Y, et al. Breast lesions: Evaluation with shear wave elastography, with special emphasis on the "stiff rim" sign. Radiology. 2014;**272**(1):63-72

Chapter 12

Shear-Wave Elastography in Diffuse Thyroid Diseases

Cristina Mihaela Cepeha, Andreea Borlea, Corina Paul,
Iulian Velea and Dana Stoian

Abstract

The diagnosis and evaluation of diffuse thyroid pathologies is often a challenge for clinicians. Ultrasonography has an essential contribution in thyroid imaging, but elastography adds more accuracy. Frequently used in the evaluation of thyroid nodules, elastography has become a necessary tool in assessing the risk of malignancy. Diffuse thyroid pathologies such as Graves' disease, chronic autoimmune thyroiditis, and subacute thyroiditis, are diagnosed based on laboratory tests completed with imaging. Recently it has been shown that elastography is useful in the evaluation and differentiation of these cases due to the differences in elasticity. This chapter describes the general principles of shear-wave elastography, examination technique, features found in diffuse thyroid disease, but also the limitations of this type of investigation for a better understanding of its use in assessing diffuse thyroid pathology.

Keywords: thyroid, elastography, shear-wave elastography, ultrasonography, diffuse

1. Introduction

Optimal thyroid function is necessary for growth and development as well as for reproductive function. Iodine deficiency is the leading cause of thyroid dysfunction. In areas unaffected by iodine deficiency, thyroid dysfunction is due to autoimmunity. Thyroid pathology can be divided into nodular and diffuse pathology. One in 20 Americans will develop a thyroid disorder in their lifetime, with women being seven times more affected than men [1, 2]. In this chapter, we will address diffuse thyroid diseases (DTD) that can be divided into non-autoimmune (subacute thyroiditis, silent thyroiditis) and autoimmune diseases such as Hashimoto thyroiditis (HT) and Graves' disease (GD) [3].

Hashimoto thyroiditis is also known as chronic autoimmune thyroiditis (CAT) is considered the most common endocrine disorder, and autoimmune pathology, as well as it represents the most common cause of hypothyroidism. HT can be divided into primary and secondary based on its etiology. Primary HT includes classic form, juvenile form [4], fibrous form, painless thyroiditis, Hashitoxicosis, and IgG4-related form [5]. Secondary HT is often iatrogenic, for example, caused by interferon [6] or monoclonal antibodies [7]. The diagnosis is established by correlating the clinical manifestations with the presence of antithyroid peroxidase (ATPO) antibodies and antithyroglobulin (ATG) antibodies correlated with the ultrasound aspect. Symptoms may vary from dysphonia, dysphagia, and dyspnea to systemic symptoms of hypothyroidism or may even be absent. The antibodies listed earlier are found in over 95% of HT cases, thus being an important diagnostic criterion [8]. The ultrasound image usually reveals hypoechogenicity and heterogeneity (**Figure 1**).

The presence of fibrous septae may explain the pseudolobulated appearance of the parenchyma. Micronodules may also be present. Increased vascularity may be observed using color Doppler. The volume of the thyroid gland is often increased, but can be normal or even decreased, atrophic in the final stages of the disease [9, 10].

Graves' disease is characterized by the presence of thyrotoxicosis, ophthalmopathy, and goiter, although not all three characteristics are always present. In iodine-sufficient areas, GD accounts for 70–80% of cases of thyrotoxicosis, being more frequent in women over 50 years old. Symptoms of hyperthyroidism include irritability, palpitations, weight loss, shortness of breath, tremor, heat intolerance, sweating, and excessive fatigue. The diagnosis is usually based on anti-TSH-receptor antibodies (TRAB) correlated with the ultrasound appearance [11–13]. The echogenicity is usually decreased, and the appearance is not homogenous. Increased volume and high blood flow may also suggest the diagnosis [10, 12, 14].

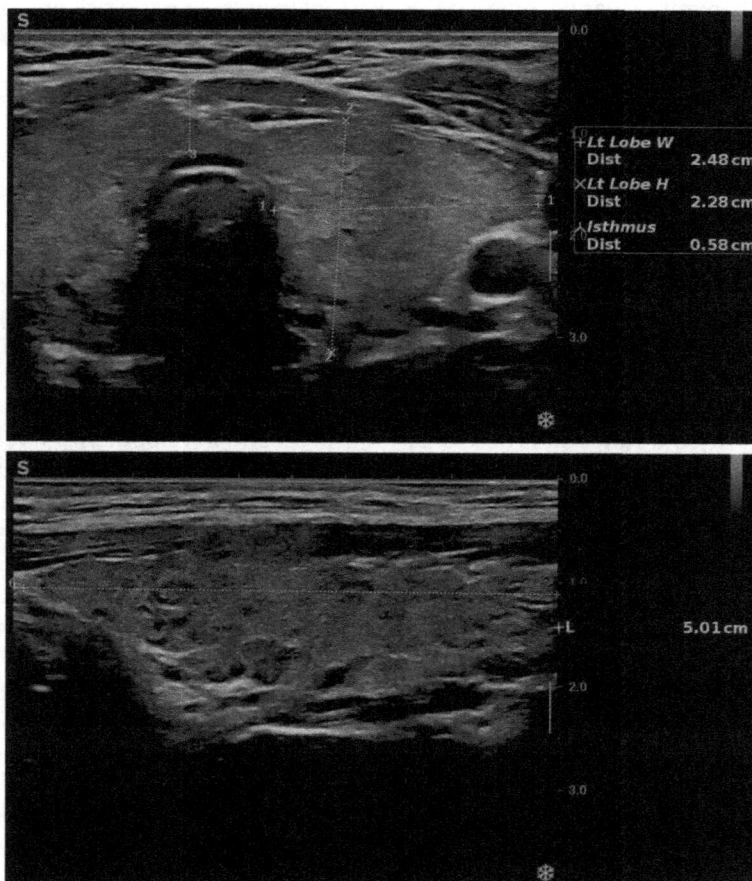

Figure 1.
US image of a patient with CAT.

Subacute thyroiditis (SA) is usually caused by a viral infection with symptoms including mild fever, swelling, and pain in the neck area, irradiating to the ear or jaw and fatigability. Thyroid stimulating hormone (TSH) is usually suppressed and inflammatory markers are elevated [15]. The presence of focal or diffuse hypoechoicity together with diminished vascularization may suggest the diagnosis if it is associated with the mentioned symptoms [16].

Post-partum thyroiditis (PPT) occurs in the first year after giving birth and may occur after an induced or spontaneous abortion. PPT prevalence may vary from 1 to 18%, but usually is reported approximatively 5%. In general, PPT has two evolutionary stages, transient thyrotoxicosis due to tissue destruction followed by the phase of hypothyroidism with or without restauration to euthyroidism [17]. Ultrasonography (US) shows the hypoechogenic inhomogeneous texture of the thyroid with decreased vascularity [18].

The ultrasonographic examination is the most sensitive imaging method for evaluating the thyroid. The most important indications of the US are: confirmation of the presence of thyroid nodules, their measurement and characterization, evaluation of diffuse tissue changes, detection of post-operative residual tumors, screening for the patients at high-risk (multiple endocrine neoplasia, history of thyroid cancer, and neck irradiation), and the guidance of the fine needle aspiration (FNA). US is widely available, non-invasive, and reproducible [19–21].

A relatively new imaging technique is elastography, which adds value by assessing tissue elasticity. There are more types of elastography, but the two most used are strain elastography (SE) and shear-wave elastography (SWE). SE evaluates the stiffness by applying external pressure which deforms the tissue. The deformation is named strain. The pressure being exerted by the operator, SE requires longer training to obtain high-quality images. To measure the stiffness, SWE uses shock waves generated by the machine. Both methods have advantages and disadvantages [22, 23]. SWE will be further described in detail, emphasizing the principles, technique, and the value of this method as well as the peculiarities of diffuse thyroid diseases.

2. Shear-wave elastography

2.1 Principles

SWE technique relies on the production and detection of shear-waves. The wave propagation velocity depends on tissue elasticity. Tissue deformation generated by the production of waves produces changes in the echo pattern. Tissue motion is monitored among the US probe in multiple locations. Shear waves are generated at low frequencies (10–2000 Hz) and their speed (~1–50 m/s) is related to tissue density [22, 24]. SWE is used for evaluation of various tissues: liver [25–27], kidney [28, 29], breast [30, 31], thyroid [32–34], prostate [35], and muscles and tendons [36]. There are three types of dynamic elastography: transient elastography (TE), point shear-wave elastography (pSWE), and 2D-SWE [37].

Transient elastography, usually used for measuring liver stiffness, uses a mechanical push. The wave velocity is proportional to tissue fibrosis. The usefulness of TE was demonstrated in many studies [38, 39].

Compared to the previous technique, point shear-wave elastography has the advantage of image guidance so the operator can choose the best acoustic window to perform the measurements. It is an acoustic radiation force impulse (ARFI)-based method that displays the elasticity as a numerical output (the average speed of shear wave within a region of interest [ROI], expressed in meters per second) [40, 41].

In 2D-SWE, multiple ARFI pulses generate shear waves on a larger area. The machine creates a colored map to display the stiffness. By convention, red is considered stiff and blue is considered soft. Quantitative results are expressed in meters/second (wave propagation speed) or kilo-Pascals (kPa). 2D-SWE is a reproductible, quantitative, and operator-independent technique (**Figure 2**) [42, 43].

2.2 Technique

The SWE evaluation is usually made after the conventional ultrasound examination. The method is non-invasive, completely painless. The subject is asked to stay in a supine position with the head tilted back for better exposure of the neck, without speaking or swallowing. The probe is positioned on one side of the neck, collecting images in longitudinal plane and SWE mode is initiated. The machine displays a color map from blue to red. The subject is asked to hold his/her breath for a few seconds. The image is frozen, and the tissue elasticity is measured and displayed.

2.3 SWE in diffuse thyroid diseases

2.3.1 Hashimoto thyroiditis

Being a common pathology, HT has been studied in detail. In recent years, the elastographic differences between this type of thyroid damage and other diffuse thyroid pathologies have also been studied. A group of Japanese researchers included in a study 229 subjects, healthy controls and patients diagnosed with CAT. The shear-wave velocity (SWV) was measured, and significant differences were observed between

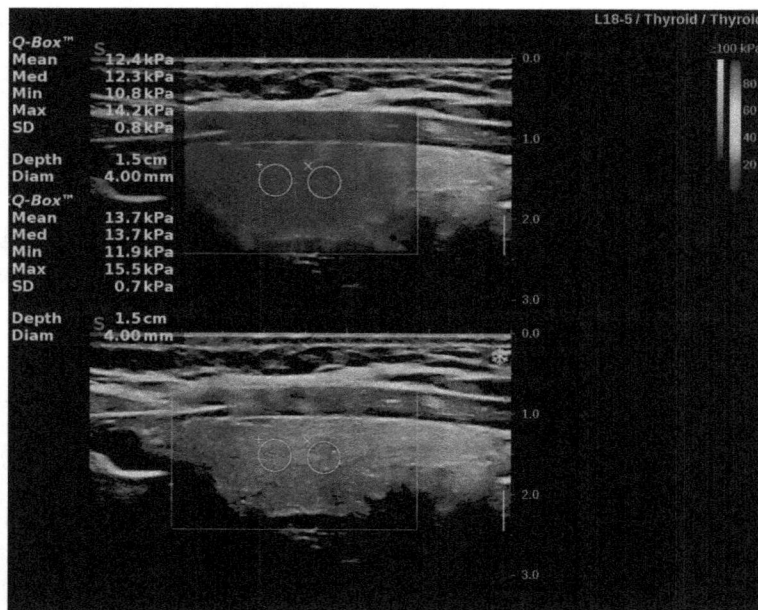

Figure 2.
Normal thyroid tissue—2D SWE.

the two groups (2.47 ± 0.57 m/s for CAT vs. 1.59 ± 0.41 m/s for the control group; $p < 0.001$). The area under the receiver operating characteristics (AUROC) for CAT was 0.899 and the SWV cut-off value was 1.96 m/s. Statistical analysis revealed 87.4% sensitivity (Se), 78.7% specificity (Sp), 74.2% positive predictive value (PPV), 94% negative predictive value (NPV), and 85.1% diagnostic accuracy. No correlation was found between SWV and ATG antibodies (Spearman's ρ = 0.101), but a weak positive correlation was found between SWV and ATPO antibodies (Spearman's correlation coefficient = 0.311) [44].

Similar results were found in a study conducted in Turkey on 50 patients diagnosed with CAT and 40 control subjects. Significant differences were found between the SWV of the two groups (2.56 ± 0.3 m/s vs. 1.63 ± 0.12 ms; $p < 0.001$). A higher cut-off value was found, 2.42 m/s, but lower Se (77%) and Sp (71%). The diagnostic accuracy was 87%, 92% PPV, 81% NPV, and AUROC 0.84 [45]. Differences between thyroid stiffness in normal healthy thyroid compared with HT were also found in a study that compared the mean maximum SWV values (2.36 ± 0.22 m/s vs. 2.08 ± 0.34 m/s; $p = 0.001$). The mean minimum SWV were not statistically different (1.83 ± 0.20 m/s in HT group vs. 1.84 ± 0.3 m/s; $p = 0.884 > 0.5$) [46].

Rahatli et al. compared SWV in three groups of patients: HT, GD, and control subjects. Significant differences were found in SWV (2.5 ± 0.2 m/s for HT group, 2.71 ± 0.22 m/s for GD group and 1.92 ± 0.14 m/s for healthy subjects; $p < 0.001$) [47].

Kara et al. conducted a study on 74 HT patients and 75 healthy controls. They propose cut-off value of 2.15 m/s (Se 85.1%, Sp 78.7%, PPV 79.7%, NPV 84.2%, and diagnostic accuracy 81.8%) and 2.45 kPa (Se 82.4%, Sp 81.3%, PPV 81.3%, NV 82.4%, and diagnostic accuracy 81.8%). The mean values of the elastic index were 25.01 ± 10.53 kPa and 2.70 ± 0.53 m/s for the HT group and 12.49 ± 3.23 kPa and 1.94 ± 0.23 m/s for the control group. A positive correlation was found between SWE values and ATG antibodies. No significant correlation was found between SWE values and ATPO antibodies [48].

Other studies have also observed differences in thyroid stiffness. Ruchala et al. studied groups of patients diagnosed with CAT, SAT, GD, and healthy controls and significant differences were found. The mean values for the CAT group were 36.15 ± 18.7 kPa, higher than values for the control group (16.18 ± 5.4 kPa), $p < 0.0001$ (**Figure 3**) [49].

2.3.2 Graves' disease

Thyroid stiffness was evaluated in a study to compare tissue elasticity in patients diagnosed with GD compared to healthy controls. The study group consisted of 51 patients with GD and 54 volunteers for the control group. The median SWE values were significantly higher compared to those of the control group (17.34 kPa and 2.28 m/s vs. 12.05 kPa and 1.92 m/s; $p < 0.001$ in both comparisons). The cut-off values were 14.5 k Pa (Se 100%, Sp 72.2%, and AUROC 0.931) and 2.15 m/s (Se85.7%, Sp 74.1%, and AUROC 0.888). The SWE values were not correlated with the age of the subject or the duration of the disease. Also, no correlation was found between SWE values and autoantibodies levels ($p > 0.05$). A negative correlation was found between SWE values and TSH values. Between fT3, fT4 levels, and SWE values were found a strong positive correlation [50].

Another study conducted in China on 207 subjects, 45 healthy volunteers and 162 patients with GD concluded that SWE is a useful tool in diagnosing GD. The control group SWE values were significantly lower than those in the GD group. Mean,

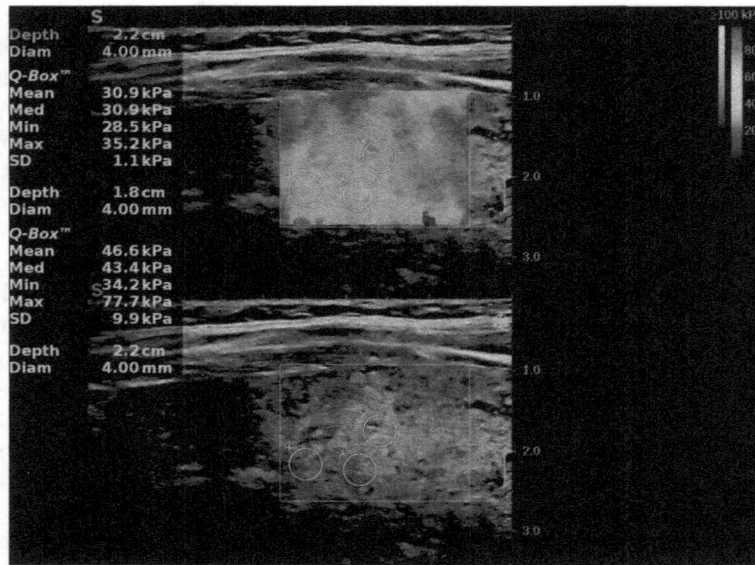

Figure 3.
SWE in CAT.

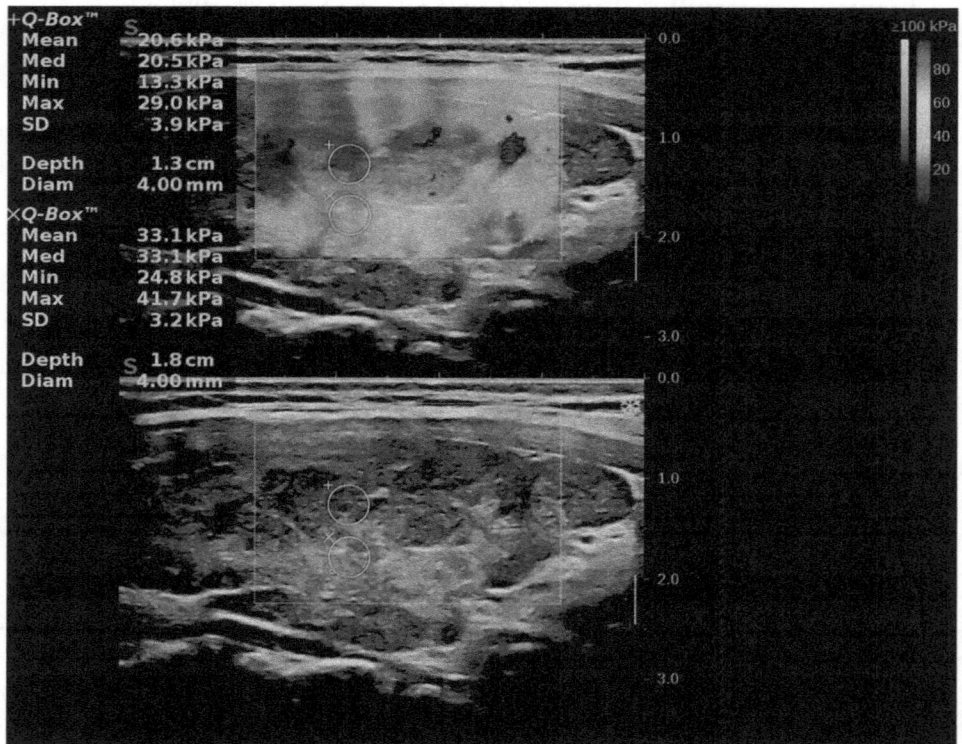

Figure 4.
SWE in GD.

minimum, and maximum values were recorded for each subject. The mean values for the control group were 8.4 ± 2.4 kPa (min); 14.3 ± 2.7 kPa (mean), and 22.1 ± 5.4 kPa (max). GD group values were 10.7 ± 6.4 kPa (min); 17.6 ± 6.4 kPa (mean), and 25.6 ± 10.6 kPa (max); $p < 0.001$. The cut-off value was 15.45 kPa (AUROC 0.656, Se 56.8%, and Sp 71.1%). In contradiction with the previously mentioned study, Li et al. found a positive correlation between SWE values and the duration of the disease, and antibodies serum levels and no correlation between SWE values and fT3, fT4, and THS [51].

Another study published in 2019 evaluated the usefulness of SWE in differentiating thyroid autoimmune diseases. In the GD group, the mean SWV was 2.61 ± 0.32 m/s (range 2.1–3.21 m/s) while in HT group, the mean SWV was 2.85 ± 0.52 m/s (range 2.31–3.82 m/s). The mean SWV value for the control group was 1.75 ± 0.37 m/s (range 1.24–2.36 m/s). The mean values for HT and GD groups were significantly higher than the control group ($p < 0.01$). However, the mean SWV values were higher in the HT group compared to the GD group [52], contrary to the results of the study conducted by Rahatli et al. where higher stiffness was in GD compared to HT [47]. Several studies reported that SWE is not suitable for differentiating GD and CAT even though, both have significantly higher values than the normal thyroid tissue (**Figure 4**) [52–55].

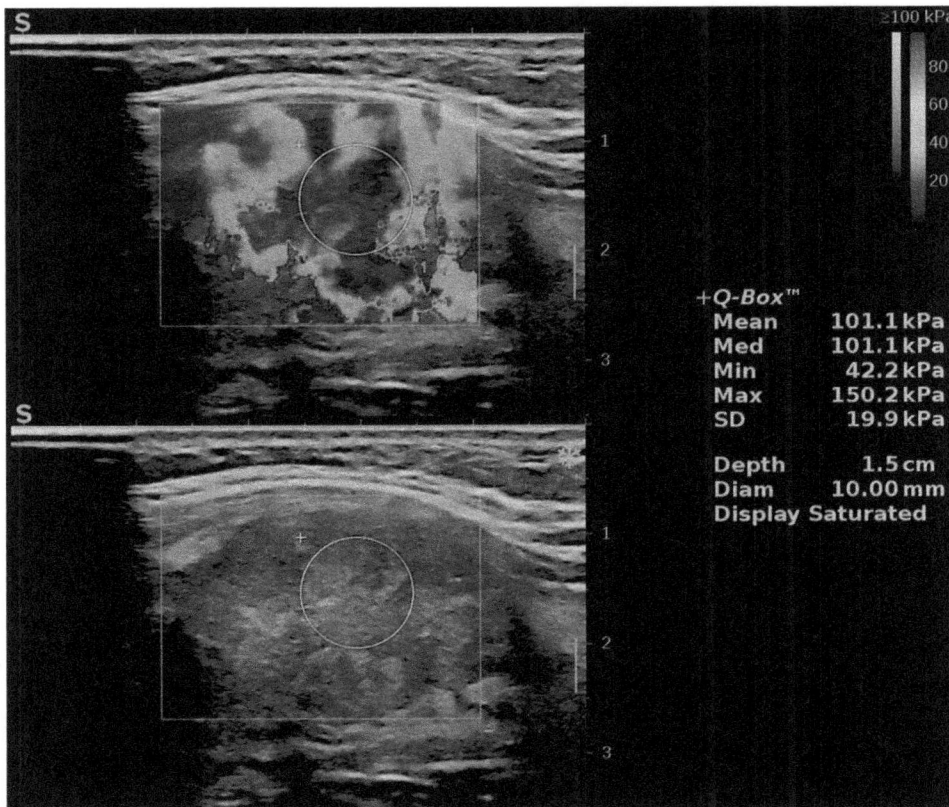

Figure 5.
SWE in subacute thyroiditis.

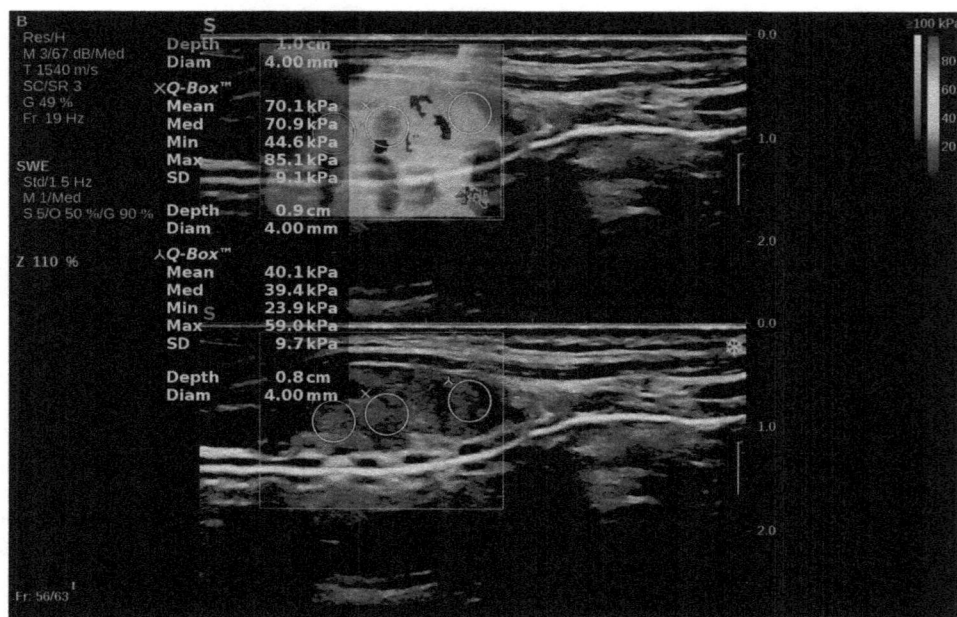

Figure 6.
Radiation-induced thyroiditis.

2.3.3 Subacute thyroiditis

Given the difference in prevalence, studies on subacute thyroiditis are fewer. Ruchala et al. comparatively studied different types of diffuse thyroid damage, including subacute thyroiditis. This study was included two patients with acute thyroiditis, 18 with SAT, 18 with CAT, and 40 healthy controls. Patients diagnosed with SAT were evaluated three times: at baseline, at 4 weeks follow-up and 10 weeks after diagnosing and treatment initiation. There were significant differences between the three measurements: 214.26 ± 32.5 kPa at the baseline, 45.92 ± 17.4 kPa at 4 weeks and 21.65 ± 5.3 kPa at 10 weeks. The thyroid stiffness was significantly higher at baseline in SAT compared to CAT (36.15 ± 18.7 kPa) or healthy control group (16.18 ± 5.4 kPa). Undertreatment, the values were restored close to normal. The SWE values for the two patients with acute thyroiditis equaled 216.6 and 241 kPa and after treatment, it decreased to 17.93 and 85.384 kPa. All evaluated categories had higher stiffness levels than healthy thyroid ($p < 0.0001$) (**Figure 5**) [49].

Liu et al. also studied thyroid stiffness in SAT. The mean SWE values were 118.01 ± 51.02 kPa. However, the time of measurement is not mentioned, only the fact that all SAT patients had hyperthyroidism at the moment of evaluation. The AUROC for differentiating SAT from CAT was 0.989. The AUROC for distinguishing SAT from GD was 0.975 [54].

Both mentioned studies concluded SWE utility in diagnosing SAT and differentiating it from CAT and GD (**Figure 6**).

To the best of our knowledge, no specific papers have been published regarding shear-wave elastography in postpartum thyroiditis or other diffuse thyroid pathologies.

3. Conclusions

The important prevalence of diffuse thyroid diseases makes their imaging assessment essential. SWE proves to be an important tool in the diagnosis and differentiation of diffuse thyroid pathology. However, new studies on larger patient groups are needed to determine exactly whether there are significant differences in elasticity between CAT and GD, as well as have of a consensus on cut-off values.

Conflict of interest

The authors declare no conflict of interest.

Author details

Cristina Mihaela Cepeha[1,2], Andreea Borlea[1,2*], Corina Paul[3], Iulian Velea[3]
and Dana Stoian[2]

1 PhD. School Department, Victor Babes University of Medicine and Pharmacy, Timisoara, Romania

2 Department of Internal Medicine II, Victor Babes University of Medicine and Pharmacy, Timisoara, Romania

3 Department of Pediatrics, Victor Babes University of Medicine and Pharmacy, Timisoara, Romania

*Address all correspondence to: borlea.andreea@umft.ro

IntechOpen

References

[1] Maniakas A, Davies L, Zafereo ME. Thyroid disease around the world. Otolaryngologic Clinics of North America. 2018;**51**:631-642. DOI: 10.1016/j.otc.2018.01.014

[2] Taylor PN, Albrecht D, Scholz A, Gutierrez-Buey G, Lazarus JH, Dayan CM, et al. Global epidemiology of hyperthyroidism and hypothyroidism. Nature Reviews Endocrinology. 2018;**14**:301-316. DOI: 10.1038/nrendo.2018.18

[3] Monaco F. Clinical perspective: Classification of thyroid diseases: Suggestions for a revision. Journal of Clinical Endocrinology and Metabolism. 2003;**88**:1428-1432. DOI: 10.1210/jc.2002-021260

[4] de Luca F, Santucci S, Corica D, Pitrolo E, Romeo M, Aversa T. Hashimoto's thyroiditis in childhood: Presentation modes and evolution over time. Italian Journal of Pediatrics. 2013;**39**:8. DOI: 10.1186/1824-7288-39-8

[5] Li Y, Bai Y, Liu Z, Ozaki T, Taniguchi E, Mori I, et al. Immunohistochemistry of IgG4 can help subclassify Hashimoto's autoimmune thyroiditis. Pathology International. 2009;**59**:636-641. DOI: 10.1111/j.1440-1827.2009.02419.x

[6] Mandac JC, Chaudhry S, Sherman KE, Tomer Y. The clinical and physiological spectrum of interferon-alpha induced thyroiditis: Toward a new classification. Hepatology. 2006;**43**:661-672. DOI: 10.1002/hep.21146

[7] Corsello SM, Barnabei A, Marchetti P, de Vecchis L, Salvatori R, Torino F. Endocrine side effects induced by immune checkpoint inhibitors. The Journal of Clinical Endocrinology and Metabolism. 2013;**98**:1361-1375. DOI: 10.1210/jc.2012-4075

[8] Caturegli P, de Remigis A, Rose NR. Hashimoto thyroiditis: Clinical and diagnostic criteria. Autoimmunity Reviews. 2014;**13**:391-397. DOI: 10.1016/j.autrev.2014.01.007

[9] Chaudhary V, Bano S. Thyroid ultrasound. Indian Journal of Endocrinology and Metabolism. 2013;**17**:219. DOI: 10.4103/2230-8210.109667

[10] Sholosh B, Borhani AA. Thyroid ultrasound part 1: Technique and diffuse disease. Radiologic Clinics of North America. 2011;**49**:391-416. DOI: 10.1016/j.rcl.2011.02.002

[11] Means JH, Littlefield J. Graves' disease. American Practitioner and Digest of Treatment. 1948;**2**:488-493. DOI: 10.1056/nejmra1510030

[12] Menconi F, Marcocci C, Marinò M. Diagnosis and classification of Graves' disease. Autoimmunity Reviews. 2014;**13**:398-402. DOI: 10.1016/j.autrev.2014.01.013

[13] Bartalena L. Diagnosis and management of Graves' disease: A global overview. Nature Reviews Endocrinology. 2013;**9**:724-734. DOI: 10.1038/nrendo.2013.193

[14] Dighe M, Barr R, Bojunga J, Cantisani V, Chammas MC, Cosgrove D, et al. Thyroid ultrasound: State of the art part 1—Thyroid ultrasound reporting and diffuse thyroid diseases. Medical Ultrasonography. 2017;**19**:79. DOI: 10.11152/mu-980

[15] Alfadda AA, Sallam RM, Elawad GE, Aldhukair H, Alyahya MM. Subacute

thyroiditis: Clinical presentation and long term outcome. International Journal of Endocrinology. 2014;**2014**:2. DOI: 10.1155/2014/794943

[16] Frates MM. Subacute granulomatous (de Quervain) thyroiditis: Grayscale and color Doppler sonographic characteristics. JUM. 2013;**32**(3):505-511. DOI: 10.7863/jum.2013.32.3.505

[17] Nguyen CT, Mestman JH. Postpartum thyroiditis. Clinical Obstetrics and Gynecology. 2019;**62**:359-364. DOI: 10.1097/GRF.0000000000000430

[18] Samuels MH. Subacute, silent, and postpartum thyroiditis. Medical Clinics of North America. 2012;**96**:223-233. DOI: 10.1016/j.mcna.2012.01.003

[19] Richman DM, Frates MC. Ultrasound of the normal thyroid with technical pearls and pitfalls. Radiologic Clinics of North America. 2020;**58**:1033-1039. DOI: 10.1016/j.rcl.2020.06.006

[20] Alexander LF, Patel NJ, Caserta MP, Robbin ML. Thyroid ultrasound: Diffuse and nodular disease. Radiologic Clinics of North America. 2020;**58**:1041-1057. DOI: 10.1016/j.rcl.2020.07.003

[21] Germano A, Schmitt W, Carvalho MR, Marques RM. Normal ultrasound anatomy and common anatomical variants of the thyroid gland plus adjacent structures—A pictorial review. Clinical Imaging. 2019;**58**:114-128. DOI: 10.1016/j.clinimag.2019.07.002

[22] Gennisson JL, Deffieux T, Fink M, Tanter M. Ultrasound elastography: Principles and techniques. Diagnostic and Interventional Imaging. 2013;**94**:487-495. DOI: 10.1016/j.diii.2013.01.022

[23] Garra BS. Elastography: History, principles, and technique comparison. Abdominal Imaging. 2015;**40**:680-697. DOI: 10.1007/s00261-014-0305-8

[24] Hoskins PR. Principles of ultrasound elastography. Ultrasound. 2012;**20**:8-15. DOI: 10.1258/ult.2011.011005

[25] Barr RG. Shear wave liver elastography. Abdominal Radiology. 2018;**43**:800-807. DOI: 10.1007/s00261-017-1375-1

[26] Guibal A, Boularan C, Bruce M, Vallin M, Pilleul F, Walter T, et al. Evaluation of shearwave elastography for the characterisation of focal liver lesions on ultrasound. European Radiology. 2013;**23**:1138-1149. DOI: 10.1007/s00330-012-2692-y

[27] Samir AE, Dhyani M, Vij A, Bhan AK, Halpern EF, Méndez-Navarro J, et al. Shear-wave elastography for the estimation of liver fibrosis in chronic liver disease: Determining accuracy and ideal site for measurement. Radiology. 2015;**274**:888-896. DOI: 10.1148/radiol.14140839

[28] Palabiyik FB, Inci E, Turkay R, Bas D. Evaluation of liver, kidney, and spleen elasticity in healthy newborns and infants using shear wave elastography. Journal of Ultrasound in Medicine. 2017;**36**:2039-2045. DOI: 10.1002/jum.14202

[29] Samir AE, Allegretti AS, Zhu Q, Dhyani M, Anvari A, Sullivan DA, et al. Shear wave elastography in chronic kidney disease: A pilot experience in native kidneys. BMC Nephrology. 2015;**16**:119. DOI: 10.1186/s12882-015-0120-7

[30] Evans A, Whelehan P, Thomson K, Brauer K, Jordan L, Purdie C, et al. Differentiating benign from malignant solid breast masses: Value of shear wave elastography according to lesion stiffness

combined with greyscale ultrasound according to BI-RADS classification. British Journal of Cancer. 2012;**107**:224-229. DOI: 10.1038/bjc.2012.253

[31] CebiOlgun D, Korkmazer B, Kilic F, Dikici AS, Velidedeoglu M, Aydogan F, et al. Use of shear wave elastography to differentiate benign and malignant breast lesions. Diagnostic and Interventional Radiology. 2014;**20**:239-244. DOI: 10.5152/dir.2014.13306

[32] Borlea A, Borcan F, Sporea I, Dehelean C, Negrea R, Cotoi L, et al. TI-RADS diagnostic performance: Which algorithm is superior and how elastography and 4D vascularity improve the malignancy risk assessment. Diagnostics. 2020;**10**:180. DOI: 10.3390/diagnostics10040180

[33] Bhatia KSS, Tong CSL, Cho CCM, Yuen EHY, Lee YYP, Ahuja AT. Shear wave elastography of thyroid nodules in routine clinical practice: Preliminary observations and utility for detecting malignancy. European Radiology. 2012;**22**:2397-2406. DOI: 10.1007/s00330-012-2495-1

[34] Borlea A, Stoian D, Cotoi L, Sporea I, Lazar F, Mozos I. Thyroid multimodal ultrasound evaluation—Impact on presurgical diagnosis of intermediate cytology cases. Applied Sciences. 2020;**10**:3439. DOI: 10.3390/app10103439

[35] Woo S, Kim SY, Cho JY, Kim SH. Shear wave elastography for detection of prostate cancer: A preliminary study. Korean Journal of Radiology. 2014;**15**:346. DOI: 10.3348/kjr.2014.15.3.346

[36] Taş S, Onur MR, Yılmaz S, Soylu AR, Korkusuz F. Shear wave elastography is a reliable and repeatable method for measuring the elastic modulus of the rectus femoris muscle and patellar

tendon. Journal of Ultrasound in Medicine. 2017;**36**:565-570. DOI: 10.7863/ultra.16.03032

[37] Ozturk A, Grajo JR, Dhyani M, Anthony BW, Samir AE. Principles of ultrasound elastography. Abdominal Radiology. 2018;**43**:773-785. DOI: 10.1007/s00261-018-1475-6

[38] Wong VW-S, Chan HL-Y. Transient elastography. Journal of Gastroenterology and Hepatology. 2010;**25**:1726-1731. DOI: 10.1111/j.1440-1746.2010.06437.x

[39] Jung KS, Kim SU. Clinical applications of transient elastography. Clinical and Molecular Hepatology. 2012;**18**:163. DOI: 10.3350/cmh.2012.18.2.163

[40] Joo I, Kim SY, Park HS, Lee ES, Kang HJ, Lee JM. Validation of a new point shear-wave elastography method for noninvasive assessment of liver fibrosis: A prospective multicenter study. Korean Journal of Radiology. 2019;**20**:1527. DOI: 10.3348/kjr.2019.0109

[41] Ferraioli G, Tinelli C, Lissandrin R, Zicchetti M, Dal Bello B, Filice G, et al. Point shear wave elastography method for assessing liver stiffness. World Journal of Gastroenterology. 2014;**20**:4787-4796. DOI: 10.3748/wjg.v20.i16.4787

[42] Xu H-X, Yan K, Liu B-J, Liu W-Y, Tang L-N, Zhou Q, et al. Guidelines and recommendations on the clinical use of shear wave elastography for evaluating thyroid nodule. Clinical Hemorheology and Microcirculation. 2019;**72**:39-60. DOI: 10.3233/CH-180452

[43] Liu B, Liang J, Zheng Y, Xie X, Huang G, Zhou L, et al. Two-dimensional shear wave elastography as promising diagnostic tool for predicting malignant thyroid nodules: A prospective

Chapter 13

Elastography Methods in the Prediction of Malignancy in Thyroid Nodules

Andreea Borlea, Laura Cotoi, Corina Paul, Felix Bende and Dana Stoian

Abstract

Ultrasonography provides a primary stratification of the malignancy risk of thyroid nodules for selecting those that need further evaluation by fine-needle aspiration cytology (FNAC). Ultrasound elastography (USE) methods have been more recently proposed as a promising tool, aiming to increase the accuracy of baseline ultrasound. By means of USE, stiffness is assessed as an indicator of malignancy. Strain elastography was the first method used in thyroid imaging, with very good accuracy in discerning thyroid cancer. More recently, 2D shear-wave elastography also confirmed to be a valuable tool with similar outcomes. The advantages, limitations, and technical details of the elastography methods currently used in assessing thyroid morphology, particularly thyroid nodules, will be presented and compared in this chapter.

Keywords: thyroid imaging, elastography, strain, shear wave, malignancy risk

1. Introduction

Thyroid nodules are among the most common thyroid pathologies, and their etiology is diverse [1, 2]. They represent masses of abnormal proliferation, formation, and structure within the thyroid parenchyma [3]. The prevalence of thyroid nodules increases with age, reaching up to 50% after 65 years, and they are more commonly found in women [4]. The diagnosis of nodules less than 1 cm, as well as lesions with a deep location, is most commonly missed at physical examination; thus, thyroid imaging techniques have drawn increasing clinical attention [5]. Conventional neck ultrasound (US) is still the preferred method for assessing thyroid morphology, including the presence and appearance of thyroid nodules [6–9].

Thyroid cancer accounts for the most common endocrine malignancy, with a slowly increasing incidence [10, 11]. Its prevalence reaches 7–15% in the group of thyroid nodules [12], and it does remain one of the cancers with the least risk of death [13]. There are certain categories considered at greater risk for cancer, such as young adults, children, and patients with a history of neck irradiation [14]. Size also seems to impact the prevalence of malignancy; nodules larger than 2 cm were more often

IntechOpen

malignant compared to smaller lesions [15], but multinodular goiters do not seem to increase the likelihood of malignancy [16].

Fine-needle aspiration cytology (FNAC) represents the procedure of choice for further examining the thyroid lesions with high-risk features documented by means of clinical or US evaluation [17]. Thyroid cytology is most commonly reported using the Bethesda classification (I-VI), with different prediction of malignancy for each category, which is meant to guide the case management decision [18]. A less aggressive approach to diagnosis and treatment was introduced starting with the 2015 American Thyroid Association (ATA) guidelines, which advise reducing FNAC indications and endorse "active surveillance" of tumors with very low risk [19].

Ultrasound elastography (USE) proved to be a valuable imaging tool in predicting the risk of malignancy of thyroid nodules [20, 21] and also in decreasing the FNAC indication [17, 22]. It assesses tissue distortion in reply to stress, assuming that a hard lesion presents an increased likelihood of cancer.

2. Ultrasound of the neck

The current recommendations regarding the stratification of risk for Thyroid nodules (TN) include a thorough anamnesis, clinical evaluation, and neck US characterization. The B-mode (2B) evaluation is performed using linear probes, with high frequency (7.5–15 MHz) for excellent details and a resolution of 0.7–1 mm up to 5-cm depth. In most of the cases, frequencies of 10–14 MHz or higher are preferred, and linear transducers with lower frequency are required in selected cases, ensuring depth penetration [23, 24].

High-resolution US is the most widely used evaluation of thyroid nodules, both for screening purposes and in presurgical settings [25–27]. US of the neck currently represents the most affordable, sensitive, and efficient imaging method for evaluating thyroid morphology, and it is widely available; its role in differentiating cancerous nodules from nonmalignant ones is crucial [19, 28–30].

Considering the large accessibility to US equipment, the current trend is to have standardized homogeneous reports, describing the general aspect of the thyroid, its volume, the presence or the absence of nodules, the number of nodules, their size, position, extracapsular relations, and the following US characteristics: internal composition (solid, cystic, or mixed), shape, margins, echogenicity, echotexture, the presence of echogenic foci, and the Doppler vascular pattern [31].

Certain US features [24, 32–35] have been described to be highly specific for malignancy, such as solid or mostly solid composition, the presence of microcalcifications, spiculated margins, markedly hypoechoic texture, extrathyroidal extension, and "taller than wide" shape, namely, the vertical diameter exceeds the transverse one. These findings are established especially for papillary carcinomas [36]. The US characteristics of follicular cancers are highly similar to follicular adenomas, and no typical appearance was described for medullary thyroid cancer (MTC), but some small studies found that half of the studied MTCs were solid, and hypoechoic and microcalcifications were more prevalent (16%) than in the benign controls [37]. Benignity-related features include smooth margins, a spongiform appearance, and completely cystic composition [38]. **Figure 1** displays the images of US low- and high-risk thyroid nodules.

After the comprehensive examination of thyroid morphology, the presence of cervical lymph nodes (LNs), their number, and appearance should be looked for,

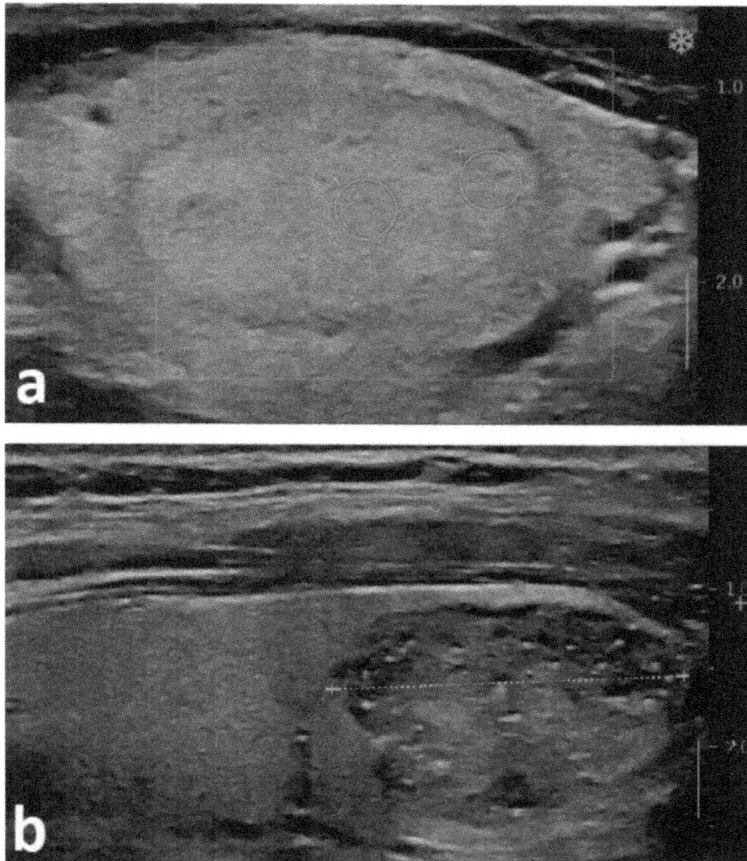

Figure 1.
B-mode image of a thyroid nodule with (a) low-risk US appearance (oval-shaped, isoechoic, peripheral halo, regular margins), benign nodule and (b) high-risk US appearance (inhomogeneous, hypoechoic, punctate echoic foci, and irregular borders), papillary thyroid cancer.

particularly in cases with intermediate- and high-risk nodules [9]. Hilum absence does not diagnose malignancy, but its presence removes its suspicion [39]. An enlarged short-axis diameter is predictive of malignancy, but it is not relevant for the long axis [39–42]. When evaluating multinodular goiters, all the lesions should be described, and their appearance should be assessed in all the cases. If more than one nodule presents features of risk, each of them should be further assessed by FNAC [7, 8, 24].

The concept of thyroid imaging reporting and data system (TI-RADS) was introduced by Horvath et al. in 2009 [43]; these quantitative US classifications are currently used for a more accurate stratification of the US risk of malignancy [44–46].

3. Elastography in the evaluation of thyroid nodules

US elastography noninvasively estimates the stiffness of a thyroid nodule by measuring the tissue displacement, respectively, the internal or external mechanic constraint induced to the tissue. The distortion appears when the nodule is compressed by a controlled external pressure, as in strain imaging, or the shear waves (SWs) induced by the US probe itself—in shear-wave elastography (SWE) [9]. It grants for "virtual palpation" of the thyroid nodules, which otherwise may not be palpable. Stiff nodules are considered to have an increased risk due to the desmoplastic transformation, disclosing firm, and tumor stroma, characterized by abundant myofibroblasts and collagen fibers [47].

Thyroid elastography was recognized starting with the 2016 American Association of Clinical Endocrinology (AACE) guidelines in the diagnosis of thyroid nodules, complementary to grayscale, and importantly, they do recommend that stiff nodules should be further evaluated by FNAC [48]. It is imperative to take into account the recommendations formulated by the 2017 World Federation for Ultrasound in Medicine and Biology (WFUMB) guidelines on the clinical use of ultrasound elastography in thyroid diseases, which validate the use of USE as an additional tool in thyroid evaluation, no matter the technique [24]. Thyroid elastography was also employed for diffuse diseases, including autoimmune thyroid disease, aiming to assess the severity of fibrosis [49]. As for multinodular goiter, elastography should be used to assess the firmness of each nodule within the thyroid, when the technique is available to the examiner [7, 24]. Together with color Doppler evaluation, it can be of help, when aiming to distinguish between one heterogeneous nodule and the aspect of multiple overlaid lesions appearing as one.

Currently available elastography techniques have various limitations related to the shear properties of the tissue. Nonetheless, in some cases, they may be complementing each other [20]. Elastography can be easily used in the assessment of the thyroid gland taking into account its conveniently superficial position, but it is still not largely embraced in practice, nor comprised in all the risk stratification systems [24].

Still, there are some open questions: Could we upgrade the risk category in nodules with high stiffness, as suggested by the previous mentioned guidelines? Is there a recommended threshold for qualitative measurements suggestive for a special risk category, as seen in breast elastography guidelines, which elastography technique should we use?

3.1 Strain elastography

Strain elastography (SE) was the first to be used, and it proved to be of great value in thyroid imaging. It displays tissue stiffness, defined as the difference in length along compression divided by the length ahead of compression. Elasticity is expressed as the Young's modulus, the relation between the stress that is applied and strain ($E = stress/strain$) [20]. The compression can be external, slightly applied manually by the operator and verified by the US machine scale (**Figure 2**); it can be generated by acoustic radiation force impulse (ARFI), or it can be internal, endogenous, by minimal physiologic movement (vascular pulsations and muscle contraction) [20, 50]. The direct quantification of stress is not attainable by the US machines, and strain is displayed relatively through elastograms [51].

3.1.1 Qualitative SE

The first approach in evaluating strain elastograms (**Figure 3**) is through qualitative pattern-based scoring systems such as the ones described by Asteria et al. [52] on a scale from 1 to 4, with scores 3 and 4 being usually considered suggestive for malignancy and the four-pattern score by Rago et al. [53], where high risk includes scores 4

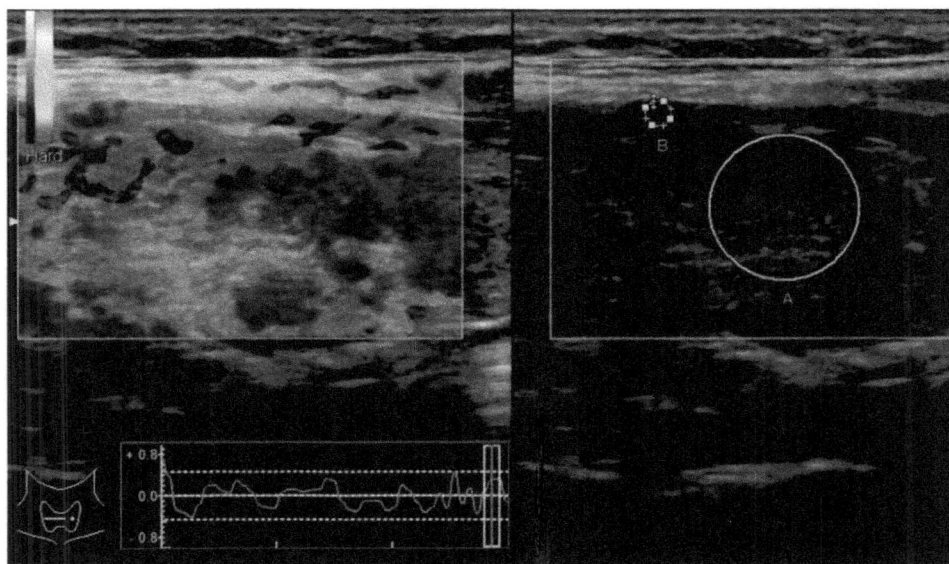

Figure 2.
Pressure scale (bottom, left) for acquiring optimal elasticity images. Elastogram obtained on a Hitachi Preirus device.

and 5. The color-map display settings are not currently standardized, and elastograms are carefully interpreted in accordance with the legend on the screen.

Qualitative elastography proved very good diagnostic quality [54, 55]. A meta-analysis that comprised 20 studies assessing the diagnostic value of SE in discriminating cancerous nodules and even its role in reducing FNACs presented a pooled specificity (Sp) of 80%, a sensitivity (Se) of 85%, the positive predictive value (PPV) of 40%, and the negative predictive value (NPV) of 97% [30, 55].

Nevertheless, some authors reported poor inter- and intraobserver agreement for qualitative elastograms [56], but the results were improved for studies using the carotid pulsations (k = 0.79) [57].

3.1.2 Semiquantitative SE

The strain ratio (SR) (**Figure 4**) provides a numeric value that offers a more objective approach, with less interobserver variability (k = 0.95 [58]) and easier to learn. This semiquantitative parameter is obtained by comparing two manually selected regions of interest (ROIs) within the same captured image, ideally located at the same depth: the first one on the target nodule and the second one on the adjacent reference thyroid parenchyma [59]. Neighboring muscle may be used in cases when thyroid gland is affected by a diffuse disease or there is not enough thyroid tissue found in the image.

SE showed encouraging results in predicting thyroid malignancy, with improved performance over time. A 2013 meta-analysis including 24 studies yielded better diagnostic performance for SE compared to conventional US features (Se = 82% and Sp = 82% for the qualitative score and Se = 89% and Sp = 82% for the strain ratio) [60]. A 2017 meta-analysis reported Se = 84% and Sp = 90% [61]. The cutoff values for the SR in real-time elastography vary in different studies and with the equipment

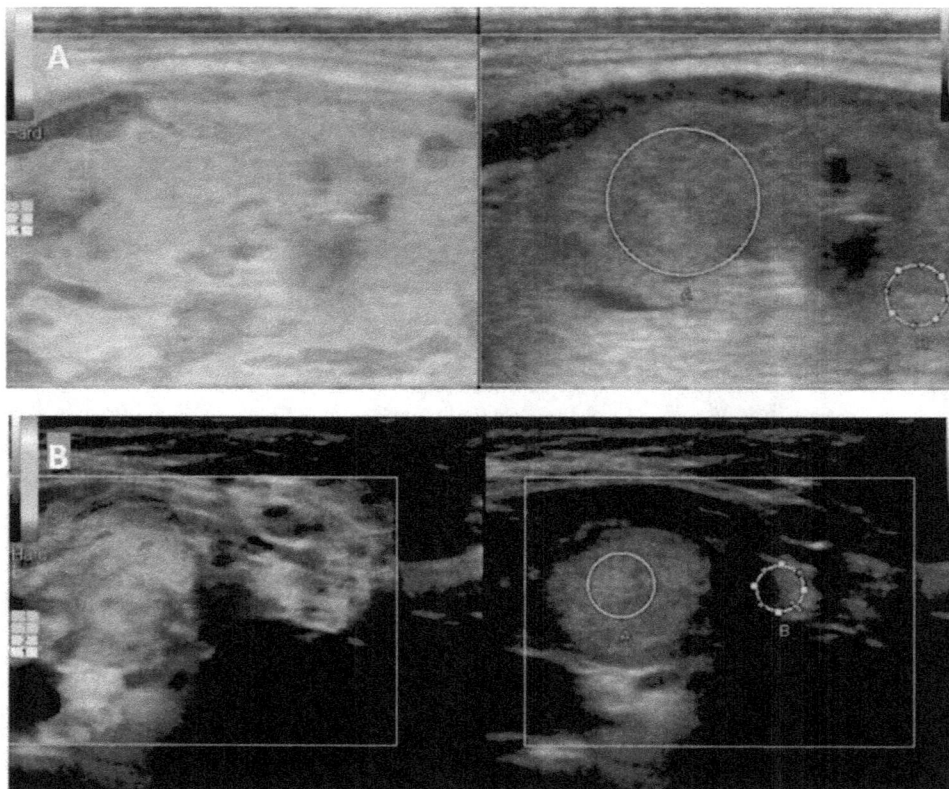

Figure 3.
Qualitative strain elastograms: A—Soft nodule, Asteria 1, benign nodule; B—Mostly stiff nodule, Asteria 3, papillary carcinoma (Hitachi Preirus equipment—The color blue displays hard tissue).

that was used: SR > 4 with 96% specificity and 82% sensitivity [62]; SR >2.7 with 93.6% accuracy [63]; SR > 2 with 93.8% accuracy [64]; SR > 2.45 with 73.9% sensitivity and 73% specificity; and SR > 4 with 95% accuracy [65].

3.1.3 2B us + SE

An approach combining conventional US and elastography was proposed. Initially, results were conflicting. Moon et al. found no significant improvement in diagnosis when combining the two imaging methods [66]. However, other studies found excellent results when adding SE to the standard US evaluation. Trimboli et al. reported for the combined assessment Se = 97% and NPV = 97% versus US-only Se = 85% and NPV = 91% [67]. Russ et al. presented a TI-RADS classification including SE parameter "stiffness" in the risk-assessment strategy, obtaining increased sensitivity (96.7% vs. 92.5%), but decreased specificity [68].

The role of strain elastography was assessed for the category of micronodules (less than 10-mm diameter). A small study including 86 patients demonstrated the value of the technique in detecting microcarcinomas with good diagnostic value in area under the receiver operating characteristic (AUROC): 0.743, with the sensitivity (Se) of 88.9% and the specificity (Sp) of 89.3%. In addition, the missed diagnosis rate was significantly lower for SE compared to conventional ultrasound ($p < 0.05$) [3].

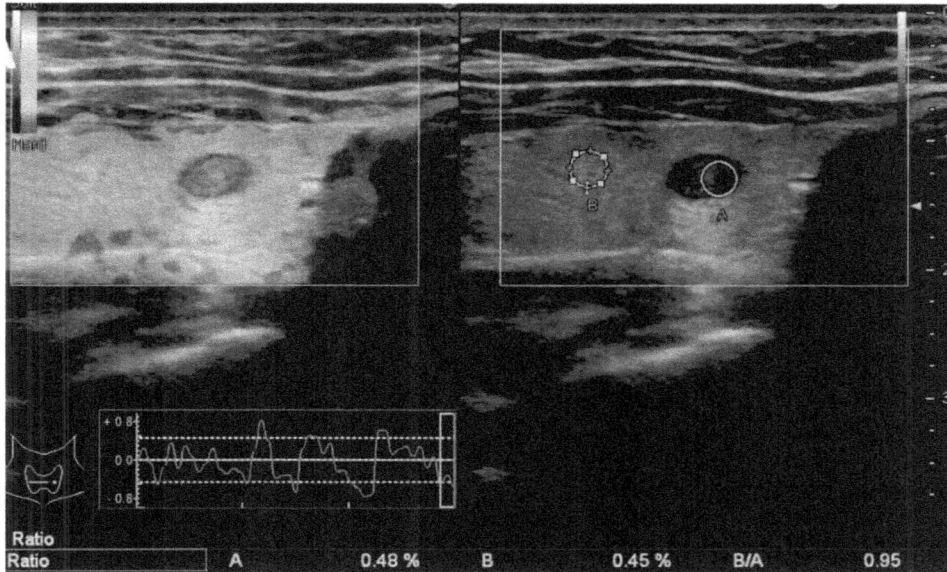

Figure 4.
Strain ratio—Nodule-to-parenchyma—Is 0.95. Soft nodule, similar strain as reference neighboring thyroid tissue; benign micronodule.

Some of the drawbacks of the technique consist in its subjectivity and its dependency on the operator and on compressibility [61]. Some authors outlined an altered performance for nodules bigger than 3 cm, as well as for very small ones, and for coalescent nodules [22, 24, 69].

Increased stiffness can be identified in benign nodules with fibrosis or coarse calcification, generating false-positive results [70, 71]. **Figure 5** illustrates an artifact generated by intranodular calcification that may falsely indicate a stiff thyroid nodule.

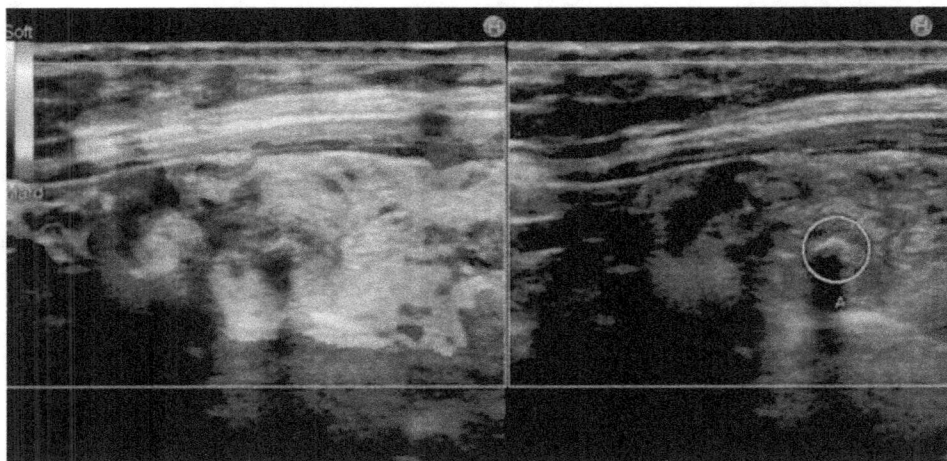

Figure 5.
SE false-positive result: Intranodular calcification in the ROI.

Presently, it is well established that follicular carcinomas may appear misleadingly elastic in SE; therefore, elastography may not be appropriate for diagnosing this particular category (44% false-negative results); other nonpapillary cancers or metastasis may also be soft [24, 70].

3.2 Shear-wave elastography

Shear-wave elastography provides the quantitative measurement that SE does not offer. It is also less dependent on the operator and, consequently, is more reproducible [72]. These dynamic techniques comprise ARFI imaging, point-SWE (pSWE), and 2D-SWE, and rely on acoustic impulses from the US probe that induce tissue movement and generate transverse shear waves. The quantitative elasticity measurement is obtained by assessing the shear wave speed, measured in meters per second or the elasticity index (Young's module) measured in kilopascals [21, 50].

Transient elastography integrates the US transducer and an exterior vibrating "punch" to create shear waves. It is largely employed (FibroScan and Echosens) for evaluating liver fibrosis but is not feasible for thyroid evaluation [73].

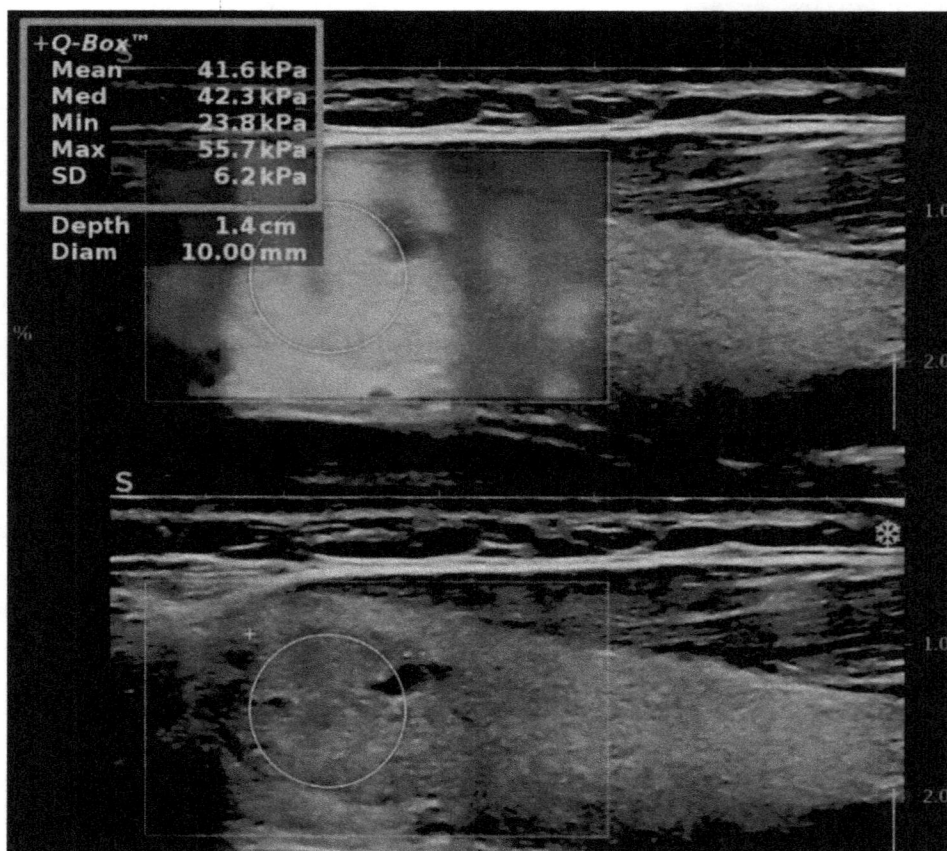

Figure 6.
2D-SWE elasticity parameters of a thyroid nodule with stiff areas displayed by the Hologic SuperSonic Mach 30 equipment, Aixplorer. Q-box parameters: EI mean = 41.6 kPa; med = 42.3 kPa; min = 23.8 kPa, max = 55.7 kPa; standard deviation (SD) = 6.2 kPa; ROI at 1.4-cm depth; ROI diameter = 10 mm.

In monoplane SWE (point-SWE—pSWE), the ARFI mechanically stimulates the tissue in the ROI applying acoustic push pulses that create local tissue displacement in the axially and shear wave (SW) velocity is estimated (m/s), providing a numerical value (Siemens, VirtualTouch Quantification, VTQ; Phillips ElastPQ) [73].

Biplane SWE (2D SWE) and 3D SWE provide a real-time imaging of a quantitative color elastogram superimposed over 2B images and an estimation of SW speed. Supersonic shear wave employs focused ultrasonic beams, which spread through the entire imaging region and show on a color map the speed of the SW or plainly the

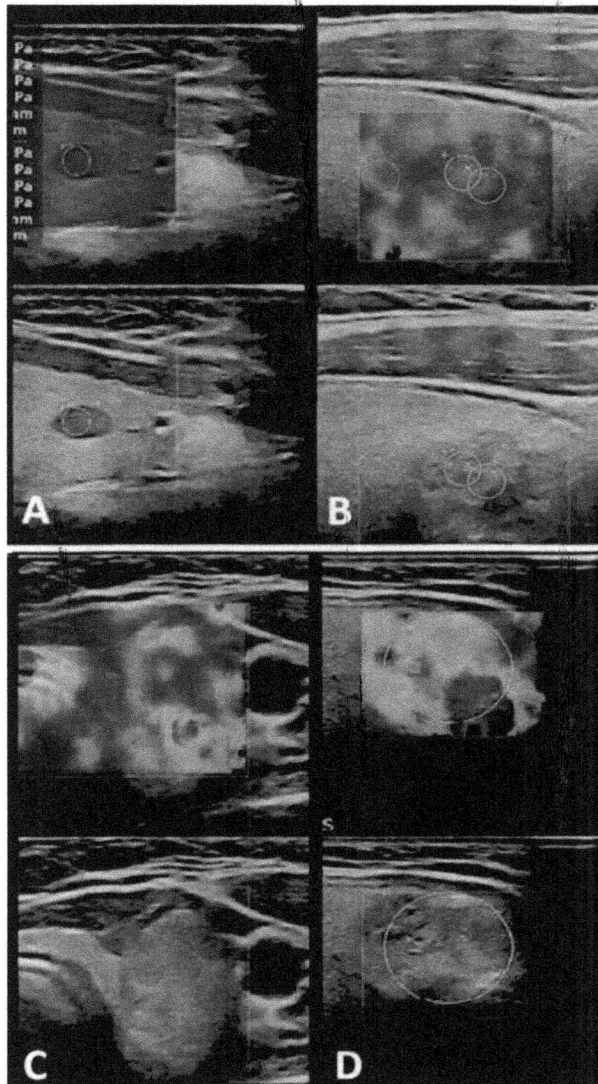

Figure 7.
2D SWE qualitative images: Negative results: A—Entirely soft nodule (homogeneously blue) and B—Mostly soft nodule (heterogeneously blue with green spots), and positive results: C—Nodule with stiff areas (heterogeneous, with patches green, yellow, and red) and D—Completely stiff nodules (heterogeneous multicolored with irregular red, orange, green, and blue areas).

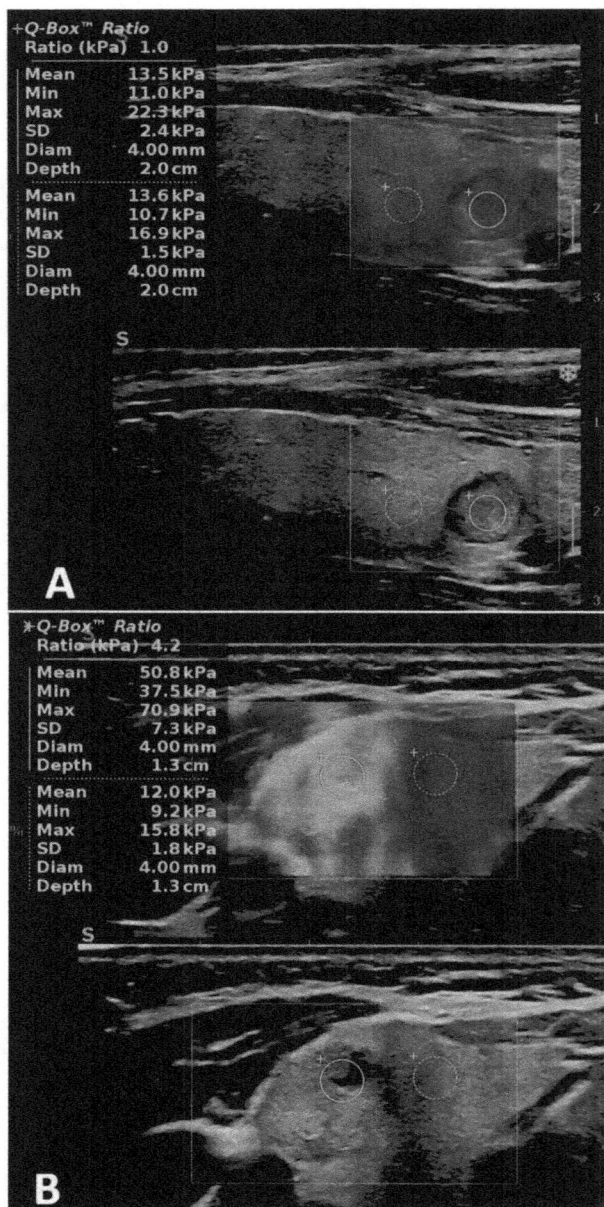

Figure 8.
The nodule-to parenchyma SWE ratio measured on a Hologic Supersonic Mach 30 device—The Q-box ratio. A— Soft nodule, elasticity similar to surrounding healthy thyroid tissue (EI mean = 13.5 kPA and Q-box ratio = 1); B—Nodule with heterogeneous elasticity map, with stiffer areas with EI mean = 50.8 kPa and Q-box ratio = 4.2.

elasticity index (kPa) for each pixel in the ROI. A set of parameters can be quantified in the ROI: the maximum, minimum, and mean E, and the standard deviation, as displayed in **Figure 6** [72, 73]. Currently accessible available technologies on US equipment include: SuperSonic Imagine—2D-SWE; Siemens—Virtual Touch Imaging Quantification, VTIQ; Toshiba—Acoustic Structure Quantification; Philips—SWE; and GE Healthcare—2D-SWE [73].

The qualitative assessment can be made also for 2D SWE. A group from China proposed a modified four-category scale adapted to the physical characteristics of SWE technique and measurements. Patterns 1 (homogeneous lesion with no meaningful color signal corresponding to high stiffness) and 2 (high stiffness signal limited to the capsule surroundings) are interpreted as low risk. Patterns 3 (marginal stiffness) and 4 (interior stiffness) are viewed as high risk; the authors described a very good diagnostic value with 89.1% sensitivity, 74.6% specificity, and the AUROC of 0.79 [74].

A standardized, systematic assessment of qualitative, color-coded elasticity maps is of great importance for discarding artifacts and ensuring reliable quantitative measurements of elasticity [21, 75]. **Figure 7** illustrates the examples of 2D SWE images for soft (A, B) and hard (C, D) thyroid nodules.

Comparable to SE, an SWE ratio can be generated by comparing the stiffness of the nodule to the bordering normal parenchyma or neighboring muscle [24]. **Figure 8** displays the SWE ratio on a SuperSonic Mach 30 machine (the Q-Box™ ratio).

The cutoff values for the elasticity index reported in SWE studies are also different. For Supersonic 2D SWE, the most accurate parameter, as described in most studies, was the E mean, and a poorer diagnostic value was obtained for the E mean. For the E mean, the following cutoffs were reported: ≥ 42.1 kPa with 76.9% sensitivity and 71.1% specificity [76]; ≥ 65 kPa with 71% accuracy [77]; ≥ 39.2 kPa with 81% accuracy [78]; ≥ 34.5 kPa with 84% sensitivity, 78% specificity, and 82% accuracy [79]; and ≥ 24.6 kPa with 84% accuracy [80]. The evaluation is not standardized; thus, the number of determinations varied between 3 and 10 per patient; the size of the ROI also varied between 2 mm and 10 mm in the reported studies.

4. Strain versus shear-wave elastography

Both SE and SWE are efficacious instruments in the stratification of malignancy risk in thyroid nodules, used complementary to grayscale assessment, as specified by the European Federation of Societies for Ultrasound in Medicine and Biology (EFSUMB) guidelines and proven by diverse studies [24], with a broad range of values for sensitivity and specificity resulting from the comparison of the two elastography methods.

Although the majority of literature data suggest that SE is slightly superior in diagnosing thyroid cancer, there is presently no consensus about which technique is superior, and both SWE and SE demonstrated to present important additional value to the classic US assessment in the preoperative examination strategy for thyroid nodules.

To date, only a few small studies have provided a head-to-head comparison of SE and SWE in the same population. More data are available for comparing the two methods. A large meta-analysis including 71 studies and 16,624 patients revealed that SE is hardly better in discriminating thyroid malignancy. The pooled results included the sensitivity of 82.9% for SE and of 78.4% for SWE and the pooled specificity of 82.8% for SE and of 82.4% for SWE [81]. Another meta-analysis assessing 22 studies revealed a pooled sensitivity of 79% (95% confidence interval (CI): 0.730–0.840) and a specificity of 87% (95% CI: 0.790–0.920) for SWE. On the other hand, a pooled sensitivity of 84% (95% CI: 0.760–0.900) and a specificity of 90% (95% CI: 0.850–0.940) were reported for SE, considerably higher than the values recorded for SWE ($p < 0.05$) [61].

2D SWE evaluation is superior when it comes to the assessment of nodules that coexist with thyroid autoimmunity, while SE has lower feasibility in this particular setting [81, 82]. The operator's experience in performing each technique is essential, especially for strain elastography evaluation, as SWE proved better reproducibility. Even so, factors such as the manual compression on the US probe may influence the measurements. In SWE, the most common evaluation errors are artifacts generated by the operator. For these reasons, although SWE is easier to learn, it is important that both the elastography techniques are always performed by experienced examiners [83].

5. Conclusions

Thyroid elastography is a promising instrument for the assessment of thyroid nodules and the detection of thyroid malignancy, regardless of the technique. It does improve the diagnostic confidence in thyroid imaging and helps achieve the final purpose: an accurate selection of the nodules that are at risk and need further management from the ones that are at low risk and benefit from follow-up.

Conflict of interest

The authors declare no conflict of interest.

Author details

Andreea Borlea*, Laura Cotoi, Corina Paul, Felix Bende and Dana Stoian
University of Medicine and Pharmacy "Victor Babes", Timisoara, Romania

*Address all correspondence to: borlea.andreea@umft.ro

IntechOpen

References

[1] Mortensen JD, Woolner LB, Bennett WA. Gross and microscopic findings in clinically normal thyroid glands. The Journal of Clinical Endocrinology and Metabolism. 1955;15(10):1270-1280

[2] Zhou Y, Chen H, Qiang J, Wang D. Systematic review and meta-analysis of ultrasonic elastography in the diagnosis of benign and malignant thyroid nodules. Gland Surgery. 2021;10(9):2734-2744

[3] Wang J, Wei W, Guo R. Ultrasonic elastography and conventional ultrasound in the diagnosis of thyroid micro-nodules. Pakistan Journal of Medical Sciences. 2019;35(6):1526-1531

[4] Grani G, Sponziello M, Pecce V, Ramundo V, Durante C. Contemporary thyroid nodule evaluation and management. The Journal of Clinical Endocrinology and Metabolism. 2020;105(9):2869-2883

[5] Egset AV, Holm C, Larsen SR, Nielsen SH, Bach J, Helweg-Larsen JP, et al. Risk of malignancy in fine-needle aspiration biopsy in patients with thyroid nodules. Danish Medical Journal. 2017;64(2):A5320

[6] Gharib H, Papini E, Paschke R, Duick DS, Valcavi R, Hegedüs L, et al. AACE/AME/ETA Task force on thyroid nodules. American Association of Clinical Endocrinologists, Associazione Medici Endocrinologi, and European Thyroid Association medical guidelines for clinical practice for the diagnosis and management of thyroid nodules: executive summary of recommendations. J Endocrinol Invest. 2010;33(5 Suppl): 51-56. PMID: 20543551

[7] Yi KH. The revised 2016 Korean thyroid association guidelines for thyroid nodules and cancers: Differences from the 2015 American Thyroid Association guidelines. Endocrinology and Metabolism. 2016;31(3):373-378. DOI: 10.3803/EnM.2016.31.3.373

[8] Alexander EK, Pearce EN, Brent GA, Brown RS, Chen H, Dosiou C, et al. 2017 guidelines of the American Thyroid Association for the diagnosis and Management of Thyroid Disease during Pregnancy and the postpartum. Thyroid. 2017;27(3):315-389. DOI: 10.1089/thy.2016.0457

[9] Russ G, Bonnema SJ, Erdogan MF, Durante C, Ngu R, Leenhardt L. European thyroid association guidelines for ultrasound malignancy risk stratification of thyroid nodules in adults: The EU-TIRADS. European Thyroid Journal. 2017;6(5):225-237

[10] Olaleye O, Ekrikpo U, Moorthy R, Lyne O, Wiseberg J, Black M, et al. Increasing incidence of differentiated thyroid cancer in south East England: 1987-2006. European Archives of Oto-Rhino-Laryngology. 2011;268(6):899-906

[11] Davies L, Welch HG. Current thyroid cancer trends in the United States. JAMA Otolaryngology. Head & Neck Surgery. 2014;140(4):317-322

[12] Pellegriti G, Frasca F, Regalbuto C, Squatrito S, Vigneri R. Worldwide increasing incidence of thyroid cancer: Update on epidemiology and risk factors. Journal of Cancer Epidemiology. 2013;2013:965212

[13] Roman BR, Morris LG, Davies L. The thyroid Cancer epidemic, 2017 perspective. Current Opinion in Endocrinology, Diabetes, and Obesity. 2017;24(5):332

[14] Kwong N, Medici M, Angell TE, Liu X, Marqusee E, Cibas ES, et al. The influence of patient age on thyroid nodule formation, multinodularity, and thyroid cancer risk. The Journal of Clinical Endocrinology and Metabolism. 2015 Dec;100(12):4434-4440. DOI: 10.1210/jc.2015-3100. [Epub Oct 14, 2015]. PMID: 26465395; PMCID: PMC4667162

[15] Shin JJ, Caragacianu D, Randolph GW. Impact of thyroid nodule size on prevalence and post-test probability of malignancy: A systematic review. The Laryngoscope. 2015;125(1):263-272

[16] Sipos JA. Advances in ultrasound for the diagnosis and Management of Thyroid Cancer. Thyroid. 2009;19(12) 1363-1372. DOI: 10.1089/thy.2009.1608

[17] Mehrotra P, McQueen A, Kolla S, Johnson SJ, Richardson DL. Does elastography reduce the need for thyroid FNAs? Clinical Endocrinology. 2012;78(6):942-949. DOI: 10.1111/cen.12077

[18] Cibas ES, Ali SZ. The 2017 Bethesda system for reporting thyroid cytopathology. Journal of the American Society of Cytopathology. 2017 Nov; 27(11):1341-1346. DOI: 10.1089/thy.2017.0500. PMID: 2909157

[19] Haugen BR, Alexander EK, Bible KC, Doherty GM, Mandel SJ, Nikiforov YE, et al. 2015 American Thyroid Association management guidelines for adult patients with thyroid nodules and differentiated thyroid Cancer: The American Thyroid Association guidelines task force on thyroid nodules and differentiated thyroid Cancer. Thyroid. 2016;26(1):1-133

[20] Bamber J, Cosgrove D, Dietrich CF, Fromageau J, Bojunga J, Calliada F, et al. EFSUMB guidelines and recommendations on the clinical use of ultrasound elastography. Part 1: Basic principles and technology. Ultraschall in der Medizin. 2013;34(2):169-184

[21] Shiina T, Nightingale KR, Palmeri ML, Hall TJ, Bamber JC, Barr RG, et al. WFUMB guidelines and recommendations for clinical use of ultrasound elastography: Part 1: Basic principles and terminology. Ultrasound in Medicine & Biology. 2015;41(5):1126-1147

[22] Oliver C, Vaillant-Lombard J, Albarel F, Berbis J, Veyrieres JB, Sebag F, et al. What is the contribution of elastography to thyroid nodules evaluation? Annales d'Endocrinologie. 2011;72(2):120-124

[23] Harris RD, Langer JE, Levine RA, Sheth S, Abramson SJ, Gabriel H, et al. AIUM thyroid and parathyroid ultrasound examination. Journal of Ultrasound in Medicine. 2013;32(7): 1319-1329

[24] Cosgrove D, Barr R, Bojunga J, Cantisani V, Chammas MC, Dighe M, et al. WFUMB guidelines and recommendations on the clinical use of ultrasound Elastography: Part 4. Thyroid. Ultrasound in Medicine and Biology. 2017;43(1):4-26

[25] Mathonnet M, Cuerq A, Tresallet C, Thalabard JC, Fery-Lemonnier E, Russ G, et al. What is the care pathway of patients who undergo thyroid surgery in France and its potential pitfalls? A national cohort. BMJ Open. 2017;7(4):e013589. DOI: 10.1136/bmjopen-2016-013589

[26] Patel KN, Yip L, Lubitz CC, Grubbs EG, Miller BS, Shen W, et al. The American association of endocrine surgeons guidelines for the definitive surgical management of thyroid disease

in adults. Annals of Surgery. 2020 Mar;271(3):e21-e93. DOI: 10.1097/ SLA.0000000000003580. PMID: 32079830

[27] Paschou S, Vryonidou A, Goulis DG. Thyroid nodules: A guide to assessment, treatment and follow-up. Maturitas. 2017 Feb;96:1-9. DOI: 10.1016/ j.maturitas.2016.11.002. [Epub Nov 9, 2016]. PMID: 28041586

[28] Guth S, Theune U, Aberle J, Galach A, Bamberger CM. Very high prevalence of thyroid nodules detected by high frequency (13 MHz) ultrasound examination. European Journal of Clinical Investigation. 2009 Aug;39(8):699-706. DOI: 10.1111/j.1365-2362.2009.02162.x. PMID: 19601965

[29] Gharib H, Papini E, Paschke R, Duick DS, Valcavi R, Heged SL, et al. American Association of Clinical Endocrinologists, Associazione Medici Endocrinologi, and European thyroid association medical guidelines for clinical practice for the diagnosis and management of thyroid nodules. Journal of Endocrinological Investigation. 2010 33;(5 Suppl):51-56. PMID: 20543551

[30] Borlea A, Cotoi L, Mozos I, Stoian D. Advanced ultrasound techniques in preoperative diagnostic of thyroid cancers. In: Knowledges on Thyroid Cancer. InTechOpen; 2019. DOI: 10.5772/ intechopen.83032

[31] Andrioli M, Carzaniga C, Persani L. Standardized ultrasound report for thyroid nodules: The Endocrinologist's viewpoint. European Thyroid Journal. 2013;2(1):37-48

[32] Hegedüs L. Clinical practice. The thyroid nodule. The New England Journal of Medicine. 2004;351(17):1764-1771

[33] Frates MC, Benson CB, Charboneau JW, Cibas ES, Clark OH, Coleman BG, et al. Management of thyroid nodules detected at US: Society of Radiologists in ultrasound consensus conference statement. Radiology. 2005;237:794-800

[34] Rago T, Vitti P. Role of thyroid ultrasound in the diagnostic evaluation of thyroid nodules. Best Practice & Research. Clinical Endocrinology & Metabolism. 2008;22(6):913-928

[35] Remonti LR, Kramer CK, Leitão CB, Pinto LCF, Gross JL. Thyroid ultrasound features and risk of carcinoma: A systematic review and Meta-analysis of observational studies. Thyroid. 2015 May;25(5):538-550. DOI: 10.1089/ thy.2014.0353. [Epub Mar 31, 2015]. PMID: 25747526; PMCID: PMC4447137

[36] Hahn SY, Han B-K, Ko EY, Shin JH, Ko ES. Ultrasound findings of papillary thyroid carcinoma originating in the isthmus: Comparison with lobe-originating papillary thyroid carcinoma. AJR. American Journal of Roentgenology. 2014;203(3):637-642

[37] Trimboli P, Nasrollah N, Amendola S, Rossi F, Ramacciato G, Romanelli F, et al. Should we use ultrasound features associated with papillary thyroid cancer in diagnosing medullary thyroid cancer? Endocrine Journal. 2012;59(6):503-508

[38] Gregory A, Bayat M, Kumar V, Denis M, Kim BH, Webb J, et al. Differentiation of benign and malignant thyroid nodules by using comb-push ultrasound shear Elastography: A preliminary two-plane view study. Academic Radiology. 2018;25(11):1388-1397

[39] Leenhardt L, Erdogan MF, Hegedus L, Mandel SJ, Paschke R, Rago T, et al. 2013 European thyroid association guidelines for cervical

ultrasound scan and ultrasound-guided techniques in the postoperative management of patients with thyroid cancer. European Thyroid Journal. 2013;**2**(3):147-159

[40] Steinkamp HJ, Cornehl M, Hosten N, Pegios W, Vogl T, Felix R. Cervical lymphadenopathy: Ratio of long- to short-axis diameter as a predictor of malignancy. The British Journal of Radiology. 1995;**68**(807):266-270

[41] Leboulleux S, Girard E, Rose M, Travagli JP, Sabbah N, Caillou B, et al. Ultrasound criteria of malignancy for cervical lymph nodes in patients followed up for differentiated thyroid cancer. The Journal of Clinical Endocrinology and Metabolism. 2007;**92**(9):3590-3594

[42] Randolph GW, Duh QY, Heller KS, LiVolsi VA, Mandel SJ, Steward DL, et al. The prognostic significance of nodal metastases from papillary thyroid carcinoma can be stratified based on the size and number of metastatic lymph nodes, as well as the presence of extranodal extension. Thyroid. 2012;**22**(11):1144-1152

[43] Horvath E, Majlis S, Rossi R, Franco C, Niedmann JP, Castro A, et al. An ultrasonogram reporting system for thyroid nodules stratifying cancer risk for clinical management. The Journal of Clinical Endocrinology and Metabolism. 2009 May;**94**(5):1748-1751. DOI: 10.1210/jc.2008-1724. [Epub Mar 10, 2009]. PMID: 19276237

[44] Castellana M, Castellana C, Treglia G, Giorgino F, Giovanella L, Russ G, et al. Performance of five ultrasound risk stratification systems in selecting thyroid nodules for FNA. A meta-analysis. The Journal of Clinical Endocrinology and Metabolism. 2019

[45] Borlea A, Borcan F, Sporea I, Dehelean CA, Negrea R, Cotoi L, et al.

TI-RADS diagnostic performance: Which algorithm is superior and how Elastography and 4D vascularity improve the malignancy risk assessment. Diagnostics. 2020;**10**(4):180

[46] Bora Makal G, Aslan A. The diagnostic value of the American College of Radiology Thyroid Imaging Reporting and Data System Classification and shear-wave Elastography for the differentiation of thyroid nodules. Ultrasound in Medicine & Biology. 2021;**47**(5):1227-1234

[47] Mai KT, Perkins DG, Yazdi HM, Commons AS, Thomas J, Meban S. Infiltrating papillary thyroid carcinoma: Review of 134 cases of papillary carcinoma. Archives of Pathology & Laboratory Medicine. 1998;**122**(2):166-171

[48] Gharib H, Papini E, Garber JR, Duick DS, Harrell RM, Hegedüs L, et al. American association of clinical endocrinologists, American college of endocrinology, and Associazione Medici Endocrinologi medical guidelines for clinical practice for the diagnosis and management of thyroid nodules - 2016 update. Endocrine Practice. 2016;**22**:1-60. Available from: www.aace.com/reprints

[49] Cepeha CM, Paul C, Borlea A, Borcan F, Fofiu R, Dehelean CA, et al. The value of strain Elastography in predicting autoimmune thyroiditis. Diagnostics. Basel, Switzerland. 2020;**10**(11):874. DOI: 10.3390/diagnostics10110874

[50] Monpeyssen H, Tramalloni J, Poirée S, Hélénon O, Correas JM. Elastography of the thyroid. Diagnostic and Interventional Imaging. 2013 May;**94**(5):535-544. DOI: 10.1016/j.diii.2013.01.023. [Epub Apr 25, 2013]. PMID: 23623210

[51] Carlsen JF, Ewertsen C, Lönn L, Nielsen MB. Strain Elastography ultrasound: An overview with emphasis on breast Cancer diagnosis. Diagnostics. 2013;3(1):117-125

[52] Asteria C, Giovanardi A, Pizzocaro A, Cozzaglio L, Morabito A, Somalvico F, et al. US-Elastography in the differential diagnosis of benign and malignant thyroid nodules. Thyroid. 2008;18(5):523-531. DOI: 10.1089/thy.2007.0323

[53] Rago T, Santini F, Scutari M, Pinchera A, Vitti P. Elastography: New developments in ultrasound for predicting malignancy in thyroid nodules. The Journal of Clinical Endocrinology and Metabolism. 2007;92(8):2917-2922

[54] Stoian D, Timar B, Craina M, Bernad E, Petre I, Craciunescu M. Qualitative strain elastography-strain ratio evaluation-an important tool in breast cancer diagnostic. Medical Ultrasonography. 2016 Jun;18(2): 195-200. DOI: 10.11152/mu.2013. 2066.182.bcd. PMID: 27239654

[55] Nell S, Kist JW, Debray TPA, de Keizer B, van Oostenbrugge TJ, Borel Rinkes IHM, et al. Qualitative elastography can replace thyroid nodule fine-needle aspiration in patients with soft thyroid nodules. A systematic review and meta-analysis. European Journal of Radiology. 2015;84(4):652-661

[56] Park SH, Kim SJ, Kim E-K, Kim MJ, Son EJ, Kwak JY. Interobserver agreement in assessing the sonographic and elastographic features of malignant thyroid nodules. AJR. American Journal of Roentgenology. 2009;193(5):W416-W423

[57] Cantisani V, Lodise P, Di Rocco G, Grazhdani H, Giannotti D, Patrizi G, et al. Diagnostic accuracy and Interobserver agreement of Quasistatic ultrasound Elastography in the diagnosis of thyroid nodules TT - Diagnostische Genauigkeit und Interobserver-Übereinstimmung der Quasistatischen-Ultraschall-Elastografie bei der diagnose von. Ultraschall in der Medizin. 2015;36(02):162-167

[58] Cantisani V, Grazhdani H, Ricci P, Mortele K, Di Segni M, D'Andrea V, et al. Q-elastosonography of solid thyroid nodules: Assessment of diagnostic efficacy and interobserver variability in a large patient cohort. European Radiology. 2014;24(1):143-150

[59] Cantisani V, Maceroni P, D'Andrea V, Patrizi G, Di Segni M, De Vito C, et al. Strain ratio ultrasound elastography increases the accuracy of colour-Doppler ultrasound in the evaluation of Thy-3 nodules. A bi-Centre university experience. European Radiology. 2016;26(5):1441-1449

[60] Razavi SA, Hadduck TA, Sadigh G, Dwamena BA. Comparative effectiveness of Elastographic and B-mode ultrasound criteria for diagnostic discrimination of thyroid nodules: A Meta-analysis. American Journal of Roentgenology. 2013;200(6):1317-1326. DOI: 10.2214/AJR.12.9215

[61] Hu X, Liu Y, Qian L. Diagnostic potential of real-time elastography (RTE) and shear wave elastography (SWE) to differentiate benign and malignant thyroid nodules: A systematic review and meta-analysis. Medicine. 2017;96(43):e8282-e8282

[62] Lyshchik A, Higashi T, Asato R, Tanaka S, Ito J, Mai JJ, et al. Thyroid gland tumor diagnosis at US elastography. Radiology. 2005 Oct;237(1):202-211

[63] Ding J, Cheng H, Ning C, Huang J, Zhang Y. Quantitative measurement for thyroid Cancer characterization based on Elastography. Journal of Ultrasound in Medicine. 2011;**30**(9):1259-1266. DOI: 10.7863/jum.2011.30.9.1259

[64] Cantisani V, D'Andrea V, Biancari F, Medvedyeva O, Di Segni M, Olive M, et al. Prospective evaluation of multiparametric ultrasound and quantitative elastosonography in the differential diagnosis of benign and malignant thyroid nodules: Preliminary experience. European Journal of Radiology. 2012;**81**(10):2678-2683

[65] Stoian D, Timar B, Derban M, Pantea S, Varcus F, Craina M, et al. Thyroid imaging reporting and data system (TI-RADS): The impact of quantitative strain elastography for better stratification of cancer risks. Medical Ultrasonography. 2015 Sep;**17**(3):327-332. DOI: 10.11152/mu.2013.2066.173.dst. PMID: 26343081

[66] Moon HJ, Sung JM, Kim E-K, Yoon JH, Youk JH, Kwak JY. Diagnostic performance of gray-scale US and elastography in solid thyroid nodules. Radiology. 2012;**262**(3):1002-1013. DOI: 10.1148/radiol.11110839

[67] Trimboli P, Guglielmi R, Monti S, Misischi I, Graziano F, Nasrollah N, et al. Ultrasound sensitivity for thyroid malignancy is increased by real-time elastography: A prospective multicenter study. The Journal of Clinical Endocrinology and Metabolism. 2012;**97**(12):4524-4530

[68] Russ G Risk stratification of thyroid nodules on ultrasonography with the French TI-RADS: Description and reflections. Ultrasonics. 2016;**35**(1):25-38

[69] Dudea SM, Botar-Jid C. Ultrasound elastography in thyroid disease. Medical Ultrasonography. 2015;**17**(1):74-96

[70] Bojunga J, Herrmann E, Meyer G, Weber S, Zeuzem S, Friedrich-Rust M. Real-time elastography for the differentiation of benign and malignant thyroid nodules: A meta-analysis. Thyroid. 2010;**20**(10):1145-1150

[71] Hong Y, Wu Y, Luo Z, Wu N, Liu X. Impact of nodular size on the predictive values of gray-scale, color-Doppler ultrasound, and sonoelastography for assessment of thyroid nodules. Journal of Zhejiang University. Science. B. 2012;**13**(9):707-716

[72] Kwak JY, Kim E-K. Ultrasound elastography for thyroid nodules: Recent advances. Ultrasonography. 2014;**33**(2):75-82. DOI: 10.14366/usg.13025

[73] Sigrist RMS, Liau J, El KA, Chammas MC, Willmann JK. Ultrasound elastography: Review of techniques and clinical applications. Theranostics. 2017;**7**(5):1303-1329

[74] Liu Q-Q, Yang Z-W, Jie T, Xing P, Tang H-L, Qiu Q-Y, et al. The application of qualitative shear wave elastography in differential diagnosis of thyroid nodules. International Journal of Clinical and Experimental Medicine. 2019;**12**(4):3569-3579

[75] Lam ACL, Pang SWA, Ahuja AT, Bhatia KSS. The influence of precompression on elasticity of thyroid nodules estimated by ultrasound shear wave elastography. European Radiology. 2016;**26**(8):2845-2852

[76] Bhatia KSS, Tong CSL, Cho CCM, Yuen EHY, Lee YYP, Ahuja AT. Shear wave elastography of thyroid nodules in routine clinical practice: Preliminary observations and utility for detecting malignancy. European Radiology. 2012;**22**(11):2397-2406

[77] Kim H, Kim JA, Son EJ, Youk JK. Quantitative assessment of shear wave ultrasound elastography in thyroid nodules: Diagnostic performance for predicting malignancy. European Radiology. 2013;**23**(9):2532-2537

[78] Liu B-X, Xie X-Y, Liang J-Y, Zheng Y-L, Huang G-L, Zhou L-Y, et al. Shear wave elastography versus real-time elastography on evaluation thyroid nodules: A preliminary study. European Journal of Radiology. 2014;**83**(7):1135-1143. DOI: 10.1016/j.ejrad.2014.02.024

[79] Duan S-B, Yu J, Li X, Han Z-Y, Zhai H-Y, Liang P. Diagnostic value of two-dimensional shear wave elastography in papillary thyroid microcarcinoma. Oncotargets and Therapy. 2016;**9**: 1311-1317

[80] Chen M, Zhang K-Q, Xu Y-F, Zhang S-M, Cao Y, Sun W-Q. Shear wave elastography and contrast-enhanced ultrasonography in the diagnosis of thyroid malignant nodules. Molecular and Clinical Oncology. 2016;**5**(6):724-730

[81] Tian W, Hao S, Gao B, Jiang Y, Zhang X, Zhang S, et al. Comparing the diagnostic accuracy of RTE and SWE in differentiating malignant thyroid nodules from benign ones: A Meta-analysis. Cellular Physiology and Biochemistry. 2016;**39**(6):2451-2463

[82] Shuzhen C. Comparison analysis between conventional ultrasonography and ultrasound elastography of thyroid nodules. European Journal of Radiology. 2012;**81**(8):1806-1811

[83] Zhao C-K, Xu H-X. Ultrasound elastography of the thyroid: Principles and current status. Ultrasonics. 2019;**38**(2):106-124. Available from: https://pubmed.ncbi.nlm.nih.gov/30690960

Chapter 14

Role of Elastography in the Evaluation of Parathyroid Disease

Dana Amzar, Laura Cotoi, Andreea Borlea, Calin Adela,
Gheorghe Nicusor Pop and Dana Stoian

Abstract

Primary hyperparathyroidism is a prevalent disease of the parathyroid glands and the third most common endocrinopathy, especially among postmenopausal women. Secondary hyperparathyroidism is a compensatory response to hypocalcemic states due to chronic renal disease, vitamin D deficiency and malabsorption syndromes, and other chronic illnesses. Elastography can be an effective tool in localizing and identifying parathyroid lesions, whether it is a parathyroid adenoma or hyperplastic parathyroid secondary to chronic kidney disease, by differentiating between possible parathyroid lesions and thyroid nodules, cervical lymph nodes, or other anatomical structures. No current guidelines recommendations are available and no established general cutoff values on the elasticity of parathyroid lesions. We have conducted several prospective studies on primary and secondary hyperparathyroidism, using ultrasound imaging and elastography, shear wave, and strain elastography to better identify the parathyroid lesions and improve the preoperative localization and diagnostic. The results were encouraging, allowing us to determine cutoff values that are different for lesions from primary hyperparathyroidism and secondary hyperparathyroidism and comparing them with normal thyroid tissue and surrounding muscle tissue.

Keywords: elastography, shear wear elastography, primary hyperparathyroidism, secondary hyperparathyroidism, hypercalcemia, parathormone, vitamin D

1. Introduction

Advancements in the medical field improved diagnostic methods, increasing the incidence of various endocrine diseases [1, 2]. Hyperparathyroidism is a common endocrine disorder, commonly as primary hyperparathyroidism. As incidence it is the third endocrinopathy after type 2 diabetes mellitus and thyroid disease [3].

When discussing primary hyperparathyroidism, parathyroid adenoma being quoted as the most common cause of primary hyperparathyroidism, parathyroid hyperplasia and parathyroid carcinoma follow [4–6].

Secondary hyperparathyroidism is a prevalent complication of chronic kidney disease, with high prevalence among patients on renal replacement therapy [7, 8].

IntechOpen

Nowadays, primary hyperparathyroidism is mostly diagnosed in asymptomatic forms, in premenopausal women mostly, by active screening, with high serum parathormone (PTH) concentrations, and consequently high serum calcium concentrations [1, 4–6, 9–11].

Secondary hyperparathyroidism is prevalent among the chronic kidney cohort, determined by the disturbances of the phosphor-calcic metabolism. Prevalence cited in the specialty literature displays high numbers among patients receiving dialysis—of 54% in the United States and Europe—43.8% in France, 46.8% in Russia, and 42.9% in the United Kingdom [7].

The pathophysiological mechanism of primary hyperparathyroidism (PHPT) shows a loss of the homeostatic control of parathormone synthesis and secretion pathway, determining an increased secretion of parathomone and/or marked proliferation of cells with normal levels of PTH. Single adenomas present a monoclonal origin, suggesting that the tumors derive from a single abnormal cell [12], while hyperplastic parathyroid tumor usually presents polyclonal origins from a genetic point of view [1].

On the other hand, secondary hyperparathyroidism (sHPT) has a multifactorial and complex mechanism driven by hypocalcaemia, vitamin D deficiency, hyperphosphatemia, and high levels of fibroblast growth factor. In this case, sHPT could be amended by treating the underlying affection, chronic renal failure, or vitamin D deficiency. However, chronical stimulation of parathyroid glands can become autonomous, resulting in persistent tertiary hyperparathyroidism [4, 13, 14].

Regardless of the etiology of hyperparathyroidism, surgery represents a legitimate, validated, and corrective treatment in both primary and secondary hyperparathyroidism. Minimally invasive parathyroidectomy (MIP) is considered as a preferred approach current recommendation, thus the requirement to correctly identify the number and localization of affected parathyroid glands in preoperative evaluation, ultrasonography being the most cost-efficient method [15–19].

Given the positive features of ultrasonography, such as the noninvasive character, high resolution in real time, reproducibility, easiness in manipulation, inoffensive to children and pregnant women, and the absence of X-Ray exposure or administration of contrast agents, making it most accessible, reliable, and cost-efficient imaging technique for identifying pathological parathyroid glands [20, 21].

Elastography is a validated, complementary method to ultrasonography, labeled as "palpation imaging," providing qualitative and quantitative information on the studied tissue such as anatomical architecture and modifications in tissue stiffness [20, 22–24]. Endorsed as a marker of pathological states in many clinical fields, contributing to the positive identification, differential diagnosis, and ultimately to the therapeutic management, establishing its role in endocrinology for both thyroid and parathyroid evaluation [25, 26], hepato-gastroenterology [20, 27–29], senology [30, 31], urology [32–34], and otorhinolaryngology [35].

Two basic principles described for ultrasound elastography: "determination of the strain or deformation of a tissue due to a force (static elastography) and analysis of the propagation speed of a shear wave (shear wave elastography)" [36]. Literature studies have obtained various parameters from these elastography techniques that characterize a modification of a tissue. Three major groups are described using those parameters:

- qualitative criteria obtained from elastograms, which are maps, presented in gray scales or color, depending on the manufacturer, displaying the distribution of elasticities. They are available on most ultrasound machines, regardless of the technique used. A rapport can be determined between the width of tissue on B-mode and elastography.

- semiquantitative criteria are estimation of deformation ratios or elasticity ratios between different regions of interest (ROI).

- quantitative criteria possible by using the shear wave technique, determining the propagation speed of the shear wave. It represents a dynamic evaluation containing multiple subtypes:

a. transient elastography (TE) giving numerical values of the elasticity index, not being able to provide ultrasonographic imagines

b. point shear-wave elastography (pSWE)

c. shear-wave elastography

The last two methods include two-dimensional shear wave elastography and three dimensional shear wave elastography, determining numerical values of the elasticity index and providing color maps [20]. The numerical value data are calculated in Young modulus in m/s or kPa [36].

Strain elastography (SE) is a quasi-static elastographic method first implemented on ultrasound systems. It necessitates an external pressure to induce the deformation of the underlying tissue, or the deformation can be generated by acoustic radiation force impulse (ARFI). The most recent elastographic technologies can use endogenous stress such as muscle contractions or vascularization beam movements [20, 37, 38].

It can determine qualitative evaluation by adding elastograms (color maps) on conventional 2 B mode and, depending on the manufacturer, it can offer real-time elastography, where the refresh rate is equal to that in gray scale or single-image display with the mean relative hardness over a time loop [20].

Shear wave elastography induces shear waves in targeted tissues using acoustic radiation force and ultrasound imaging techniques to track the propagating shear waves. The shear waves induce a perpendicular oscillation to the direction of the wave propagation, expressed by shear modulus G and measured by shear wave speed (cS), which can be then further recorded in m/s or converted by using the Young's modulus E in kilopascals (kPa). The wave speed is then spatially mapped and directly related to the local stiffness of the evaluated tissue. This manner allows real-time monitoring of shear wave deformation in 2D and measures the shear wave speed or Young's modulus E and generates quantitative elastograms [2, 22, 39].

Elastography was used in both primary and secondary hyperparathyroidism, with an important clinical impact, proven in our previous studies [11, 25, 40–42]. Is has been proven to accurately predict the parathyroid tissue when compared with thyroid or muscle tissue.

This chapter aims to identify the characteristics of parathyroid adenomas in primary hyperparathyroidism and the attributes of hyper-plastic parathyroid glands in patients with chronic kidney on renal replacement therapy and to identify if the elastography can add value to the presurgical identification and differential diagnosis.

2. Ultrasound and elastographic evaluation of parathyroid disease

2.1 2B-ultrasonography evaluation

Gray scale ultrasound (US) has become a very accessible imaging technique in the endocrinology field, especially for thyroid and parathyroid evaluation, becoming the gold standard in these domains. The noninvasive character, the low cost, the repeatability, and especially the real-time assessment are some of the many advantages of this imagistic technique [43, 44].

The ultrasound evaluation of both thyroid and parathyroid glands involves a large ultrasound framework. Anatomical structures must be well observed and identified both in longitudinal and transverse modes [23, 45, 46]. Additional auxiliary techniques, including the rotation of the head to improve the ultrasound framework on the neck structures or swallowing, could improve the correct identification of anatomical structures and of ectopic parathyroid glands [45].

The sensitivity of ultrasound identification of parathyroid tumors varies from 70 to 80% [47] with higher positive identification for parathyroid hyperplasia 30–90% [48], but precision is dependent on the location and size of the tumor [16], by body habitus and gland morphology, and by the experience of the evaluator [46]. Increased false-positive ultrasound results are caused by structures mimicking parathyroid adenomas such as thyroid nodules, lymph nodes, muscles, vessels, and esophagus [15].

2.1.1 Adding color Doppler mode

Parathyroid adenomas typically present a peripheral vascular rim and an abnormally increased blood flow than the thyroid gland [49]. Therefore, by adding color Doppler mode in the ultrasound evaluation can increase the accuracy and sensitivity of ultrasound by 54% [50].

2.2 Ultrasound elastography: description and method

Elastography can be a helpful complementary imaging technique in the evaluation of parathyroid disease, adding additional information on tissue stiffness.

Neoplastic, fibrous, or atherosclerotic transformation in tissues is translated by tissue stiffness in elastographic evaluation [38]. The development of neoplastic tissue can be identified even in early stages, as from the physiopathological point of view, we can have an increased production of connective tissue, changes in cell density, and increased blood flow, all these changes determining a change in the tissue matrix, thus a change in the elasticity of the tissue [2]. Elastography can identify the differences between benign and malignant tissues from the early development of the disease, offering high sensitivity and resolution for deep-situated structures [51].

Elastography evaluates tissue stiffness by applying an external stress and calculating the distortion degree. The distortion in elastography is obtained by applying external pressure, manually or via ultrasound transducer. In acoustic radiation force impulse (ARFI), the distortion is induced by using crossing deformation, with converged ultrasound beams or by emitting of short duration focused acoustic beam that will generate shear waves that diffuse transversally through the tissue [52]. It thus determines qualitative information about tissue stiffness through color maps and color codes and quantitative information through numerical values [38].

An elastographic evaluation follows a 2B-mode ultrasound evaluation of the parathyroid glands. It can be performed in all patients; it is cost-efficient and adds valuable information. The elastography module is available on multiple ultrasound machines such as Aixplorer Mach 30 machine (SuperSonic Imagine, France), Philips, Fujifilm, Hitachi Preirus (Hitachi Medical Corporation, Tokyo, Japan) machine.

Elastography on the parathyroid is performed using a linear, high-resolution transducer of 15–4, respectively, 18–5 MHz chosen depending on the clarity of the image, profound parathyroid glands being evaluated with 15–4 probe, obtaining better images. The patient was examined in a supine position with neck hyperextension, maintaining regular superficial breathing. The following parathyroid parameters are to be evaluated—localization, form, parathyroid dimensions, and total volume of the gland.

Two elastographic procedures will be discussed in the chapter—2D shear wave elastography and real-time elastography.

The procedure depends on the type of elastography performed, for example, for shear wave elastography, the examiner must maintain a precise adherence for minimal 6 seconds to the probe on the examined area, with careful attention not to apply any manual compression, permitting the transducer to induce the acoustic vibrations in the parathyroid tissue. After image stabilization, a real-time elastogram will overlap on the B-mode image, obtaining an elastogram or color map (**Figure 1**). Afterimage stabilization, quantitative measurements can be performed on a frozen image.

Quantitative information, described as the elasticity index (EI) obtained on the frozen elastogram image, using a quantification box (Q-box), placed in the regions of interest (ROI). After software computing evaluates the mean SWE, minimum SWE, maximum SWE, and standard deviation, the elasticity parameters are displayed. All measurements are numerically expressed in kilopascals (kPa). As there is no scale setting recommended for the parathyroid examination, we recommend using a thyroid scale (0–100 kPa).

Another elastographic technique that requires external pressure in order to induce a deformation of the examined tissue that is further quantified by the machine software. This method is called real-time elastography (RTE) or strain elastography (SE).

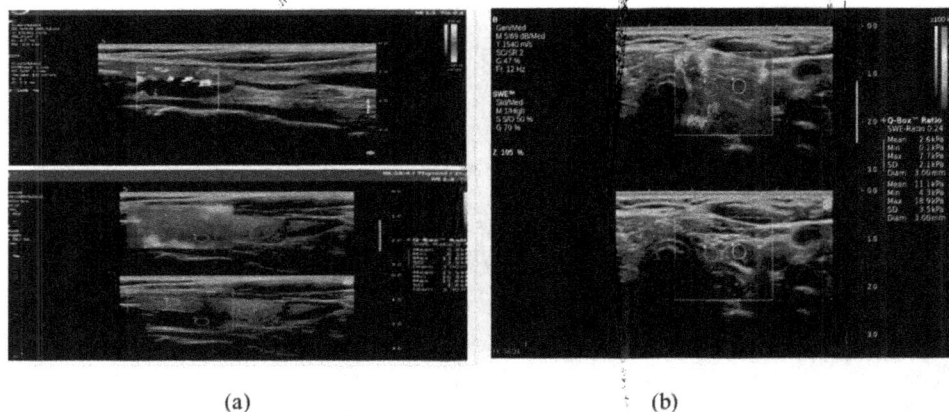

(a)   (b)

Figure 1.
(a) 2B-mode ultrasound evaluation of parathyroid adenoma, with complementary color Doppler mode; (b) Elastogram of parathyroid adenoma overlying B mode image and color map of tissue elasticity, with Q-box on the region of interest and quantitative evaluation [53] .

The examiner must apply controlled external pressure, usually manually pressure, which determines a mechanical deformation. An elastographic map is overlayed on the 2B greyscale that is displayed as a color map (red for liquid, green for soft tissue, blue for hard tissue), permitting the examined to obtain qualitative information about tissue stiffness for the examined area (**Figure 2**) [38].

Semiquantitative values can be obtained using strain elastography by comparing tissue strain in the region of interest (ROI) of the targeted tissue with another adjacent tissue, calculating a strain ratio (SR) ratio.

2.3 Strain elastography

The experience with strain elastography on parathyroid disease is primarily focused on parathyroid adenomas as parathyroid hyperplasia is more difficult to evaluate with this form of elastography [54]. The evaluation scale used to evaluate parathyroid lesions is the Rago criteria, frequently used for thyroid pathology. Rago criteria [38, 55], described for thyroid pathology, especially nodular goiter, was used to assess the qualitative strain elastography evaluation, as it follows: a score 1 means that the elasticity in the whole lesion is soft tissue, a score 2 means that the tissue is mostly soft, a score 3 is defined by soft tissue in the peripheral part of lesion, a score 4 implies that the examined lesion is entirely stiff, and a score 5 involves stiffness that exceeds beyond the examined lesion's margins, infiltrating in the enclosing tissues.

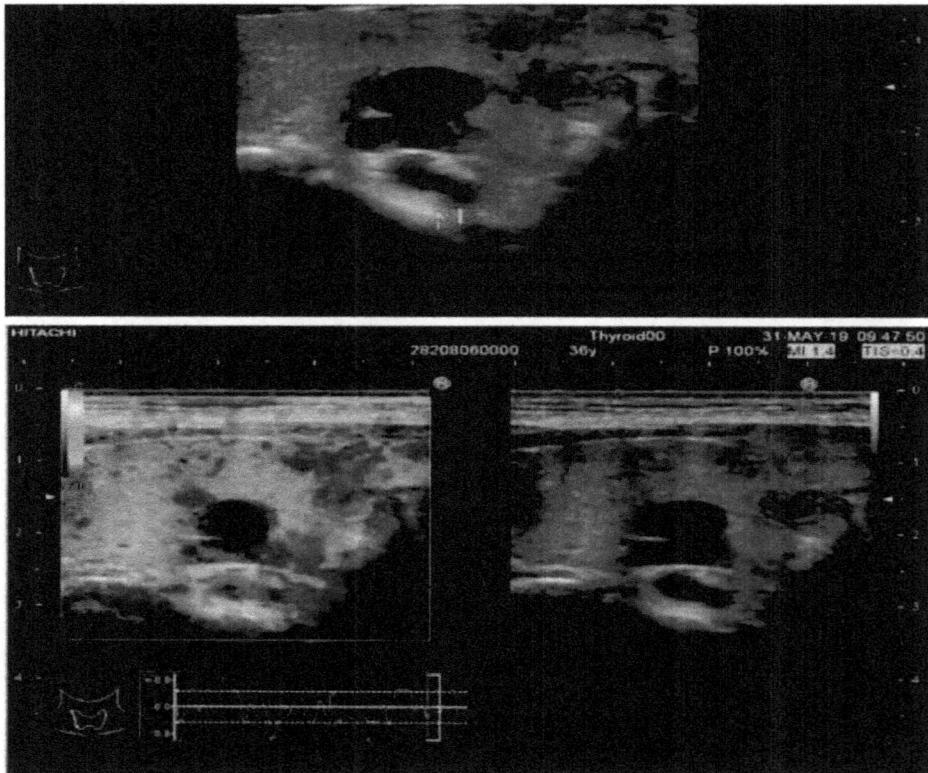

Figure 2.
Ultrasound evaluation and strain elastography of parathyroid adenoma [54].

The leading disadvantage of this qualitative technique is the depth of the evaluated tissue or lesion, determining an incomplete, unusable, and uninterpretable color map for higher depths. Most of the parathyroid adenomas evaluated in the paper previously published were of score 1 according to the Rago criteria (**Figure 3**) [25].

The first study conducted evaluated strain elastography on primary hyperparathyroidism on 20 consecutives patients evaluating qualitative and semiquantitative values. Out of the total 20 cases, two parathyroid adenomas could not be evaluated and for the rest a score 1 according to the Rago criteria was found [25].

The size and localization of the parathyroid adenoma were also quantified, so on ultrasound evaluation, the mean parathyroid adenoma dimensions were 0.776 ± 0.50 cm, the maximum size found was 2.46 cm, and the minimum was 0.34 mm. Most of the parathyroid adenomas were found near the right superior thyroid lobe (nine adenomas), three were located near the right inferior thyroid lobe, three were located near the left superior lobe, and five near the left inferior lobe. As for ultrasound appearance 13 parathyroid adenomas had cystic appearance (65%), 5 parathyroid adenomas homogeneously solid and hypoechoic appearance (25%), and 2 adenomas had a mixed appearance (10%)—mostly cystic and one with an elongated shape.

Semiquantitative information was also achieved using strain elastography, by comparing tissue strain the parathyroid adenoma parenchyma and thyroid or muscle tissue. No significant differences were found between the strain ratio determined using SE for the parathyroid adenoma and the thyroid tissue (nine out of twenty cases)

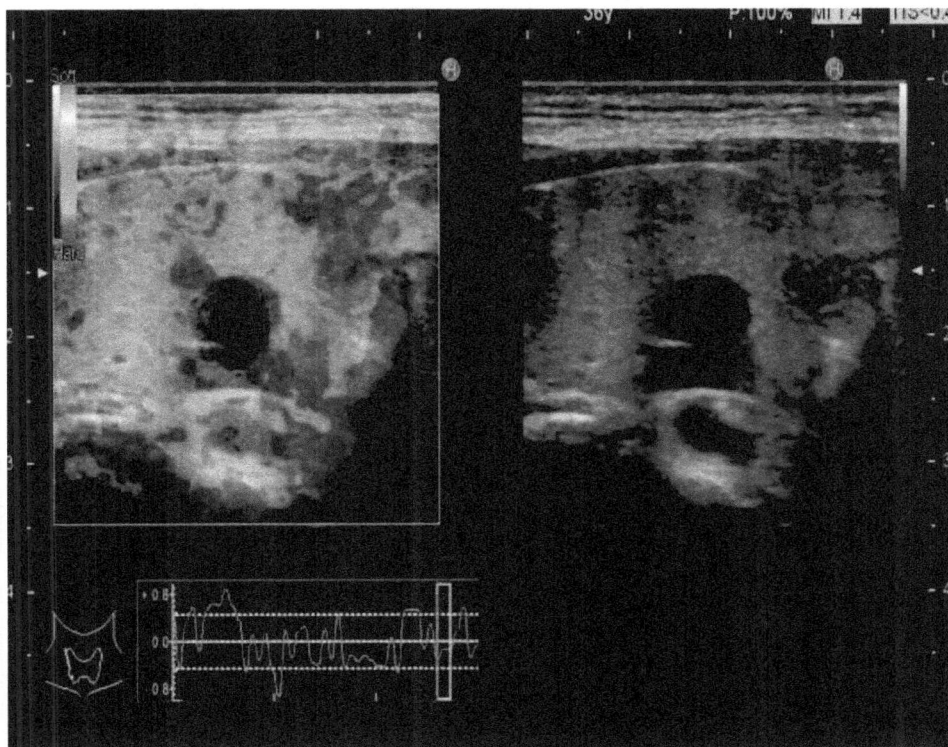

Figure 3.
Color map with strain elastography with Hitachi machine showing a score 1 on Rago criteria [54].

with a mean SR of 1.465 ± 1.458, respectively, strain ratio of the parathyroid adenoma compared with the strain ratio of the thyroid tissue with autoimmune disease (11 out of 20 cases) with a mean SR = 1.656 ± 1.746, p = 0.481 [25].

Other literature studies have compared the elasticity of parathyroid pathology using strain elastography, identifying that parathyroid adenomas appear as stiff lesions (median SR = 3.56) and parathyroid hyperplasia has a lower stiffness and a higher elasticity score (median SR = 1.49) [56].

A study based on another type of elastographic evaluation–Elastoscan Core Index (ECI) evaluating parathyroid adenomas and lymph nodes found that the ECI index was significantly higher in malignant lesions than in benign lesions. They concluded that combining ECI index with conventional US, particularly with shape and vascularization, can improve the differentiation of parathyroid lesions from lymph nodes and thyroid nodules [57].

2.4 Shear-wave elastography

We conducted several studies on primary and secondary hyperparathyroidism, comparing the results to evaluate the differences between the two clinical entities, as the pathophysiological mechanism is quite different.

Our first study [25] (previously published) evaluated the values of shear wave elastography on primary hyperparathyroidism. Twenty consecutive patients with primary hyperparathyroidism presenting a solitary adenoma were included. The parathyroid tissue was compared with thyroid and muscle tissue, as normal parathyroid adenomas cannot be evaluated using ultrasonography. The best parameter identified for evaluating parathyroid adenomas was mean SWE, with the highest specificity, sensitivity, and accuracy. The results are displayed in **Table 1** [25].

Statistical analysis has found significant difference between parathyroid elasticity (kPa) compared with thyroid and muscle elasticity (p < 0.001).

A second study [40] (previously published) was conducted on patients on renal replacement therapy with consequential secondary hyperparathyroidism. A cohort of 120 patients was evaluated, founding 59 with secondary parathyroid hyperplasia. A total of 97 hyperplastic parathyroid glands were evaluated, comparing normal thyroid and muscle tissue with hyperplastic parathyroid tissue. Statistical differences were found in this cohort and identified the best parameter to evaluate the elasticity of parathyroid tissue and the cut-off values (**Table 2**) [40].

After analyzing the two cohorts, a natural question has appeared—are there any differences between primary and secondary hyperparathyroidism on elastographic evaluation?

The third study answered this question—evaluating a total of 68 patients divided into two groups of 27 patients diagnosed with primary and 41 patients diagnosed with secondary hyperparathyroidism (**Figures 4** and **5**).

The baseline characteristics of the primary and secondary hyperparathyroidism study are presented in **Table 3** [41].

When comparing the results of the two studied lots, we found statistically significant differences in sex distribution between the two lots (p < 0.001, Fischer-exact Test).

Keeping the different pathophysiology pathways for primary and secondary hyperparathyroidism in mind, we conducted diagnostic tests to evaluate the elastographic differences between the two types of hyperparathyroidism [41].

	SWE-min PTX/T	SWE-mean PTX/T	SWE-max PTX/T	SWE-min PTX/M	SWE-mean PTX/M	SWE-max PTX/M
Area under curve (AUC) value	0.957	0.950	0.765	0.998	0.997	0.955
Specificity	85%	90.0%	70.0%	95.0%	95.0%	80.0%
Sensitivity	95%	95.0%	80.0%	100%	100%	100%
PPV	86.4%	90.5%	72.7%	95.2%	95.2%	83.3%
NPV	94.4%	94.7%	77.8%	100%	100%	100%
Accuracy	90.0%	92.5%	75.0%	97.5%	97.5%	90.0%
p value	<.0.001	<0.001	<0.001	<0.001	<0.001	<0.001
Cut-off value	<3.14 kPa	<7.28 kPa	<9.14 kPa	<5.32 kPa	<10.47 kPa	<15.16 kPa

Table 1.
Sensitivity, specificity, ROC curve for measured elastographic index SWE-min, SWE-max, and SWE-mean for primary hyperparathyroidism.

	SWE min PTX/T	SWE mean PTX/T	SWE max PTX/T	SWE min PTX/M	SWE mean PTX/M	SWE max PTX/M
AUC value	0.943	0.940	0.858	0.957	0.949	0.882
Specificity	86.6%	90.7%	75.3%	95.9%	90.7%	84.5%
Sensitivity	94.8%	94.8%	83.5%	86.6%	93.8%	78.4%
PPV	87.6%	91.1%	77.1%	95.9%	91%	83.5%
NPV	94.4%	94.6%	82.0%	87.7%	93.6%	79.6%
Accuracy	90.7%	92.26%	79.4%	91.2%	91.75%	81.45%
Cutoff value	< 6.02 kPa	< 9.74 kPa	< 15.3 kPa	< 7.94 kPa	< 9.98 kPa	< 17.3 kPa

Table 2.
Sensitivity, specificity, AUROC for measured SWE min, SWE max, and SWE mean for secondary hyperparathyroidism [40].

A statistically significant difference (p < 0.001) was found when comparing the results of SWE-mean parathyroid tissue between primary and secondary hyperparathyroidism, with higher values for the secondary hyperparathyroidism group **(Figure 6)**.

There are multiple research studies on the elastographic evaluation of primary hyperparathyroidism, but this method is less approached for secondary hyperparathyroidism.

Different threshold values for parathyroid adenomas have been established by various authors in the field of primary hyperparathyroidism, depending on the elastography techniques used. By using shear wave virtual touch imaging quantification, higher values have been found for parathyroid adenomas (2.16 ± 0.33 m/s) compared

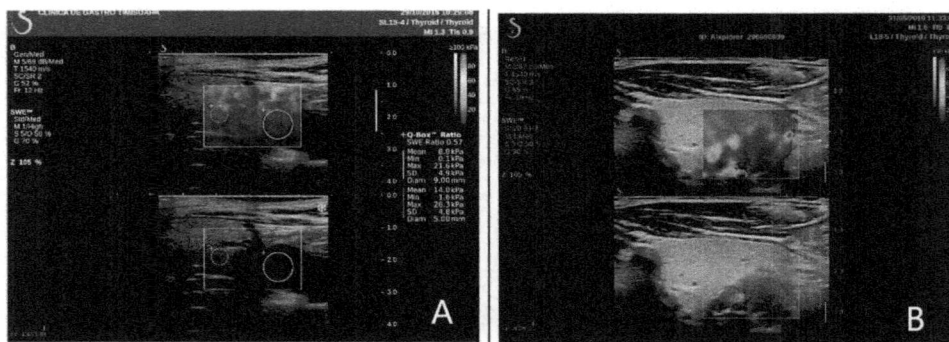

Figure 4.
Elastograms using 2D SWE. In image A – Elastogram overlaying gray scale ultrasound of a right inferior parathyroid adenoma; In image B – Elastogram overlaying gray scale image of a right inferior parathyroid hyperplasia in secondary hyperparathyroidism [41].

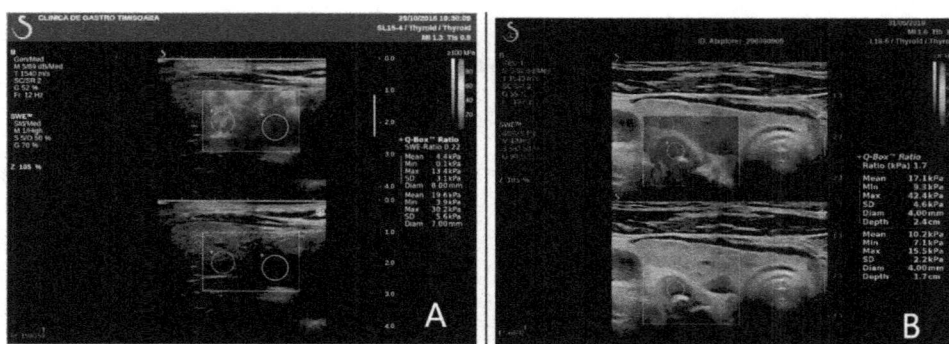

Figure 5.
Elasticity index evaluation for parathyroid and thyroid tissue. In image A – Elastographic evaluation of a right inferior parathyroid adenoma from primary hyperparathyroidism; In image B – Elastograohic evaluation of a left inferior parathyroid hyperplasia from secondary hyperparathyroidism [41].

with parathyroid hyperplasia (1.75 ± 0.28 m/s), identifying a cutoff value superior to 1.92 m/s for parathyroid adenomas [44]. Another study presented their results between the elastographic differences between thyroid and parathyroid tissue, using the same elastograohic method as the previous. Their conclusion was that the elastographic index of parathyroid adenomas is lower than of the thyroid tissue, presenting a shear wave velocity of 2.01 m/s, respectively 2.77 m/s [58].

Another representative study performed an analysis using the ARFI imaging 2D SWE, comparing parathyroid adenomas with malignant and benign thyroid pathology. They have identified that parathyroid adenomas present a higher elasticity index than benign thyroid pathology (3.09 ± 0.75 m/s versus SWV of 2.20 ± 0.39 m/s) and an even higher elasticity than malignant thyroid lesions with a mean SWV of 3.59 ± 0.43 m/s [59].

In the 2D SWE elastography field, a study conducted on parathyroid adenomas and benign thyroid nodules has identified that parathyroid adenomas present a significantly lower elasticity index than benign thyroid nodules (mean SWE 5.2 ± 7.2 kPa, respectively mean SWE of 24.3 ± 33.8 kPa) [60]. The results are similar with our conclusion using the same elastographic method.

Characteristics	Primary hyperparathyroidism	Secondary hyperparathyroidism	p-value
Male-to-female ratio	2/25	22/19	<0.001
Age (years)	61 [48.67]	58 [50–65.5]	0.763
Parathormone (PTH) (pg/ml)	160.6 [115.0–206.3]	1117 [785.95–1407]	<0.001
Serum phosphorus (mg/dl)	2.60 [2.30–3.12]	6.00 [5.15–7.77]	<0.001
Total serum calcium (mg/dl)	10.50 [10.10–11.40]	9.00 [8.35–9.35]	<0.001
Serum vitamin D (ng/ml)	21.33 [15.55–25.52]	35.80 [24.20–44.70]	<0.001
Parathyroid volume (ml)	0.120 [0.068–0.240]	0.251 [0.109–0.332]	0.107
Maximum diameter (mm)	8.30 [6.20–12.00]	9.50 [7.25–11.75]	0.543
Dialysis years	—	5.10 [4.00–8.10]	NA
Kt/v	—	1.350 [1.30–1.46]	NA

Table 3.
Baseline characteristics of patients evaluated with primary and secondary hyperparathyroidism.

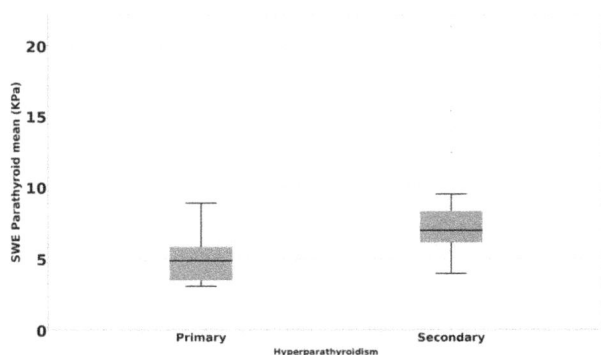

Figure 6.
Shear wave differences between mean value SWE for primary hyperparathyroidism and secondary hyperparathyroidism. [41].

Some elastographic studies on parathyroid hyperplasia have been published, but they not focused on patients with chronic kidney disease on hemodialysis. There are currently no other threshold values for secondary hyperparathyroidism, apart those presented [40, 41].

2.5 Strain versus shear-wave elastography

Strain elastography is a very useful elastographic technique that requires external pressure in order to produce deformation of subjacent tissue that has been validated in the field of thyroid and breast evaluation.

Even if strain elastography can be without any doubt a very useful qualitative tool by using the color mapping, 2D-SWE elastography can offer a better identification of parathyroid tissue.

There are certain limitations of the elastography in the evaluation of parathyroid glands, the most important is the difficulty in evaluating ectopic and supranumerary parathyroid glands, especially when located in the thymus or posterior mediastinum. When using elastography, a low value, near to zero could indicate the presence of a liquid lesion or a depth lesion, inaccessible to the linear probe. It is very important to verify the signal intensity, to distinguish between liquid lesions and depth lesion, and to opt for a linear probe with lower frequencies is available. Another limitation to consider is that the trachea or the carotid movement could generate artifacts, in this case, elastographic noise can be decreased by increasing the gain. One of the most important aspects in the elastographic evaluation is the external pressure applied to the probe that can produce false-positive values. This is a limitation because it is operator-dependent, less present in shear-wave elastography than in strain elastography. Another aspect to be considered is the choice of the elastography scale, as there is no recommendation for parathyroid evaluation, we have used in our studies a scale between 0 and 100 kPa.

3. Conclusions

The clinical implications of elastography in the evaluation of primary or secondary hyperparathyroidism are undeniable. As a complementary method to conventional ultrasonography, elastography is a simple, noninvasive, repeatable, and reproducible method that can improve diagnosis and preoperative evaluation of the patient with either primary or secondary hyperparathyroidism.

Even if there are certain limitations to the technique, such as operator experience and some techniques are more operator-dependent that others, we have to take in mind that it is a complementary technique and that is noninvasive, highly reproducible, easy to manipulate, presents a high resolution in real time, it is harmless to children and pregnant women with absence of X-ray exposure or need of contrast agents, making it a very accessible and cost-efficient imaging technique for complementary evaluation of parathyroid disease.

We have found significant differences between primary and secondary hyperparathyroidism, identifying a cutoff elastographic value for parathyroid adenomas below 5.96 kPa [41].

One of the essential questions of the studies has been answered, the following question was to determine a general cutoff value for parathyroid tissue. Thus, we have considered into analysis both parathyroid adenomas and parathyroid hyperplasia values, permitting us to establish a mean SWE cutoff value for parathyroid tissue below 9.58 kPa [41].

Further studies could help establish the elastographic differences between pathological parathyroid tissue and thyroid nodules. Current literature studies had determined that there is a major difference between malignant and benign thyroid nodules, the first being stiffer than the ladder. Furthermore, benign thyroid nodules present a higher elasticity index than normal thyroid tissue. We can imagine that if parathyroid tissue should be compared with benign or malignant thyroid tissue, a significant elasticity difference should be found.

Elastography is a proven and validated method in many clinical areas and recognized by the current guideline, including thyroid disease [61, 62]. It most certainly presents a major role in the localization of the parathyroid disease as useful tool for both qualitative, but mainly quantitative evaluation of parathyroid tissue. Significant elastographic differences between parathyroid adenoma and parathyroid hyperplasia have been identified, but in both cases, the parathyroid tissue is significantly lower than the healthy thyroid tissue and the surrounding muscle tissue.

Acknowledgements

We would like to thank all our contributors—Prof Dr. Ioan Sporea, Prof Dr. Adalbert Schiller, and Dr. Oana Schiller for the guidance and for allowing us to conduct our studies in their services.

Conflict of interest

The authors declare no conflict of interest.

Notes

The current chapter represents a summary of our experience with the elastography techniques applied in the field of parathyroid disease. Six papers were published on this subject. Images and statistical values were previously published in our studies.

Author details

Dana Amzar[2], Laura Cotoi[1*], Andreea Borlea[1], Calin Adela[1], Gheorghe Nicusor Pop[3] and Dana Stoian[2]

1 PhD School Department, "Victor Babes" University of Medicine and Pharmacy Timisoara, Timisoara, Romania

2 Endocrinology Department, "Victor Babes" University of Medicine and Pharmacy Timisoara, Timisoara, Romania

3 Department of Functional Sciences, "Victor Babes" University of Medicine and Pharmacy Timisoara, Centre for Modeling Biological Systems and Data Analysis, Timisoara, Romania

*Address all correspondence to: laura_cotoi@yahoo.com and cotoi.laura@umft.ro

IntechOpen

References

[1] Bilezikian JP, Cusano NE, Khan AA, Liu J-M, Marcocci C, Bandeira F. Primary hyperparathyroidism. Nature Reviews Disease Primers. 2016;**2**:16033

[2] Barr RG, Nakashima K, Amy D, Cosgrove D, Farrokh A, Schafer F, et al. WFUMB guidelines and recommendations for clinical use of ultrasound elastography: Part 2: Breast. Ultrasound in Medicine and Biology. 2015;**41**(5):1148-1160

[3] Hindié E, Ugur Ö, Fuster D, O'Doherty M, Grassetto G, Ureña P, et al. 2009 EANM parathyroid guidelines. European Journal of Nuclear Medicine and Molecular Imaging. 2009;**36**(7):1201-1216

[4] Mizamtsidi M, Nastos C, Mastorakos G, Dina R, Vassiliou I, Gazouli M, et al. Diagnosis, management, histology and genetics of sporadic primary hyperparathyroidism: Old knowledge with new tricks. Endocrine Connections. 2018;**7**(2):R56-R68

[5] Kebebew E, Clark OH. Parathyroid adenoma, hyperplasia, and carcinoma: Localization, technical details of primary neck exploration, and treatment of hypercalcemic crisis. Surgical Oncology Clinics of North America. 1998;**7**(4):721-748

[6] Rahbari R, Holloway AK, He M, Khanafshar E, Clark OH, Kebebew E. Identification of differentially expressed microRNA in parathyroid tumors. Annals of Surgical Oncology. 2011 Apr;**18**(4):1158-1165. DOI: 10.1245/s10434-010-1359-7. Epub 2010 Nov 18. PMID: 21086055; PMCID: PMC3449317

[7] Hedgeman E, Lipworth L, Lowe K, Saran R, Do T, Fryzek J. International burden of chronic kidney disease and secondary hyperparathyroidism: A systematic review of the literature and available data. International Journal of Nephrology. 2015;**2015**:184321. DOI: 10.1155/2015/184321. Epub 2015 Mar 31. PMID: 25918645; PMCID: PMC4396737

[8] Jean G, Lafage-Proust MH, Souberbielle JC, Lechevallier S, Deleaval P, Lorriaux C, et al. Severe secondary hyperparathyroidism in patients on haemodialysis is associated with a high initial serum parathyroid hormone and beta-CrossLaps level: Results from an incident cohort. PLoS One. 2018;**13**(6):1-15

[9] Bandeira F, Griz L, Chaves N, Carvalho NC, Borges LM, Lazaretti-Castro M, et al. Diagnosis and management of primary hyperparathyroidism - a scientific statement from the Department of Bone Metabolism, the Brazilian Society for Endocrinology and metabolism. Arquivos Brasileiros de Endocrinologia e Metabologia. 2013;**57**(6):406-424

[10] Eufrazino C, Veras A, Bandeira F. Epidemiology of primary hyperparathyroidism and its non-classical manifestations in the City of Recife. Brazil. Clin Med Insights Endocrinol Diabetes. 2013;**6**:69-74

[11] Cotoi L, Stoian D. Ultrasonographic and Elastographic diagnostic of parathyroid lesions – A literature review. Austin Journal of Endocrinology and Diabetes. 2019;**6**(2-2019):1068

[12] Arnold A, Staunton CE, Kim HG, Gaz RD, Kronenberg HM. Monoclonality and abnormal parathyroid hormone genes in parathyroid adenomas. England Journal of Medicine. 1988 Mar 17;**318**(11):658-662. DOI: 10.1056/NEJM198803173181102. PMID: 3344017

[13] Arrangoiz R, Cordera F, Lambreton F, De LEL, Moreno E. Current thinking on primary hyperparathyroidism. JSM Head and Neck Cancer Cases and Reviews. 2016;**1**(August):1-15

[14] Allgrove J. Parathyroid disorders. American Family Physician. 2001;**11**(5):357-363. ISSN 0957-5839, DOI: 10.1054/cupe.2001.0206

[15] Gasser RW. Clinical aspects of primary hyperparathyroidism: Clinical manifestations, diagnosis, and therapy. Wiener Medizinische Wochenschrift (1946). 2013;**163**(17-18):397-402

[16] Mariani G, Gulec S, Rubello D, Boni G, Puccini M, Pelizzo MR, et al. Preoperative localization and radioguided parathyroid surgery. Journal of Nuclear Medicine. 2003;**44**(9):1443-1458

[17] Lorenz K, Bartsch DK, Sancho JJ, Guigard S, Triponez F. Surgical management of secondary hyperparathyroidism in chronic kidney disease—A consensus report of the European Society of Endocrine Surgeons. Langenbeck's Archives of Surgery. 2015;**400**(8):907-927

[18] Korosi A. Practice guidelines for chronic kidney disease. Annals of Internal Medicine. 2004 Jun 1;**140**(11):934; author reply 934-5. DOI: 10.7326/0003-4819-140-11-200406010-00025. PMID: 15172915

[19] Russo D, Battaglia Y. Clinical significance of FGF-23 in patients with CKD. International Journal of Nephrology. 2011;**2011**:1-5

[20] Bamber J, Cosgrove D, Dietrich CF, Fromageau J, Bojunga J, Calliada F, et al. EFSUMB guidelines and recommendations on the clinical use of ultrasound elastographypart 1: Basic principles and technology. Ultraschall in der Medizin. 2013;**34**(2):169-184

[21] Park AY, Son EJ, Han K, Youk JH, Kim JA, Park CS. Shear wave elastography of thyroid nodules for the prediction of malignancy in a large scale study. European Journal of Radiology. 2015;**84**(3):407-412

[22] Gennisson JL, Deffieux T, Fink M, Tanter M. Ultrasound elastography: principles and techniques. Diagnostic and Interventional Imaging. 2013 May;**94**(5):487-495. DOI: 10.1016/j.diii.2013.01.022. Epub 2013 Apr 22. PMID: 23619292

[23] Parameter AP. AIUM practice Parameter for the performance of a thyroid and parathyroid ultrasound examination. Journal of Ultrasound in Medicine. 2016;**35**(9):1-11

[24] Cosgrove D, Barr R, Bojunga J, Cantisani V, Chammas MC, Dighe M, et al. WFUMB guidelines and recommendations on the clinical use of ultrasound Elastography: Part 4. Thyroid. Ultrasound in Medicine and Biology. 2017;**43**(1):4-26

[25] Cotoi L, Amzar D, Sporea I, Borlea A, Navolan D, Varcus F, et al. Shear wave Elastography versus strain Elastography in diagnosing parathyroid adenomas. International Journal of Endocrinology. 2020;**2020**:1-11

[26] Stoian D, Ivan V, Sporea I, Florian V, Mozos I, Navolan D, et al. Advanced ultrasound application – Impact on presurgical risk stratification of the thyroid nodules. Therapeutics and Clinical Risk Management. 2020;**16**:21-30

[27] Sporea I, Lie I. Shear wave elastography. Ultraschall Medicine. 2012 Aug;**33**(4):393-394. PMID: 23045734

[28] Bota S, Herkner H, Sporea I, Salzl P, Sirli R, Neghina AM, Peck-Radosavljevic M. Meta-analysis: ARFI elastography versus transient elastography

for the evaluation of liver fibrosis. Liver International. 2013 Sep;**33**(8):1138-1147. DOI: 10.1111/liv12240. Epub 2013 Jul 16. PMID: 23859217

[29] Garra BS. Elastography: history, principles, and technique comparison. Abdominal Imaging. 2015 Apr;**40**(4):680-697. DOI: 10.1007/s00261-014-0305-8. PMID: 25637125

[30] Stoian D, Timar B, Craina M, Bernad E, Petre I, Craciunescu M. Qualitative strain elastography-strain ratio evaluation-an important tool in breast cancer diagnostic. Medical Ultrasonography. 2016;**18**(2):195-200

[31] Youk JH, Gweon HM, Son EJ. Shear-wave elastography in breast ultrasonography: The state of the art. Ultrasonography. 2017;**36**(4):300-309

[32] Correas JM, Tissier AM, Khairoune A, Khoury G, Eiss D, Hélénon O. Ultrasound elastography of the prostate: State of the art. Diagnostic and Interventional Imaging. 2013;**94**(5):551-560

[33] Rus G, Faris IH, Torres J, Callejas A, Melchor J. Why are viscosity and nonlinearity bound to make an impact in clinical elastographic diagnosis? Sensors (Switzerland). 2020;**20**(8):1-35

[34] Rus G, Melchor JM, Faris I, Callejas A, Riveiro M, Molina F, et al. Mechanical biomarkers by torsional shear ultrasound for medical diagnosis. The Journal of the Acoustical Society of America. 2018;**144**:1747. DOI: 10.1121/1.5067744

[35] Bhatia KS, Cho CC, Tong CS, Yuen EH, Ahuja AT. Shear wave elasticity imaging of cervical lymph nodes. Ultrasound in Medicine and Biology. 2012 Feb;**38**(2):195-201. DOI: 10.1016/j.ultrasmedbio.2011.10.024. Epub 2011 Dec 16. Erratum in: Ultrasound Med Biol. 2012 Oct;**38**(10):1849. PMID: 22178167

[36] Franchi-Abella S, Elie C, Correas JM. Ultrasound elastography: Advantages, limitations and artefacts of the different techniques from a study on a phantom. Diagnostic and Interventional Imaging. 2013;**94**(5):497-501

[37] Monpeyssen H, Tramalloni J, Poirée S, Hélénon O, Correas JM. Elastography of the thyroid. Diagnostic and Interventional Imaging. 2013;**94**(5):535-544

[38] Stoian D, Bogdan T, Craina M, Craciunescu M, Timar R, Schiller A. Elastography: A new ultrasound technique in nodular thyroid pathology. In: Ahmadzadehfar H, editor. Thyroid Cancer-Advances in Diagnosis and Therapy [Internet]. London: IntechOpen; 2016 [cited 2022 Jul 10]. DOI: 10.5772/64374. Available from: https://www.intechopen.com/chapters/51576

[39] Sigrist RMS, Liau J, El Kaffas A, Chammas MC, Willmann JK. Ultrasound elastography: Review of techniques and clinical applications. Theranostics. 2017;7:1303-1329

[40] Cotoi L, Borcan F, Sporea I, Amzar D, Schiller O, Schiller A, et al. Shear wave elastography in diagnosing secondary hyperparathyroidism. Diagnostics. 2019;**9**(4):1-16

[41] Amzar D, Cotoi L, Sporea I, Timar B, Schiller O, Schiller A, et al. Shear wave Elastography in patients with primary and secondary hyperparathyroidism. Journal of Clinical Medicine. 2021;**10**(4):697

[42] Cotoi L, Amz D, Sporea I, Borlea A, Schiller O, Schiller A, et al. Parathyroid Elastography — Elastography evaluation algorithm. Timişoara Medicală. 2020;**2020**(1):1-16

[43] Ruchała M, Szczepanek E. Endokrynologia polska. Endokrynologia Polska. 2010;**61**(3):330-344

[44] Polat AV, Ozturk M, Akyuz B, Celenk C, Kefeli M, Polat C. The diagnostic value of shear wave elastography for parathyroid lesions and comparison with cervical lymph nodes. Medical Ultrasonography. 2017;**19**(4):386-391

[45] Sung JY. Parathyroid ultrasonography: The evolving role of the radiologist. Ultrasonography. 2015;**34**(4):268-274

[46] Kunstman JW, Kirsch JD, Mahajan A, Udelsman R. Parathyroid localization and implications for clinical management. Journal of Clinical Endocrinology and Metabolism. 2013;**98**(3):902-912

[47] Geatti O, Shapiro B, Orsolon PG, Proto G, Guerra UP, Antonucci F, Gasparini D. Localization of parathyroid enlargement: experience with technetium-99m methoxyisobutylisonitrile and thallium-201 scintigraphy, ultrasonography and computed tomography. European Journal of Nuclear Medicine. 1994 Jan;**21**(1):17-22. DOI: 10.1007/BF00182301. PMID: 8088281

[48] Casara D, Rubello D, Pelizzo M, Shapiro B. Clinical role of 99mTcO4/MIBI scan, ultrasound and intra-operative gamma probe in the performance of unilateral and minimally invasive surgery in primary hyperparathyroidism. European Journal of Nuclear Medicine. 2001;**28**(9):1351-1359

[49] Rickes S, Sitzy J, Neye H, Ocran KW, Wermke W. High-resolution ultrasound in combination with colour-Doppler sonography for preoperative localization of parathyroid adenomas in patients with primary hyperparathyroidism. Ultraschall in der Medizin. 2003 Apr;**24**(2):85-89. DOIO: 10.1055/s-2003-38667. PMID: 12698372

[50] Lane MJ, Desser TS, Weigel RJ, Jeffrey RB Jr. Use of color and power Doppler

sonography to identify feeding arteries associated with parathyroid adenomas. American Journal of Roentgenology. 1998 Sep;**171**(3):819-823. DOI: 10.2214/ajr.171.3.9725323. PMID: 9725323

[51] Dietrich CF, Barr RG, Farrokh A, Dighe M, Hocke M, Jenssen C, et al. Strain Elastography - how to Do it ? Authors introduction to Elastography what Elastography techniques are used ? Definition of color coding, why ? Strain-based Elastography – How does it work ? Technical principles of tissue Elastography. Ultrasound International Open. 2017;**3**:E137-E149

[52] G C, D M. Strain Elastosonography of thyroid nodules: A new tool for malignancy prediction? Overview of literature. Endocrinology & Metabolic Syndrome. 2016;**5**(3):12-15

[53] Cotoi L, Amzar D, Sporea I, Borlea A, Navolan D, Varcus F, et al. Shear wave Elastography versus strain Elastography in diagnosing parathyroid adenomas. Borretta G, editor. International Journal of Endocrinology [Internet] 2020;**2020**:3801902. DOI: 10.1155/2020/3801902

[54] Cotoi L, Amzar D, Sporea I, Borlea A, Navolan D, Varcus F, et al. Shear wave elastography versus strain elastography in diagnosing parathyroid adenomas. International Journal of Endocrinology. 2020 Mar 17;**2020**:3801902. DOI: 10.1155/2020/3801902. PMID: 32256571; PMCID: PMC7103049

[55] Rago T, Santini F, Scutari M, Pinchera A, Vitti P. Elastography: New developments in ultrasound for predicting malignancy in thyroid nodules. Journal of Clinical Endocrinology and Metabolism. 2007;**92**(8):2917-2922

[56] Ünlütürk U, Erdoğan MF, Demir O, Culha C, Güllü S, Başkal N. The role of

ultrasound elastography in preoperative localization of parathyroid lesions: a new assisting method to preoperative parathyroid ultrasonography. Clinical Endocrinology (Oxf). 2012 Apr;**76**(4):492-498. DOI: 10.1111/j.1365-2265.2011.04241.x. PMID: 21955171

[57] Isidori AM, Cantisani V, Giannetta E, Diacinti D, David E, Forte V, et al. Multiparametric ultrasonography and ultrasound elastography in the differentiation of parathyroid lesions from ectopic thyroid lesions or lymphadenopathies. Endocrine. 2017 Aug;**57**(2):335-343. DOI: 10.1007/s12020-016-1116-1. Epub 2016 Oct 5. PMID: 27709473

[58] Azizi G, Piper K, Keller JM, Mayo ML, Puett D, Earp KM, et al. Shear wave elastography and parathyroid adenoma: A new tool for diagnosing parathyroid adenomas. European Journal of Radiology. 2016;**85**(9):1586-1593

[59] Batur A, Atmaca M, Yavuz A, Ozgokce M, Bora A, Bulut MD, et al. Ultrasound elastography for distinction between parathyroid adenomas and thyroid nodules. Journal of Ultrasound in Medicine. 2016;**35**(6):1277-1282

[60] Stangierski A, Wolinski K, Ruchala M. Shear wave elastography in the diagnostics of parathyroid adenomas–new application of the method. Endocrine. 2018;**60**(2):240-245

[61] Gharib H, Papini E, Paschke R, Duick DS, Valcavi R, Hegeds L, et al. American Association of Clinical Endocrinologists, Associazione Medici Endocrinologi, and European thyroid association medical guidelines for clinical practice for the diagnosis and management of thyroid nodules. Journal of Endocrinological Investigation. 2010;**33**(5 SUPPL):1-50

[62] Perros P, Boelaert K, Colley S, Evans C, Evans RM, Gerrard Ba G, et al. Guidelines for the management of thyroid cancer. Clinical Endocrinology (Oxf). 2014 Jul;**81**(Suppl 1):1-122. DOI: 10.1111/cen.12515. PMID: 24989897

Chapter 15

Use of Shear Wave Elastography in Pediatric Musculoskeletal Disorders

Celik Halil Ibrahim and Karaduman Aynur Ayşe

Abstract

Muscle shear-wave elastography (SWE) is an exciting and rapidly evolving ultrasound technique that allows quantification of muscle stiffness with a non-invasive, non-painful and non-irradiating examination. It has the potential of wider clinical use due to relatively low-cost, providing real-time measurement and, especially for the pediatric population, taking less time and sedation/anesthesia-free. Research indicate that muscle SWE shows promise as an adjunct clinical tool for differentiating between a normal and an abnormal muscle, monitoring the effectiveness of therapeutic interventions, altering the therapeutic intervention, or deciding treatment duration. This chapter will aim to provide an overview of the knowledge about the using of muscle SWE in common pediatric musculoskeletal disorders such as Duchenne Muscular Dystrophy, Cerebral Palsy, Adolescent Idiopathic Scoliosis, and Congenital Muscular Torticollis in the light of current evidence.

Keywords: shear-wave elastography, ultrasound elastography, muscle stiffness, muscle elasticity, musculoskeletal disorders

1. Introduction

Palpation is an ancient diagnostic method that has been used in medical practice for thousands of years since Hippocrates' day. Nevertheless, palpation is still valuable and often preferred today to assess the mechanical properties of a tissue in many clinical settings. However, some disadvantages such as limited tissue accessibility and inherent subjectivity may cause hesitations in its use [1]. To overcome these disadvantages by providing a more objective assessment of tissue mechanical properties, Magnetic Resonance Imaging Elastography and Ultrasound Elastography (USE) are the options offered by today's technology. However, the latter has the potential for wider clinical use because it is relatively low-cost, it provides real-time measurement, it takes less time, especially for the pediatric population, and it is sedation/anesthesia-free. The rapidly evolving evidence appears to be very promising that USE may be used to assess the mechanical properties of a tissue, especially muscle stiffness, that is, the degree of muscle resistance to deformation [2–4].

To briefly explain the basic principle, USE measures deformation in response to force/stress applied to the muscle. There are various USE techniques (strain elastography, Acoustic radiation force impulse [ARFI], Transient elastography, and Shear-wave elastography [SWE]), depending on the way of stress application and the measurement of deformation. SWE quantitatively measures muscle stiffness based on shear-wave propagation within the tissue and seems to be ahead of other USE techniques due to some prominent features such as less user-dependency, providing quantitative results besides elastogram, and higher reliability and repeatability [1, 4].

SWE shows promise as an adjunct clinical tool for differentiating between a normal and an abnormal muscle, monitoring the effectiveness of therapeutic interventions, altering the therapeutic intervention, or deciding treatment duration. Therefore, SWE, which measures individual muscle stiffness, can provide significant benefits, especially for physiotherapists because many rehabilitation strategies aim to change the muscle structure.

This chapter aims to present an overview of the knowledge about the use of muscle SWE in common pediatric musculoskeletal disorders such as Duchenne Muscular Dystrophy and Adolescent Idiopathic Scoliosis in the light of current evidence.

2. Shear-wave elastography in pediatric musculoskeletal disorders

2.1 Duchenne muscular dystrophy

Duchenne Muscular Dystrophy (DMD), which is the most common childhood neuromuscular disease with a prevalence of 1/3600–9300, is an X-linked recessive hereditary disease characterized by progressive muscle degeneration and weakness [5, 6]. The natural course of DMD includes pathological muscle changes, including a decrease in the number of normal muscle cells, dystrophic changes in myofibrils, and the replacement of normal muscle cells by adipose and fibrous tissues [7].

It is difficult to evaluate pathological changes in muscles and ultimately disease progression in patients with DMD because repeated muscle biopsies are invasive and not easily obtained [8, 9]. Therefore, it is emphasized that there is a need for reliable and non-invasive objective assessment tools that can be used routinely to evaluate disease progression and the efficacy of therapeutic interventions [10]. In response to this need, it has been emphasized in recent years that SWE is a promising clinical assessment tool to evaluate muscle pathology and disease progression in DMD [10–13].

Lacourpaille et al. and Pichiecchio et al. have found that lower and upper extremity muscle stiffness was higher in children with DMD compared with healthy controls and that SWE was able to distinguish between normal and dystrophic muscles [11, 12]. In another study, it was shown that muscle stiffness increased significantly in children with DMD after a 12-month follow-up period while muscle stiffness was stable in controls, and it was stated that SWE has the potential to be used in monitoring DMD progression [13]. Lin et al. reported that the stiffness of the tibialis anterior and the gastrocnemius medialis muscles decreased from ambulatory to early non-ambulatory stages, whereas the stiffness of the rectus femoris muscle increased. This result pointed out that individual muscles have different alteration patterns in stiffness as the ambulatory function declined and that SWE may be useful in the classification and prediction of ambulation status in children with DMD [10]. Additional information on muscle SWE studies in children with DMD is provided in **Tables 1** and **2**.

2.2 Cerebral palsy

Cerebral palsy (CP), a neurodevelopmental disorder caused by non-progressive immature brain disturbances, affects 2.11 of every 1000 children in high-income

Authors	Participants	Muscles	Findings
Lacourpaille [12]	14 children with DMD (age: 13.3 ± 5.9 y); 13 healthy controls (age: 12.8 ± 5.5 y)	TA, GM, VL, BB, TB, ADM	Significantly higher muscle stiffness in DMD patients compared with controls for all muscles, except for ADM.
Lacourpaille [13]	10 children with DMD (age range: 7–22 y); 9 healthy controls (age range: 7–22 y)	TA, GM, BB, TB, ADM	Significant increase in TA, GM, and TB stiffness over 12 months follow-up in patients with DMD while stiffness was stable in controls.
Pichiecchio [11]	5 preschool children with DMD (age range: 3.2–4.9 y); 5 healthy controls (age range: 3.3–3.9 y)	GM, RF, VM, VL, AM, TA, GMax	Muscle stiffness of the DMD patients was moderately higher than controls in the RF, VL, AM, and GMax muscles, whereas VM, TA and GM muscles of DMD patients were only minimally more stiff.
Lin [10]	39 children with DMD (age: 10.4 ± 3.8 y); 36 healthy controls (age: 9.2 ± 4.1 y)	RF, TA, GM	The stiffness of the RF and GM muscles was significantly higher in DMD patients compared with the control group. The stiffness of the TA and GM muscles decreased from ambulatory to early non-ambulatory stages, whereas the stiffness of the RF muscle increased from ambulatory to late non-ambulatory stages in DMD patients.

GMax, gluteus maximus; AM, adductor magnus; ADM, abductor digiti minimi; BB, biceps brachii; GM, gastrocnemius medialis; GL, gastrocnemius lateralis; RA, rectus abdominis; RF, rectus femoris; TA, tibialis anterior; TB, triceps brachii; VL, vastus lateralis; VM, vastus medialis.

Table 1.
Studies using muscle shear-wave elastography in Duchenne muscular dystrophy.

countries and is often considered to be the most common childhood motor disability [14, 15]. In CP, spasticity caused by an upper motor neuron lesion often leads to muscle weakness, muscle stiffness, and contractures, which eventually restrict general mobility [16]. Recent studies have emphasized the increased intensity of the connective tissue and extracellular matrix in spastic muscles, indicating that muscle stiffness may be a critical factor in the worsening of motor disorder over time in children with CP [17, 18]. These research findings may explain our clinical observations that many children with CP have an increase in muscle stiffness and a decrease in joint range of motion and in the efficiency of walking as they age into adolescence and adulthood. Therefore, it is not surprising that many studies have evaluated muscle stiffness with SWE in children with CP.

Muscle SWE studies comparing healthy children and children with CP have reported that muscle (GM, GL, BB, and SoL) stiffness is significantly higher in children with CP [16, 19–21]. Lee et al. [22] and Boulard et al. [23] have noted that muscle stiffness was higher in the more-affected limb than in the less-affected limb of children with CP. In addition, positive correlation has been reported between muscle stiffness and spasticity [20, 24, 25]. SWE has been used not only to distinguish between spastic and normal muscles but also to evaluate intervention effectiveness. All but one [26] of the studies investigating the effectiveness of botulinum toxin A (BTX) injection have reported a significant decrease in muscle stiffness a month after the injection [24, 25, 27]. In addition, it was stated that muscle stiffness values after 3 months is not significantly different from baseline values due to the duration of the

Muscles		Lacourpaille 2015 [12]	Pichiecchio 2018 [11]	Lin 2021 [10]
TA	DMD	23.1 ± 14.7 kPa	11.64 ± 1.35 kPa	2.87 ± 0.77 m/s
	HC	12.5 ± 3.1 kPa	13.54 ± 3.99 kPa	2.70 ± 0.42 m/s
GM	DMD	21.9 ± 12.7 kPa	12.9 ± 3.45 kPa	2.19 ± 0.57 m/s
	HC	14.5 ± 3.5 kPa	12.18 ± 5.56 kPa	1.85 ± 0.28 m/s
VL	DMD	21.5 ± 18.8 kPa	14.26 ± 1.34 kPa	—
	HC	9.6 ± 2.2 kPa	7.8 ± 2.74 kPa	—
VM	DMD	—	15.30 ± 2.43 kPa	—
	HC	—	11.56 ± 3.29 kPa	—
RF	DMD	—	14.44 ± 2.64 kPa	2.10 ± 0.72 m/s
	HC	—	8.10 ± 1.19 kPa	1.77 ± 0.28 m/s
GMax	DMD	—	13.92 ± 2.76 kPa	—
	HC	—	9.92 ± 1.31 kPa	—
AM	DMD	—	14.10 ± 1.31 kPa	—
	HC	—	9.74 ± 3.09 kPa	—
BB	DMD	34.9 ± 23.3 kPa	—	—
	HC	18.9 ± 6.4 kPa	—	—
TB	DMD	8.7 ± 2.1 kPa	—	—
	HC	7.3 ± 1.4 kPa	—	—
ADM	DMD	14.1 ± 7.8 kPa	—	—
	HC	11.9 ± 5.0 kPa	—	—

Table 2.
Muscles stiffness values in Duchenne Muscular Dystrophy.

effect of botulinum toxin [26]. In a study examining the relationship between hip muscle stiffness and hip dislocation, it was reported that there was a correlation between the Reimers Migration Index and the stiffness of the adductor magnus and the iliopsoas muscles [28]. Additional information on muscle SWE studies in children with CP is provided in **Tables 3** and **4**.

2.3 Adolescent idiopathic scoliosis

Adolescent idiopathic scoliosis (AIS), the most common type of scoliosis, is a 3D spinal deformity characterized by the deviation of the spine in the sagittal, frontal, and transverse plane [29]. The etiology of AIS has remained unclear until today even though many hypotheses have been put forward to explain the origin of this deformity [30].

Asymmetric loading on the vertebrae may be one of the causes contributing to the etiology of AIS [31]. Therefore, studies evaluating muscle stiffness with SWE and investigating muscle imbalance have been conducted to clarify the etiology of scoliosis. It has been suggested that this asymmetrical load may be caused by the paravertebral and lateral abdominal muscles consisting of the transversus abdominis (TrA), obliquus internal (OI), and obliquus external (OE) [32, 33]. Liu et al. reported no significant difference in paravertebral muscle stiffness between the concave and

Authors	Participants	Muscle(s) and Stiffness Values		Findings
Lallemant-Dudek [19]	16 children with CP (age: 8.3 ± 2.8 y); 29 healthy controls (age: 12.1 ± 3.3 y)	GM Stretched GCM; CP: 8.8 ± 4.1 m/s Controls: 2.9 ± 0.7 m/s GCM at rest CP: 3.1 ± 1.8 m/s Controls:1.8 ± 0.6 m/s	BB did not provide original data	Intra-rater ICC: 0.90 and inter-rater ICC: 0.92 in healthy controls. Stretched GM was significantly stiffer in CP than in controls. GM at rest did not show any difference between groups, nor did BB either at rest nor stretched.
Vola [20]	21 children with CP (age range: 3–16 y); 21 healthy controls (age range: 3–14 y)	SoL CP: 8.1 ± 2.3 kPa Controls: 4.8 ± 1.7 kPa		Muscle stiffness is significantly higher in children with CP compared with controls. High positive correlation ($r = 0.74$) between muscle stiffness and spasticity (MAS).
Lee [22]	8 children with CP (age: 9.4 ± 3.7 y)	GM more affected: 5.05 ± 0.55 m/s, less-affected: 4.46 ± 0.57 m/s	TA more affected: 3.86 ± 0.79 m/s, less-affected: 3.22 ± 0.40 m/s	Muscle stiffness of the GM and TA in the more-affected limb was higher than in the less-affected limb.
Brandenburg [16]	13 children with CP (age range: 2–12 y); 13 healthy controls (age range: 2–12 y)	GL CP: 15.0 (11.6, 17.5) kPa Controls: 7.8 (6.1, 11.0) kPa		Muscle stiffness is significantly higher in children with CP compared with controls.
Boulard [23]	11 children with CP (age: 11.1 ± 1.7 y)	GM more-affected: 10.2 ± 2.6 kPa less-affected: 7.9 ± 1.5 kPa		Muscle stiffness of the stretched GM in the more-affected limb was higher than in the less-affected limb.
Bilgici [21]	17 children with CP (age: 9.25 ± 2.68 y); 25 healthy controls (age: 10.40 ± 2.76 y)	GM CP: 3.17 ± 0.81 m/s Controls: 1.45 ± 0.25 m/s		Muscle stiffness is significantly higher in children with CP compared with controls.
Doruk Analan [28]	25 children with CP (age: 4.07 ± 2.25 y);	AM, IP AM: 2.65 ± 1.03 m/s IP: 2.61 ± 0.85 m/s		AM and IP muscle stiffness show correlation with the Reimers Migration Index (0.70 and 0.71, respectively).

IP, Iliopsoas; AM, adductor magnus; BB, biceps brachii; GM, gastrocnemius medialis; GL, gastrocnemius lateralis; SoL, Soleus; TA, tibialis anterior; MAS, Modified Ashworth Scale; kPa, kilopascal.

Table 3.
Studies using muscle shear-wave elastography in cerebral palsy-1.

the convex side of scoliosis [32]. In a study examining the stiffness of the lateral abdominal muscles (TrA, OI, and OE), it was stated that there were no differences between healthy control and AIS groups in terms of muscles stiffness at rest and during isometric contraction and also there was no muscles stiffness asymmetry between the concave and the convex sides of scoliosis [33]. In addition, the same

Authors	Participants	Muscle(s) and Stiffness Values		Findings
Bilgici [24]	12 children with CP (age: 8.58 ± 2.48 y);	GM Before: 3.20 ± 0.14 m/s After: 2.45 ± 0.21 m/s		Significant decrease in muscle stiffness a month after BTX injection. Muscle stiffness is correlate with MAS (r = 0.578).
Brandenburg [26]	10 children with CP (age range: 2.1–8.8 y);	GL (The article provided the change values, not the original values.)		Notable, but non-significant, decrease in muscle stiffness 1 month after BTX injection. Baseline muscle stiffness is not significantly different from 3 month after BTX injection.
Bertan [27]	17 children with CP (age: 4.6 ± 1.2 y); 16 children with CP (Control group) (age: 4.4 ± 1.2 y)	GM Before and after values for CP: 2.32 ± 0.50 and 2.08 ± 0.47 m/s Before and after values for controls: 2.34 ± 0.53 and 2.32 ± 0.48 m/s	GL Before and after values for CP: 2.07 ± 0.37 and 1.90 ± 0.31 m/s Before and after values for CP: 2.10 ± 0.48 and 1.98 ± 0.40 m/s	Significant decrease in muscle stiffness of GM and GL 1 month after BTX injection in study group while no significant decrease in the control group.
Dağ [25]	24 children with CP (age: 6 ± 2.8 y);	GM Before: 45.9 ± 6.5 kPa After: 25.0 ± 5.7 kPa		Significant decrease in muscle stiffness 1 month after BTX injection. Muscle stiffness is correlate with MAS and MTS (r = 0.77 and 0.79, respectively).

GM, gastrocnemius medialis; GL, gastrocnemius lateralis; MAS, Modified Ashworth Scale; MTS, Modified Tardieu Scale; BTX, botulinum toxin; kPa, kilopascal.

Table 4.
Studies using muscle shear-wave elastography in cerebral palsy-2.

research group found that stiffness measurements of the lateral abdominal muscles were carried out with high reliability/agreement during contraction, while the reliability of the stiffness measurements ranged from moderate to excellent at rest [34]. Another issue that attracts the attention of researchers is the involvement of respiratory muscles in scoliosis. By altering the biomechanics of the rib cage, scoliosis can affect the intercostal muscles (ICMs), thoracic expansion, and ultimately respiration. However, Pietton et al. investigated the stiffness of the ICMs in healthy control and AIS groups and reported that there was no significant difference between groups, although the AIS group displayed a trend toward higher stiffness of the ICMs than in the healthy group [35]. Additional information on muscle SWE studies in children with CP is provided in **Table 5**.

2.4 Congenital muscular torticollis

Congenital muscular torticollis (CMT) is a common muscular disorder occurring at or shortly after delivery as a result of the unilateral shortening of the

Authors	Participants	Muscle(s) and stiffness values	Findings
Linek [34]	35 children and adolescents with AIS (age: 12.8 ± 2.8 y)	OE, OI, TrA OE:21.1 ± 9.19 kPa OI:14.6 ± 4.24 kPa TrA:13.8 ± 4.22 kPa	At rest, the reliability of stiffness measurements ranged from moderate to excellent in all examined muscles (ICC: 0.56–0.94). During contraction, muscles stiffness was measured with high reliability/ agreement (ICC:0.63–0.91).
Linek [33]	108 children and adolescents with AIS (age range: 10–17 y); 151 healthy controls (age range: 10–17 y)	OE, OI, TrA For AIS; OE:16.6 ± 5.64 kPa OI:15.5 ± 4.63 kPa TrA:14.1 ± 3.50 kPa For healthy controls; OE:16.2 ± 5.67 kPa OI:15.2 ± 4.03 kPa TrA:13.9 ± 3.06 kPa	There were no differences between control and AIS groups in the muscles stiffness at rest and during isometric contraction. There were no muscles stiffness asymmetry between convex and concave body sides.
Liu [32]	40 children and adolescents with AIS (age: 10–18 y)	paravertebral muscles Concave side: 18.27 kPa Convex side: 14.31 kPa	No significant difference in muscle elasticity between the concave and the convex sides.
Pietton [35]	16 children and adolescents with AIS (age: 13 ± 2.5 y); 19 healthy controls (age: 12.6 ± 1.7 y)	ICMs AIS: 2.2 ± 0.3 m/s Healthy controls: 2.1 ± 0.4 m/s	SWE is feasible and reliable in the assessment of the ICMs of healthy individuals and those with scoliosis (ICC: 0.85 and 0.83, respectively). Although the AIS group showed a tendency toward higher ICMs stiffness than in the healthy group, there was no significant difference between groups.

OE = external oblique muscle; OI = internal oblique muscle; TrA = transversus abdominis muscle; ICMs, intercostal muscles; kPa, kilopascal.

Table 5.
Studies using muscle shear-wave elastography in adolescent idiopathic scoliosis.

sternocleidomastoid muscle (SCM), which results in clinical symptoms including head lateral tilt toward the ipsilateral side and head rotation to the opposite side [36, 37]. Long-lasting severe CMT can lead to asymmetric cranial and facial structures. Although the exact etiology of CMT remains unclear, endomysial fibrosis with collagen deposition and the migration of fibroblasts to individual muscle fibers are involved in the pathogenesis of CMT [38]. Ultimately, muscle fibrosis and increased stiffness can reduce the elasticity and function of the muscles, which leads to the range of motion deficit and contracture. Although CMT is a muscle-derived condition, the insufficient number of muscle SWE studies addressed the SCM stiffness indicates a large gap in the literature.

It was reported that the stiffness of the affected SCM was positively correlated with the degree of PROM deficit of neck rotation in the affected side [39–41] and affected SCM stiffness was significantly higher than that of the

Authors	Participants	Muscle(s) and stiffness values	Findings
Park [39]	20 infants with CMT (age: 0.71 ± 0.25 mo); 12 healthy controls (age: 0.65 ± 0.27 mo)	SCM infants with CMT: 3.65 ± 0.75 m/s Healthy controls: 1.50 ± 0.30 m/s	In the CMT group, the stiffness of the affected SCM was significantly higher than that of the unaffected SCM and than that in the control group. The stiffness of the affected SCM was positively correlated with the degree of PROM deficit of neck rotation in the affected side ($r = 0.77$). The intrarater reliability: ICC = 0.923.
Hwang [41]	22 infants with CMT (age: 1.16 ± 0.66 mo)	SCM Initial assessment: 2.33 ± 0.47 m/s After 3 months: 1.56 ± 0.63 m/s	The SCM stiffness decreased significantly from the initial evaluation to 3 months after the start of the physiotherapy. The initial SCM stiffness showed negative correlations with the degree of cervical rotation and lateral flexion, respectively ($r = -0.642$ and $r = -0.643$)
Zhang [40]	46 late-referral infants with CMT (age: 8.13 ± 1.77 mo)	SCM Affected SCM: 205.53 ± 46.34 kPa Unaffected SCM: 27.91 ± 4.90 kPa	SCM stiffness was positively correlated with the degree of the PROM deficit in neck rotation ($r = 0.82$). The intrarater reliability: ICC = 0.981

SCM, sternocleidomastoid muscle; PROM, passive range of motion; kPa, kilopascal.

Table 6.
Studies using muscle shear-wave elastography in congenital muscular torticollis.

unaffected SCM and than that in the control group [39]. Hwang et al. also reported that SCM stiffness decreased significantly after 3 months of physiotherapy [41]. These studies point out the potential of muscle SWE in the diagnosis and treatment of CMT. Additional information on muscle SWE studies in CMT is provided in **Table 6**.

2.5 Healthy children

Muscle SWE studies in healthy children are important for the reliability and repeatability of the measurement methods and to understand the effect of some individual factors such as sex and age on muscle stiffness. Brandenburg et al. reported that sex, age, BMI, extremity dominancy, and calf circumference were not associated with muscle stiffness in children [42]. Liu et al. compared the gastrocnemius medialis muscle stiffness of different age groups and found that there was no significant difference between sexes and muscle stiffness was the greatest in the older group, followed by the middle-aged group and then the children group [43]. Although these two studies give some clues, we think that further muscle SWE studies in healthy children are required and these studies are important especially for the measurement reliability, standardization of the measurement method, and establishing norm values for muscle stiffness. Additional information on muscle SWE studies in healthy children is provided in **Table 7**.

Authors	Participants	Muscle(s) and stiffness values	Findings
Liu [43]	27 children (age: 7.46 ± 1.46 y), 31 middle-aged individuals (age: 34.65 ± 3.19 y), and 28 older people (age: 62.25 ± 2.72 y).	GM Children: 24.28 ± 7.72 kPa Middle-aged individuals: 28.39 ± 6.85 kPa Older people: 34.89 ± 8.48 kPa	In all groups, passive muscle stiffness increased as the ankle DF increased. There was no significant difference between sexes. No significant difference in muscle stiffness between the three groups in terms of PF angles. The difference in muscle stiffness among the three groups became significant as DF increased. In terms of the ankle angles of DF, the muscle stiffness was the greatest in the older group, followed by the middle-aged group and then the children group (that is, stiffness increases with age).
Brandenburg [42]	20 healthy children (age range: 2–12 y),	GL R: 7.7 ± 2.5 kPa L: 7.8 ± 3.3 kPa	Sex, age, BMI, extremity dominancy, and calf circumference did not significantly correlate with muscle stiffness.

GM, gastrocnemius medialis; GL, gastrocnemius lateralis; DF, dorsi flexion; PF, plantar flexion; BMI, body mass index; R, right; L, left; kPa, kilopascal.

Table 7.
Studies using muscle shear-wave elastography in healthy children.

3. Conclusions

Muscle SWE is an exciting and rapidly evolving US technique that allows quantification of muscle stiffness with a non-invasive, non-painful, and non-irradiating examination. It has the potential of wider clinical use because it is relatively low-cost, it provides real-time measurement, it takes less time, especially for the pediatric population, and it is sedation/anesthesia-free. SWE shows promise as an adjunct clinical tool for differentiating between normal and abnormal muscles, monitoring the effectiveness of therapeutic interventions, altering the therapeutic intervention, or deciding treatment duration. Therefore, SWE, which measures individual muscle stiffness, can provide significant benefits, especially for physiotherapists because many rehabilitation strategies aim to change muscle structure. However, some remarkable points such as the insufficient number of studies, the small sample size, the differences in measurement settings and methods between studies, and the lack of norm values for different muscles indicate the necessity for further studies.

Conflict of interest

The authors declare that they have no conflict of interest.

Author details

Celik Halil Ibrahim* and Karaduman Aynur Ayşe*
Faculty of Health Sciences, Department of Physiotherapy and Rehabilitation, Lokman
Hekim University, Ankara, Turkey

*Address all correspondence to: ibrahim.celik@lokmanhekim.edu.tr; ayse.
karaduman@lokmanhekim.edu.tr

IntechOpen

References

[1] Bamber J, Cosgrove D, Dietrich CF, Fromageau J, Bojunga J, Calliada F, et al. EFSUMB guidelines and recommendations on the clinical use of ultrasound elastography. Part 1: Basic principles and technology. Ultraschall in der Medizin-European. Journal of Ultrasound. 2013;**34**(02):169-184

[2] Brandenburg JE, Eby SF, Song P, Zhao H, Brault JS, Chen S, et al. Ultrasound elastography: The new frontier in direct measurement of muscle stiffness. Archives of Physical Medicine and Rehabilitation. 2014;**95**(11): 2207-2219

[3] Miller T, Ying M, Sau Lan Tsang C, Huang M, Pang MY. Reliability and validity of ultrasound elastography for evaluating muscle stiffness in neurological populations: A systematic review and meta-analysis. Physical Therapy. 2021;**101**(1):pzaa188

[4] Goo M, Johnston LM, Hug F, Tucker K. Systematic review of instrumented measures of skeletal muscle mechanical properties: Evidence for the application of shear wave elastography with children. Ultrasound in Medicine & Biology. 2020;**46**(8): 1831-1840

[5] Mercuri E, Muntoni F. Muscular dystrophies. The Lancet. 2013; **381**(9869):845-860

[6] Mendell JR, Shilling C, Leslie ND, Flanigan KM, al-Dahhak R, Gastier-Foster J, et al. Evidence-based path to newborn screening for Duchenne muscular dystrophy. Annals of Neurology. 2012;**71**(3):304-313

[7] Desguerre I, Mayer M, Leturcq F, Barbet J-P, Gherardi RK, Christov C. Endomysial fibrosis in Duchenne

muscular dystrophy: A marker of poor outcome associated with macrophage alternative activation. Journal of Neuropathology & Experimental Neurology. 2009;**68**(7):762-773

[8] Mazzone E, Martinelli D, Berardinelli A, Messina S, D'Amico A, Vasco G, et al. North star ambulatory assessment, 6-minute walk test and timed items in ambulant boys with Duchenne muscular dystrophy. Neuromuscular Disorders. 2010;**20**(11):712-716

[9] Stuberg WA, Metcalf W. Reliability of quantitative muscle testing in healthy children and in children with Duchenne muscular dystrophy using a hand-held dynamometer. Physical Therapy. 1988; **68**(6):977-982

[10] Lin C-W, Tsui P-H, Lu C-H, Hung Y-H, Tsai M-R, Shieh J-Y, et al. Quantifying lower limb muscle stiffness as ambulation function declines in Duchenne muscular dystrophy with acoustic radiation force impulse shear wave elastography. Ultrasound in Medicine & Biology. 2021; **47**(10):2880-2889

[11] Pichiecchio A, Alessandrino F, Bortolotto C, Cerica A, Rosti C, Raciti MV, et al. Muscle ultrasound elastography and MRI in preschool children with Duchenne muscular dystrophy. Neuromuscular Disorders. 2018;**28**(6):476-483

[12] Lacourpaille L, Hug F, Guével A, Péréon Y, Magot A, Hogrel JY, et al. Non-invasive assessment of muscle stiffness in patients with Duchenne muscular dystrophy. Muscle & Nerve. 2015;**51**(2):284-286

[13] Lacourpaille L, Gross R, Hug F, Guével A, Péréon Y, Magot A, et al. Effects of Duchenne muscular dystrophy

on muscle stiffness and response to electrically-induced muscle contraction: A 12-month follow-up. Neuromuscular Disorders. 2017;**27**(3):214-220

[14] Rosenbaum P, Paneth N, Leviton A, Goldstein M, Bax M, Damiano D, et al. A report: The definition and classification of cerebral palsy April 2006. Developmental Medicine and Child Neurology. Supplement. 2007;**109** (suppl. 109):8-14

[15] Oskoui M, Coutinho F, Dykeman J, Jetté N, Pringsheim T. An update on the prevalence of cerebral palsy: A systematic review and meta-analysis. Developmental Medicine & Child Neurology. 2013;**55**(6):509-519

[16] Brandenburg JE, Eby SF, Song P, Kingsley-Berg S, Bamlet W, Sieck GC, et al. Quantifying passive muscle stiffness in children with and without cerebral palsy using ultrasound shear wave elastography. Developmental Medicine & Child Neurology. 2016; **58**(12):1288-1294

[17] Howard JJ, Graham K, Shortland AP. Understanding skeletal muscle in cerebral palsy: A path to personalized medicine? Developmental Medicine & Child Neurology. 2021. Sep 9. DOI: 10.1111/dmcn.15018. Epub ahead of print. PMID: 34499350

[18] Smith LR, Lee KS, Ward SR, Chambers HG, Lieber RL. Hamstring contractures in children with spastic cerebral palsy result from a stiffer extracellular matrix and increased in vivo sarcomere length. The Journal of Physiology. 2011;**589**(10):2625-2639

[19] Lallemant-Dudek P, Vergari C, Dubois G, Forin V, Vialle R, Skalli W. Ultrasound shearwave elastography to characterize muscles of healthy and cerebral palsy children. Scientific Reports. 2021;**11**(1):1-7

[20] Vola E, Albano M, Di Luise C, Servodidio V, Sansone M, Russo S, et al. Use of ultrasound shear wave to measure muscle stiffness in children with cerebral palsy. Journal of Ultrasound. 2018;**21**(3): 241-247

[21] Bilgici MC, Bekci T, Ulus Y, Ozyurek H, Aydin OF, Tomak L, et al. Quantitative assessment of muscular stiffness in children with cerebral palsy using acoustic radiation force impulse (ARFI) ultrasound elastography. Journal of Medical Ultrasonics. 2018;**45**(2): 295-300

[22] Lee SS, Gaebler-Spira D, Zhang L-Q, Rymer WZ, Steele KM. Use of shear wave ultrasound elastography to quantify muscle properties in cerebral palsy. Clinical Biomechanics. 2016;**31**: 20-28

[23] Boulard C, Gautheron V, Lapole T. Mechanical properties of ankle joint and gastrocnemius muscle in spastic children with unilateral cerebral palsy measured with shear wave elastography. Journal of Biomechanics. 2021;**124**: 110502. DOI: 10.1016/j.jbiomech.2021. 110502. Epub 2021 Jun 7. PMID: 34126561

[24] Bilgici MC, Bekci T, Ulus Y, Bilgici A, Tomak L, Selcuk MB. Quantitative assessment of muscle stiffness with acoustic radiation force impulse elastography after botulinum toxin A injection in children with cerebral palsy. Journal of Medical Ultrasonics. 2018;**45**(1):137-141

[25] Dağ N, Cerit MN, Şendur HN, Zinnuroğlu M, Muşmal BN, Cindil E, et al. The utility of shear wave elastography in the evaluation of muscle stiffness in patients with cerebral palsy after botulinum toxin A injection.

Journal of Medical Ultrasonics. 2020;
47(4):609-615

[26] Brandenburg JE, Eby SF, Song P, Bamlet W, Sieck GC, An K-N. Quantifying effect of onabotulinum toxin a on passive muscle stiffness in children with cerebral palsy using ultrasound shear wave elastography. American Journal of Physical Medicine & Rehabilitation. 2018;**97**(7):500

[27] Bertan H, Oncu J, Vanli E, Alptekin K, Sahillioglu A, Kuran B, et al. Use of shear wave elastography for quantitative assessment of muscle stiffness after botulinum toxin injection in children with cerebral palsy. Journal of Ultrasound in Medicine. 2020;**39**(12): 2327-2337

[28] Doruk Analan P, Aslan H. Association between the elasticity of hip muscles and the hip migration index in cerebral palsy. Journal of Ultrasound in Medicine. 2019;**38**(10):2667-2672

[29] Konieczny MR, Senyurt H, Krauspe R. Epidemiology of adolescent idiopathic scoliosis. Journal of Children's Orthopaedics. 2013;**7**(1):3-9

[30] Kouwenhoven J-WM, Castelein RM. The pathogenesis of adolescent idiopathic scoliosis: Review of the literature. Spine. 2008;**33**(26):2898-2908

[31] Stokes I. Mechanical effects on skeletal growth. Journal of Musculoskeletal and Neuronal Interactions. 2002;**2**(3):277-280

[32] Liu Y, Pan A, Hai Y, Li W, Yin L, Guo R. Asymmetric biomechanical characteristics of the paravertebral muscle in adolescent idiopathic scoliosis. Clinical Biomechanics. 2019;**65**:81-86

[33] Linek P, Pałac M, Wolny T. Shear wave elastography of the lateral

abdominal muscles in C-shaped idiopathic scoliosis: A case–control study. Scientific Reports. 2021;**11**(1):1-12

[34] Linek P, Wolny T, Sikora D, Klepek A. Supersonic shear imaging for quantification of lateral abdominal muscle shear modulus in pediatric population with scoliosis: A reliability and agreement study. Ultrasound in Medicine & Biology. 2019;**45**(7):1551-1561

[35] Pietton R, David M, Hisaund A, Langlais T, Skalli W, Vialle R, et al. Biomechanical evaluation of intercostal muscles in healthy children and adolescent idiopathic scoliosis: A preliminary study. Ultrasound in Medicine & Biology. 2021;**47**(1):51-57

[36] Sargent B, Kaplan SL, Coulter C, Baker C. Congenital muscular torticollis: Bridging the gap between research and clinical practice. Pediatrics. 2019;**144**(2): e20190582

[37] Ben Zvi I, Thompson DN. Torticollis in childhood—A practical guide for initial assessment. European Journal of Pediatrics. 2021;**1–9**. DOI: 10.1007/ s00431-021-04316-4. Epub ahead of print. PMID: 34773160

[38] Chen HX, Tang SP, Gao FT, et al. Fibrosis, adipogenesis, and muscle atrophy in congenital muscular torticollis. Medicine (Baltimore). 2014; **93**(23):e138. DOI: 10.1097/ MD.0000000000000138

[39] Park GY, Kwon DR, Kwon DG. Shear wave sonoelastography in infants with congenital muscular torticollis. Medicine. 2018;**97**(6):p e9818. DOI: 10.1097/MD.0000000000009818

[40] Zhang C, Ban W, Jiang J, Zhou Q, Li J, Li M. Two-dimensional ultrasound and shear wave elastography in infants with late-referral congenital muscular

torticollis. Journal of Ultrasound in
Medicine. 2019;38(9):2407-2415

[41] Hwang D, Shin YJ, Choi JY, Jung SJ,
Yang S-S. Changes in muscle stiffness in
infants with congenital muscular
torticollis. Diagnostics. 2019;9(4):158

[42] Brandenburg JE, Eby SF, Song P,
Zhao H, Landry BW, Kingsley-Berg S,
et al. Feasibility and reliability of
quantifying passive muscle stiffness in
young children by using shear wave
ultrasound elastography. Journal of
Ultrasound in Medicine. 2015;34(4):
663-670

[43] Liu X, Yu H-K, Sheng S-Y, Liang
S-M, Lu H, Chen R-Y, et al. Quantitative
evaluation of passive muscle stiffness by
shear wave elastography in healthy
individuals of different ages. European
Radiology. 2021;31(5):3187-3194

Chapter 16

Shear Wave Elastography for Chronic Musculoskeletal Problem

Tomonori Kawai

Abstract

Shear wave elastography is a new noninvasive tool for the analysis of the biomechanical properties of the muscles in healthy and pathological conditions. Shear wave elastography is currently considered as a promising real-time visualization tool for quantifying explicitly the mechanical properties of soft tissues in sports medicine including muscle strain injury (MSI). This chapter shows utilizing diagnostic tools of magnetic resonance imaging, B mode ultrasound (US), and shear wave elastography in both acute and chronic phases. Also, the proposal for this chapter is to indicate the possibility of utilizing shear wave elastography for musculoskeletal injury, not only properties of the muscle but also fascial tissues. It introduces the relationship between previous muscle strain injury and local soft tissue stiffness, and we assessed the mechanical properties of soft tissues from a clinical perspective.

Keywords: shear wave elastography, muscle strain, connective tissue, fascia, chronic injury

1. Introduction

In the sports medicine field, in order to evaluate musculoskeletal conditions such as muscle strain injury (MSI), magnetic resonance imaging (MRI) is commonly used in the diagnosis and prognosis of MSI. MRI uses the power of a magnetic field to determine the amount of water present in cells and tissues in the body.

The basic mechanism of MRI is that water has two hydrogen atoms, which are composed of a central proton and surrounding electrons. When a high-frequency current is pulsed to an object, the protons are stimulated and become imbalanced by acting against the gravitational pull of the magnetic field. When the radiofrequency field is turned off, the MRI sensors can detect the energy emitted when the protons rearrange to the magnetic field.

The time it takes for the protons to realign to a magnetic field depends on the environment and nature of the chemistry of the molecule to detect pathological changes [1]. MRI usually includes two types: T1-weighted and T2-weighted images, which are basically sets of settings. In T1-weighted images, the major adipose tissue appears white and the water and liquid components appear black. On the contrary, adipose tissue and fluid components appear white on T2-weighted images and can be used to detect the presence of pathological or morphological changes. Therefore, it can be used to assess fibrotic scar tissue when returning to sports or in the chronic phase of muscle injury to show anatomical features of the tissue [2].

While ultrasound (US) is used in musculoskeletal injury, the US uses high-frequency sound waves to evaluate organs and structures including muscle or other soft tissues. High-spatial-resolution modality provides details of a structure especially superficial area. There are some advantages of using both US and MRI evaluation. MRI is better in evaluating morphological changes, such as scar tissue and deep or large areas. On the other hand, the US is excellent at assessing small areas in detail. Because of its excellent contrast, high spatial resolution, and ability to view soft tissues with multiplanar evaluation, MRI currently appears to be the best imaging method for early-phase diagnosis and follow-up cases of muscle injuries. While the US can be a well-detected imaging method to assess adjunct tissues and can determine real-time conditions of muscle injuries.

1.1 Shear wave elastography

There are some kinds of diagnostic US, such as B mode US or shear wave elastography (SWE) for evaluating the musculoskeletal problems. B mode US is easy accessibility and relatively low cost, plus the possibility of real-time evaluation. Therefore, B mode US is widely used in the musculoskeletal field. However, B mode US cannot exactly investigate the biomechanical properties of tissues; therefore, it is difficult to assess the relationship with structural disorganization. In contrast, SWE is a novel noninvasive diagnostic ultrasound modality for analyzing the biomechanical properties of the soft tissues in healthy and pathological conditions.

Acoustic emission impulses are utilized to excite the tissue and measure the distribution of shear wave propagation speed by the shear wave as regards the mechanism of SWE [3]. SWE visualizes shear wave propagation and can quantify tissue stiffness based on the speed of propagation. SWE primarily assesses elasticity, also known as stiffness; the term of stiffness is basically recognized as the extent to which an object resists deformation in response to an applied force, and the speed of shear wave propagation is determined by both the elasticity and viscosity of the tissue [4]. As a result, it evaluates mechanical properties that indicate the deformity as an indicator of the quality of the object's form and shape. Normal muscle is considered a linear relationship between shear wave modulus and muscle tone. Therefore, normal muscle shows optimal stiffness on SWE (**Figure 1**) [5]. However, the score of SWE is influenced by the components of collagenous fiber tissue such as epimysium or endomysium; therefore, the definitive optimal stiffness is difficult to determine.

By contrast, B-mode US uses a monitor to convert the intensity of reflected waves into a two-dimensional tomographic image in the cross section parallel to the direction of the ultrasonic wave.

Because B-mode US is operator-independent, relatively reproducible, and quantitative method, SWE is currently considered as a promising real-time visualization tool for explicitly quantifying the mechanical properties of soft tissues in sports medicine [6].

B-mode US has a limitation that it is difficult to show the biomechanical properties of tissues.

Therefore, there is a difficulty to assess certain relationships between structural disorganization and clinical features [7]. On the other hand, SWE can obtain additional morphological information with elastic value of tissue structures and

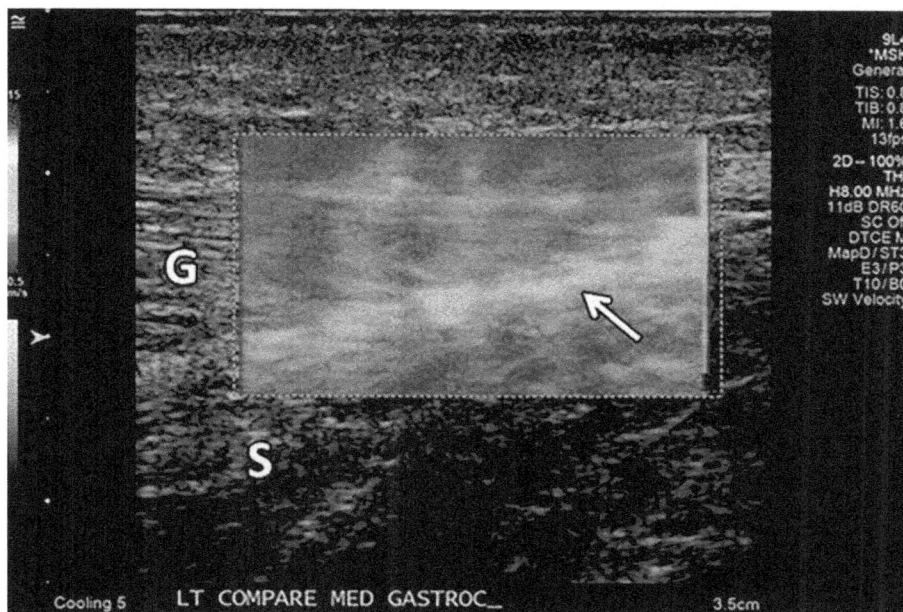

Figure 1.
Normal calf muscles are seen with normal echotexture on SWE [3].

mechanical properties in regard to tissue degeneration, tissue healing, or injury in the wide variety of tissues and injury phases.

Soft tissues, which are referred to muscle, fat, fibrous tissue, blood vessels, or other supporting tissue of the body, are generally recognized viscoelastic, inhomogeneous, and anisotropic [8]. Viscoelastic tissues have both elastic and viscous fluid properties that vary from tissue to tissue [9]. In order to evaluate elasticity, it assumes linear, elastic, solid tissues, a first-order approximation is possible without the force from viscous fluid properties. Elastography systems are based on the prerequisite assumption that object material tissues are elastic, incompressible, homogeneous, and isotropic [10]. Since the elasticity of soft tissues is nonlinear and dependent on the tissue density, strain magnitude, or applied excitation frequency, the evaluation of soft tissues still has been challenging with using diagnostic US.

Utilization of SWE for the musculoskeletal system should be taken into several considerations. Firstly, in order to evaluate swear wave values, a transducer of SWE is put on the surface of the body. As musculoskeletal tissue is heterogeneity, skeletal muscle fibers are surrounded by fascial tissues and passed through by nerve, arteries, veins, and lymphatic vessels. Besides the skin, which is a relatively tight organ, and dermis are superficial to the skeletal muscle fibers [11].

Secondly, the individual muscle fibers are thought to be parallel or oblique to the long axis of the muscle. Muscle fiber types, pennate, unipennate, or multipennate, may affect shear wave measurements; therefore, transductor positioning should be taken according to the muscle fiber architecture.

Thirdly, shear wave value may not change with depth within superficial muscles; however, if the muscle is deeper than 4 cm, the unit of measurement will be difficult to normalize [12].

Lastly, shear wave value, stiffness, can be affected by muscle activities. Changes in SWS measurements with muscle activation are shown during muscle contraction [13].

265

Plus, SWE measurements are different between active and passive muscles [14]. The more increased tension in the tissue, the more stiffness is measured [15]. Controlling the muscle activation and sustaining the perfect resting positioning are difficult in human in vivo study; therefore, the positioning is special care due to technical errors.

Evaluating for stiffness in MSI used to be difficult because it required a high mechanical load in a view of safety for the participants; however, SWE can have a low invasive approach besides visible in a resting position. In this regard, SWE takes an advantage to other diagnostic tools.

Furthermore, the measurement can be affected by some internal factors. Shear wave values tend to be higher in men than women. In addition, shear wave values are gradually increased according to age [16].

2. Imaging of musculoskeletal injury

2.1 Musculoskeletal injury

The general process of most MSI cases, and it leads to the typical inflammatory process. Muscle inflammation basically occurs in the following three phases: damage, repair, and remodeling; especially repair and remodeling phases happen almost at the same time. Muscle inflammation is a normal and inevitable process, which is healing tissues, and ensures optimal tissue regeneration in order to lead to proper muscle function. In the inflammatory phase, it begins with the destruction of the injured tissue. This reaction leads to an influx of extracellular calcium and the activation of calcium-dependent proteases and phospholipases. Furthermore, this destructed reaction will secrete the serum proteins deriving from disrupted tissue increase as creatine kinase, present in the cytosol of the muscle cell, and found in excessive mechanical stress or muscle degenerative diseases.

In the regeneration phase, the fibrotic scar tissue formation is built and the mature tissue recovers its muscle function as normal reaction [17]. In this phase, an increase in elastography stiffness can occur.

Recovering functional muscle tissue depends on proper joint motion at the remodeling phase. Proper fiber alignment can be one of the important factors for muscle function.

Fibroblasts play an important role in muscle tissue repair by secreting extracellular matrix (ECM) proteins including: collagen types I and III, fibronectin, elastin, proteoglycans, laminin, and growth factors. However, if fibroblasts excessively secret in ECM, the tissue alters the mechanical characteristics of the muscle, which leads to the development of fibrosis and incomplete muscle recovery [18]. Fibrotic tissue such as fibrotic scar tissue is characterized by the accumulation of ECM, primarily type I collagen. Fibrotic scar tissue is usually induced by chronic connective tissue injuries; however, the relationship between scar tissue and injuries has been still controversial [19]. Therefore, this relationship should be required further investigation and considerations.

2.2 In acute phase on MRI

MRI is commonly used for the diagnosis and recovery of muscle injuries [20].

T2 mapping may be useful from a musculoskeletal injury. Using a series of diffusion-weighted images and subsequent muscle fiber tracking, diffusion tensor imaging provides diffusion quantification of anisotropic tissues such as muscle tissues.

It has been shown that diffusion tensor imaging can be useful for identifying muscle fiber direction, detecting the subclinical changes after a muscle injury, and differentiating injured muscles from normal control muscles [21].

In the general clinical practice especially in sports medicine, MRI observation is suggested to monitor recovery following the injury and decide to return to play. It is basically observed increased signal intensity on fluid-sensitive sequences consistent with edema may persist after resolution of clinical symptoms 6 weeks after the onset of injury. However, even though almost all athletes that are clinically recovered and successfully returned to play showed increased signal intensities on fluid-sensitive sequences, MRI feature only should not be the decision to return to play because it is moderate correlation between clinical assessment using functional tests and MRI findings, plus it showed that functional testing was more accurate than MRI assessment [22].

2.3 In acute phase on B mode US and SWE

B mode US offers dynamic muscle assessment in acute musculoskeletal injury. It is a fast, relatively inexpensive, easier tool for the injuries. And also, it allows serial evaluation for the healing process, and it can be used to perform real-time interventions. In addition, B mode US takes an advantage to MRI in regard that it can demonstrate relevant anatomy surrounding an injury. In acute injury, it is sometimes difficult to show the tissues on MRI images due to inflammation reactions such as an edema [23].

Normal muscle fibers are properly arranged in parallel to fibrofatty septa. The muscle fibers and fascicles are usually hypo echogenicity compared with adjacent fascial tissues. Thick hyperechoic areas are dense fibrous content, which basically contains collagen fiber.

B mode US shows that normal muscle is hypoechoic muscle bundles and the linear hyperechoic perimysium are arranged in layers (**Figure 2**).

From a clinical perspective, in grade 1 MSI injuries, B mode US images may be either negative or exhibit focal or diffuse areas of increased echogenicity within the muscle at the site of injury. As Grade 1 MSI is known with or without actual fiber disruption, it may include injuries exhibiting minimal focal fiber disruption occupying less than 5% of the cross-sectional area of the muscle. The site of injury is represented by a well-defined focal hypoechoic or anechoic area within the muscle. However, there is no consensus about this definition. Therefore, the exact classification is unclear between grade 1 and grade 2 MSI [24]. In grade 2 MSI, the presence of areas of partial fiber disruption is less than 100% of the cross-sectional area of the muscle. Discontinuous fiber arrangement is usually seen in the echogenic perimysium striae around either the myotendon junction or the myofascial junction. Obvious intramuscular hematoma is normally seen in grade 2 MSI in initial almost 24–48 h. In this inflammation phase, hematomas may solidify and display increased echogenicity in comparison to the surrounding muscle. Up to 48 h, hematomas will develop into a well-defined hypoechoic fluid collection with an echogenic margin. In grade 3 MSI, total disruption or discontinuous fiber arrangement is observed on the B mode US. Perifascial fluid may be depicted on the B mode US and with hypoechoic area, which is the presence of extravascular blood in the inflammation phase.

The evaluation of B mode US should be careful because the linear configuration of the septae makes them susceptible to anisotropy artifact leading to decreased echogenicity or absence of conspicuity of septae.

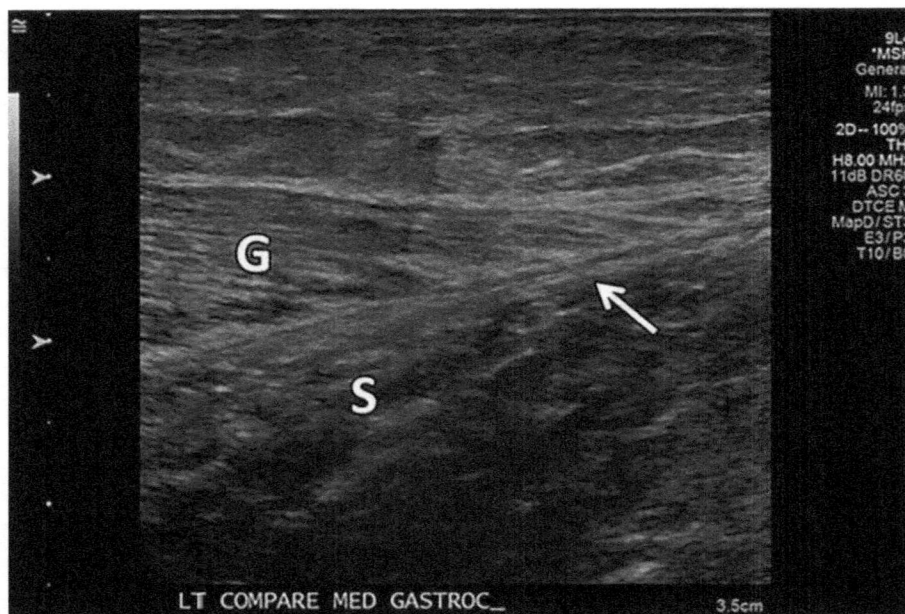

Figure 2.
Normal calf muscles are seen with proper layered fiber arrangement on B mode US [3].

The evaluation of SWE, when MSI occurred, the stiffness as shear wave value is decreased for 4–8 weeks. Then the stiffness is gradually increased, and it can generally return to a similar value as the uninjured side. This phenomenon is well explained that muscle tissue is properly in the acute phase of the healing process (**Figures 3** and **4**) [25].

Furthermore, another study shows that the stiffness of the postoperative tendon initially decreases and gradually increases following the recovery phases [26].

Improper healing tissue can be potential for re-injury; therefore; these results will be the parameter for return to play [27].

After MSI injury, MRI evaluation is basically used for injury evaluation in the acute phase.

Importantly, the T2 value is highest at 5 days on MRI while shear wave value is highest at 2 days on SWE.

2.4 In chronic phase on MRI

In the early stages of MSI, scar tissue formation can be visible as low signal intensity on T1-weighted images and high signal intensity on fluid-sensitive MRI. Scar tissue is observed almost 6 weeks after MSI, which can display low signal intensity on T1-weighted and high signal intensity on fluid-sensitive MRI at early stages.

It is typical for scar tissue to display as low signal intensity with MRI pulse sequences at the late stages. In the clinical practice, it may be misdiagnosed due to residual scar tissue and lead to over- or under-identification of new injuries [28].

During the healing phase up to a couple of months after MSI, differences in the hydrogen and proton environment due to obtained structural tissue changes including

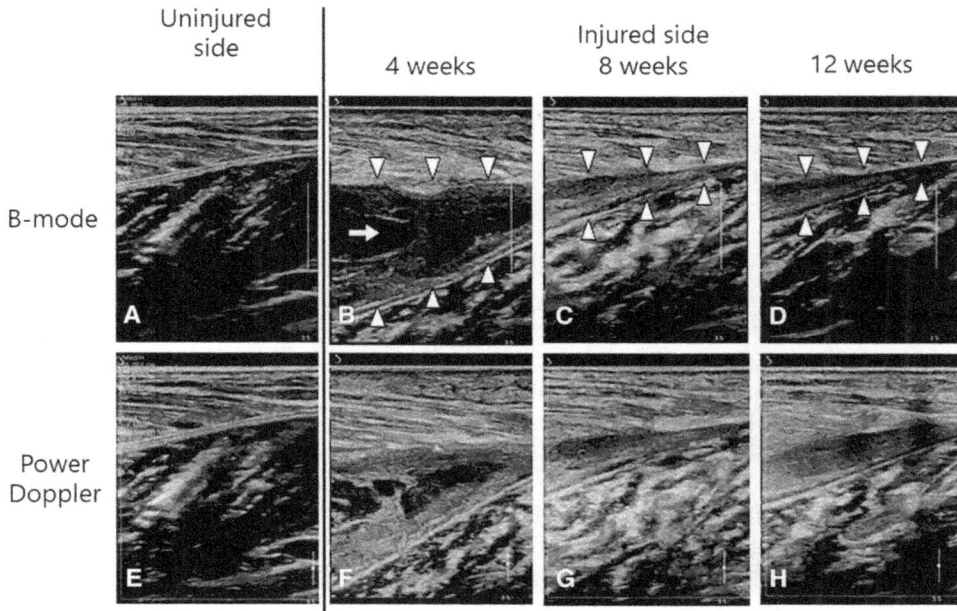

Figure 3.
The healing process of gastrocnemius muscle imaging B mode US [25].

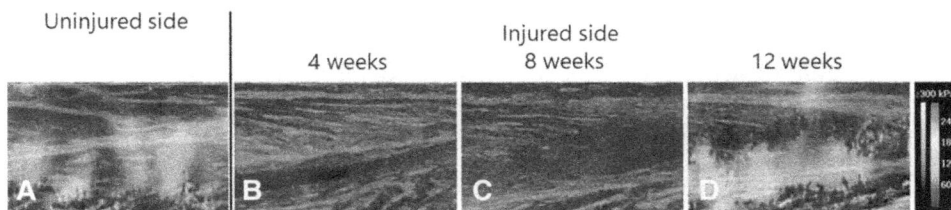

Figure 4.
The healing process of gastrocnemius muscle imaging and SWE [25].

hemorrhage may contribute to susceptibility artifacts. It may be observed during follow-up evaluation. A study shows that MRI could evaluate morphologic changes of musculotendon remodeling following MSI by using quantification of the scar tissue volumes [29].

2.5 In chronic phase on B mode US

The US can observe the healing process of injured tissues depending on the nature of the original injury. The B mode US may appear hyperechogenic during the healing phase. Normal tissue healing is considered a reduction in size or resolution of the region of increased echogenicity [30]. Even though the B mode US can evaluate the chronic phase of injured tissue, it is less sensitive than MRI to residual morphologic changes after MSI for the higher soft-tissue contrast and high to extracellular fluid in MRI [31]. In clinical practice, the detection of small echogenic scar tissue by using the B mode US is difficult for a less experienced practitioner. As mentioned above, the relationship between demonstration of scar tissue and re-injury is still controversial. However, excessive scar tissue may be symptomatic that is described as "feeling tight." It may disturb neural tension, which leads to re-injury [32].

Scar tissue is often shown as irregular thickening of the fascial tissue compared with the uninjured side on the B mode US [33].

Skeletal muscles are also composed of connective tissue, which resists and transmits the force generated by myofibrils to the tendon and bone structures to generate physical movement. When skeletal muscles are injured, any one of these components including fascial tissue can be damaged [18].

2.6 In chronic phase on SWE

SWE can take an advantage to evaluate tissue properties in chronic phase compared with B mode US. SWE can evaluate the absolute elasticity value of soft tissue structures and obtain useful quantitative information about the mechanical properties in the chronic phase.

In the chronic phase of MSI, the stiffness is significantly higher in the chronic phase compared with the acute phase [25].

In the chronic phase of tendon rupture injury, the stiffness of the tissue gradually increased following the healing process with or without surgical repair [34].

From these results, SWE can be a useful tool for evaluating in the phase of transition of acute to chronic phase.

Tendinopathy is considered to occur from mechanical, degenerative, and overuse diseases. It is associated with degeneration and disorganization of the collagenous structure, changes in the proteoglycan and water contents, increased cellularity, fatty infiltration, and neovascularization due to repetitive mechanical stress [35]. A study of tendinopathy shows tendon stiffness is correlated with the patients' symptom scores, demonstrating the promise of shear wave elastography during follow-up for tendinopathies [36].

Interestingly, by evaluating SWE, injured area of fascial tissue increased stiffness between injured leg and uninjured leg in 11 injured professional rugby players, mean average of shear wave modulus on injured side (17.34 ± 9.04 kPa) and maximum shear wave modulus on injured side (33.53 kPa) compared with mean average of shear wave modulus on uninjured side (12.7 ± 4.96 kPa) and maximum shear wave modulus on uninjured side (20.86 kPa) (**Figures 5** and **6**) [37].

Chronic cumulative injury can affect the fascial tissue in addition to the chronic phase of direct trauma. Cumulative mechanical stress leads to fibrotic tissue, thickness of tendinous tissue could be related to the injury [38]. Repetitive cumulative stress, especially eccentric contraction, causes microscopic tissue damage and increases inflammation. ECM of tissue changes plays an important role in tissue stiffness changes [39]. Change in property of ECM by cumulative stress may affect the stiffness in the chronic musculoskeletal injury.

Considering the results, in chronic musculoskeletal injury, it affects not only the muscle tissue but also a wide variety of tissues including fascial tissue. Even though a wide variety of ultrasound imaging has been used in fascial tissue, there is a lack of standardization [40]. SWE can be a more accurate diagnostic tool compared with B-mode, and the combination of SWE and B-US can be a strong diagnostic tool for fascial pathology [41].

To measure the fascial tissue, SWE provides the images reflecting the shear wave value as a tightness of the area of interest.

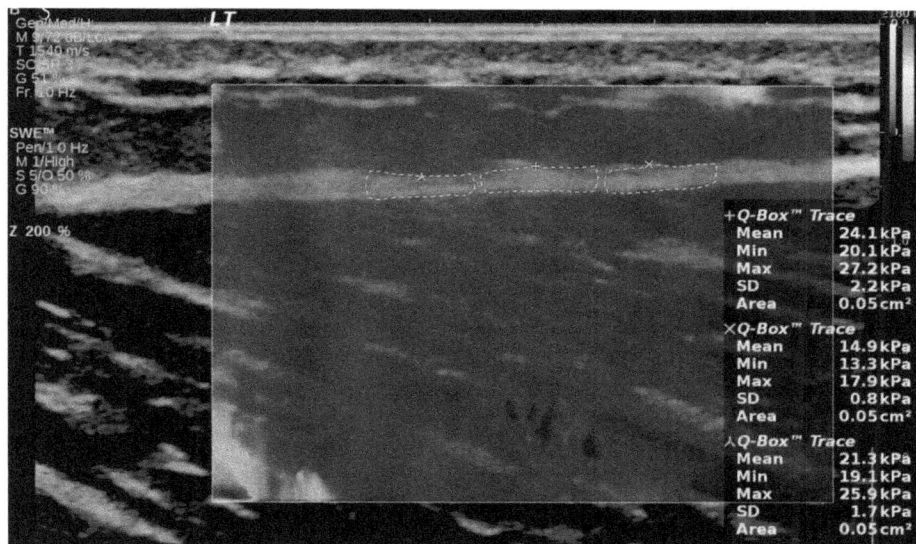

Figure 5.
The stiffness of fascial tissue of injured side by using Q box trace mode, and the unit was given automatically by machine in kilopascal units. Injured side stiffness is higher than that of uninjured side.

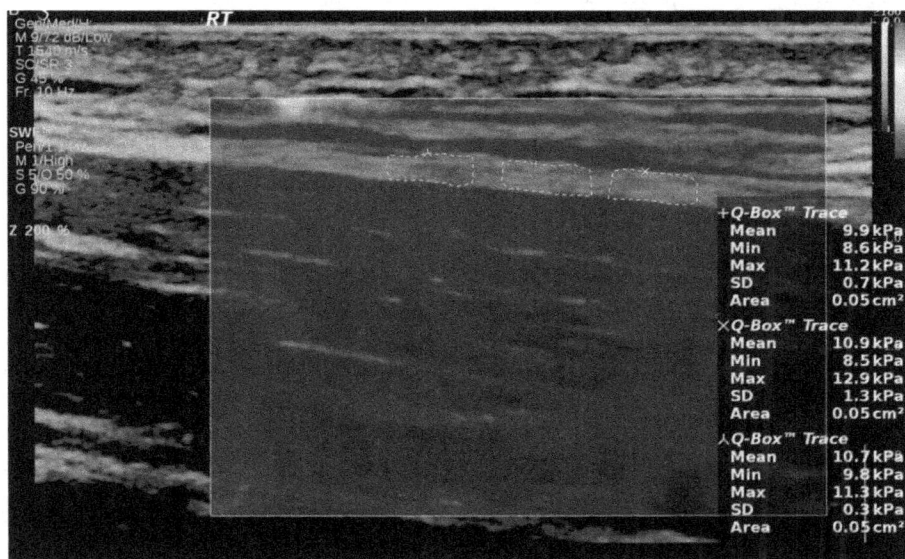

Figure 6.
The stiffness of fascial tissue of uninjured side by using Q box trace mode, and the unit was given automatically by machine in kilopascal units.

As considering the tissue property depending on viscoelastic property, utilization of SWE can be a useful tool for evaluating a wide variety of tissues in chronic musculoskeletal injury.

To explain fascial tissue, the term Fascia is used to be recognized as "a sheet or band of soft connective tissue that attaches, surrounds and separates internal organs and skeletal muscles." However, according to the recognition of physiological and pathophysiological behaviors of a range of connective tissues, the definition is widely considered. With current understanding of mechanical aspects of connective tissue function, fascia is considered in the view of micro to macro as fibril to fascial system. From a morphological view, fascia is described as a sheet or any other dissectible aggregations of connective tissue that forms beneath the skin to attach, enclose, and separate muscles and other internal organs.

There are several types of fascial tissues in the fascial system. The fascial system consists of adipose tissue, adventitia, neurovascular sheaths, aponeuroses, deep and superficial fasciae, dermis, epineurium, joint capsules, ligaments, membranes, meninges, myofascial expansions, periostea, retinacula, septa, tendons. The fascial system is also considered to be included endotendon, peritendon, epitendon, and paratenson, visceral fasciae, and all the intramuscular and intermuscular connective tissues, including endomysium, perimysium, epimysium. The fascial system consists of various components, and it is built on three-dimensional soft seamless collagenous fibers. The loose and dense fibrous connective tissue fills the whole body and allows the integration of body systems.

With injured fascial tissues, it will have a very similar healing process to muscle injury. Micro or macro changes occurred by excessive or repetitive loading or direct trauma of fascial tissue. The pathological changes will modify mechanical function that compromises initial tissue or function. In the acute inflammation phase of fascial tissue, immune response proceeds by phagocytose from the injured cell. It releases proinflammatory cytokines and macrophages to promote immune cell infiltration. If the excessive loading is chronically prolonged, continuing inflammation develops, which leads to the presence of cytotoxic cytokines affected tissues. From this reaction, interleukin-1β, tumor necrosis factor (TNF) and transforming growth factor beta (TGFβ-1)) can promote fibrosis by excessive fibroblast proliferation and collagen matrix deposition that consequently develops fibrotic tissue. A study indicates that substance P stimulates TGFβ-1, which leads to fibrotic tissue development [42]. That phenomenon shows in the chronic phase of fascial injury.

Most pathological cases of fascial tissue demonstrated that a decreased tissue stiffness is present, while some cases demonstrated an increased stiffness due to fibrotic tissues.

However, the viscoelasticity is varied from tissue to tissue. The stiffness of tissue can be affected by the viscoelastic properties of ECM, especially the aponeurotic tissue containing loose connective tissue in which the ECM has ground substances, such as glycosaminoglycans (GAGs) especially hyaluronan (HA)-containing fluid between each layer [43]. The fascial component of the ECM is the main site of the inflammatory responses that occur in tissues. Thus, when the tissue reacts to an inflammatory response, the viscosity of the tissue can be increased, which could lead to increased viscoelasticity of the fascial tissue.

Evaluation of the stiffness of fascial tissue using SWE is considered as viscoelastic, inhomogeneous tissues [44]. The shear modulus value, stiffness, of fascial tissue is affected not only by the fibrotic tissue itself, but also ground substances and fluid components [45]. Therefore, stiffness is affected not only by pure elastic properties, but also by viscosity properties in the fascial tissue [46].

Fascial tissue can be affected by viscoelastic properties more than muscle [47].

Fascial tissue should include loose connective tissue, which contains rich ground substances between each layer. These properties affect the movement of loose connective tissue within and under the tissues [48].

In the chronic condition of MSI, the concentration and molecular weight of HA are altered. In this regard, binding interactions with other macromolecules may affect the sliding movement of fascial tissues [49]. Generally speaking, elastic tissues are hydrophilic and function using a tissue sliding system. However, fibrotic tissues exhibit an altered tissue sliding system, which affects the rehydration and expansion [50]. Therefore, in chronic MSI with scar tissue, there may be less function of rehydration; consequently, it will be stiffer tissue than healthy tissue. Even though SWE is considered not operator-dependent, the viscosity component will affect the results of measurement. Therefore, viscoelastic tissue such as fascial tissue must take special consideration in chronic musculoskeletal conditions.

This phenomenon may affect our daily activities for some reasons.

First, fascial tissues are rich in nerve receptors and free and encapsulated nerve endings including Pacinian corpuscles and Ruffini endings. Those receptors detect and react to mechanical stimulations [51]. As the tissue is stimulated, the nerve endings react and provide sensory feedback that translates into the human ability to detect and coordinate movement and achieve neuromuscular control. Chronic musculoskeletal issues, especially with fibrotic scar tissue, can alter the movement in daily activities.

Secondly, changes in the viscoelasticity of the tissues, basically modulated by ground substances, alter pain sensitivity as activation of nociceptors [48]. The more adhered tissue such as an inflamed tissue, the less lubricated that leads to the alteration of the tissue sliding. Thus, nociceptors can translate mechanical stimuli into pain sensation; consequently, incorrect sensory feedback will modify proprioceptors to nociceptors. Finally, myofascial network transmits to other tissues for muscle force [52]. Stiffened tissue affects this transmission and may change muscle mechanics [53]. Therefore, impaired myofascial force transmission by stiffened tissue may have a negative effect on the proper muscle biomechanics.

3. Conclusion

SWE is a newly developed diagnostic tool and is widely used in the musculoskeletal system.

SWE is a promising diagnostic modality for MSI and the accurate measurement of muscle and fascial tissues' properties, which has a major impact in clinical practice. In this chapter, diagnostic tools of magnetic resonance imaging, B mode ultrasound, and shear wave elastography in both acute and chronic phases are compared. There are pros and cons for utilization between the tools; however, there is new insight by using SWE in MSI not only properties of muscle but also fascial tissues. SWE generally evaluates tissue stiffness as viscoelasticity. SWE visualizes the propagation of shear waves and can quantify tissue "stiffness" by the speed of propagation. In the chronic MSI cases, viscoelasticity comes from ground substances, which are contained more in fascial tissue. The stiffness increases in fascial tissue more than muscle; therefore, in the chronic case of MSI, not only muscle but also a wide variety of connective tissues can be considered. However, utilization of SWE should be careful due to technical pitfalls or internal factors. All in all, SWE is a promising diagnostic modality for MSI and the accurate measurement of muscle and fascial tissues properties, which has a major impact in clinical practice. There are few studies that investigate for chronic musculoskeletal problem including fascial tissue problem by using SWE especially in clinical trials. Furthermore, the shear wave value is different according to active muscle contraction. Therefore, further studies for chronic musculoskeletal problem will be expected in a wide variety of conditions.

Conflict of interest

The authors declare no conflict of interest.

Author details

Tomonori Kawai
Faculty of Human Sciences, Department of Sports and Health Sciences, University of East Asia, Ichinomiya, Yamaguchi, Japan

*Address all correspondence to: tomochiro@toua-u.ac.jp

IntechOpen

References

[1] Berger A. Magnetic resonance imaging. BMJ. 2002;**324**(7328):35. DOI: 10.1136/bmj.324.7328.35

[2] Verrall GM, Slavotinek JP, Barnes PG, Fon GT, Esterman A. Assessment of physical examination and magnetic resonance imaging findings of hamstring injury as predictors for recurrent injury. The Journal of Orthopaedic and Sports Physical Therapy. 2006;**36**(4):215-224. DOI: 10.2519/jospt.2006.36.4.215

[3] Taljanovic MS, Gimber LH, Becker GW, et al. Shear-wave elastography: Basic physics and musculoskeletal applications. Radiographics. 2017;**37**(3):855-870. DOI: 10.1148/rg.2017160116

[4] Chan O, Del Buono A, Best TM, Maffulli N. Acute muscle strain injuries: A proposed new classification system. Knee Surgery, Sports Traumatology, Arthroscopy. 2012;**20**:2356-2362. DOI: 10.1007/s00167-012-2118-z

[5] Eby SF, Song P, Chen S, Chen Q, Greenleaf JF, An K-N. Validation of shear wave elastography in skeletal muscle. Journal of Biomechanics. 2013;**46**:2381-2387

[6] Finnoff JT, Hall MM, Adams E, et al. American Medical Society for Sports Medicine (AMSSM) position statement: Interventional musculoskeletal ultrasound in sports medicine. PM&R. 2015;**7**:151-168. DOI: 10.1016/j.pmrj.2015.01.003

[7] Docking SI, Ooi CC, Connell D. Tendinopathy: Is imaging telling us the entire story? The Journal of Orthopaedic and Sports Physical Therapy. 2015;**45**:842-852. DOI: 10.2519/jospt.2015.5880

[8] Bercoff J, Tanter M, Muller M, Fink M. The role of viscosity in the impulse diffraction field of elastic waves induced by the acoustic radiation force. IEEE Transactions on Ultrasonics, Ferroelectrics, and Frequency Control. 2004;**51**:1523-1536. DOI: 10.1109/tuffc.2004.1367494

[9] Bercoff J, Tanter M, Fink M. Supersonic shear imaging: A new technique for soft tissue elasticity mapping. IEEE Transactions on Ultrasonics, Ferroelectrics, and Frequency Control. 2004;**51**:396-409. DOI: 10.1109/tuffc.2004.1295425

[10] Barr RG, Ferraioli G, Palmeri ML, Goodman ZD, et al. Elastography assessment of liver fibrosis: Society of radiologists in ultrasound consensus conference statement. Radiology. 2015;**276**:845-861. DOI: 10.1148/radiol.2015150619. Epub 2015 Jun 16

[11] Chino K, Kawakami Y, Takahashi H. Tissue elasticity of in vivo skeletal muscles measured in the transverse and longitudinal planes using shear wave elastography. Clinical Physiology and Functional Imaging. 2017;**37**(4):394-399. DOI: 10.1111/cpf.12315. Epub 2015 Dec 22

[12] Alfuraih AM, O'Connor P, Hensor E, et al. The effect of unit, depth, and probe load on the reliability of muscle shear wave elastography: Variables affecting reliability of SWE. Journal of Clinical Ultrasound. 2018;**46**(2):108-115. DOI: 10.1002/jcu.22534

[13] Nordez A, Gennisson JL, Casari P, et al. Characterization of muscle belly elastic properties during passive stretching using transient elastography. Journal of Biomechanics. 2008;**41**:2305-2311. DOI: 10.1016/j.jbiomech.2008.03.033. Epub 2008 Jun 9

[14] Chernak LA, DeWall RJ, Lee KS, et al. Length and activation dependent variations in muscle shear wave speed. Physiological Measurement. 2013;**34**(6):713-721. DOI: 10.1088/0967-3334/34/6/713

[15] Yavuz A, Bora A, Bulut MD, Batur A, et al. Acoustic radiation force impulse (ARFI) elastography quantification of muscle stiffness over a course of gradual isometric contractions: A preliminary study. Medical Ultrasonography. 2015;**17**(1):49-57. DOI: 10.11152/mu.2013.2066.171.yvz

[16] Eby SF, Cloud BA, Brandenburg JE, et al. Shear wave elastography of passive skeletal muscle stiffness: Influences of sex and age throughout adulthood. Clinical Biomechanics. 2015;**30**:22-27. DOI: 10.1016/j.clinbiomech.2014.11.011

[17] Järvinen TA, Järvinen M, Kalimo H. Regeneration of injured skeletal muscle after the injury. Muscle, Ligaments and Tendons Journal. 2014;**3**:337-345

[18] Kääriäinen M, Järvinen T, Järvinen M, et al. Relation between myofibers and connective tissue during muscle injury repair. Scandinavian Journal of Medicine & Science in Sports. 2000;**10**:332-337. DOI: 10.1034/j.1600-0838.2000.010006332.x

[19] Reurink G, Almusa E, Goudswaard GJ, et al. No association between fibrosis on magnetic resonance imaging at return to play and hamstring reinjury risk. American Journal of Sports Medicine. 2015;**43**:1228-1134. DOI: 10.1177/0363546515572603. Epub 2015 Mar 6

[20] Kerkhoffs GMMJ, van Es N, Wieldraaijer T, et al. Diagnosis and prognosis of acute hamstring injuries in athletes. Knee Surgery, Sports Traumatology, Arthroscopy.

2013;**21**:500-509. DOI: 10.1007/s00167-012-2055-x. Epub 2012 May 24

[21] May DA, Disler DG, Jones EA, et al. Abnormal signal intensity in skeletal muscle at MR imaging: Patterns, pearls, and pitfalls. Radiographics. 2000;**20**:S295-S315. DOI: 10.1148/radiographics.20.suppl_1.g00oc18s295

[22] Schneider-Kolsky ME, Hoving JL, Warren P, et al. A comparison between clinical assessment and magnetic resonance imaging of acute hamstring injuries. The American Journal of Sports Medicine. 2006;**34**:1008-1015. DOI: 10.1177/0363546505283835

[23] Connell DA, Schneider-Kolsky ME, Hoving JL, et al. Longitudinal study comparing sonographic and MRI assessments of acute and healing hamstring injuries. AJR. American Journal of Roentgenology. 2004;**183**(4):975-984. DOI: 10.2214/ajr.183.4.1830975

[24] Lee JC, Mitchell AW, Healy JC, Thorstensson A. Imaging of muscle injury in the elite athlete. The British Journal of Radiology. 2012;**85**(1016):1173-1185. DOI: 10.1259/bjr/84622172. Epub 2012 Apr 11

[25] Yoshida K, Itoigawa K, Maruyama Y, et al. Healing process of gastrocnemius muscle injury on ultrasonography using B-mode imaging, power doppler imaging, and shear wave elastography. Journal of Ultrasound in Medicine. 2019;**38**(12):3239-3246. DOI: 10.1002/jum.15035. Epub 2019 Jun 4

[26] Zhang L, Wan W, Wang Y, et al. Evaluation of elastic stiffness in healing achilles tendon after surgical repair of a tendon rupture using in vivo ultrasound shear wave elastography. Medical Science Monitor. 2016;**22**:1186-1191. DOI: 10.12659/MSM.895674

[27] Eming SA, Martin P, Tomic-Canic M. Wound repair and regeneration: Mechanisms, signaling, and translation. Science Translational Medicine. 2014;**6**(265):265sr6. DOI: 10.1126/scitranslmed.3009337

[28] Blankenbaker DG, Tuite MJ. Temporal changes of muscle injury. Seminars in Musculoskeletal Radiology. 2010;**14**(2):176-193. DOI: 10.1055/s-0030-1253159

[29] Slider A, Heiderscheit BC, Thelen DG, Enright T, Tuite MJ. MR observations of longterm musculotendon remodeling following a hamstring strain injury. Skeletal Radiology. 2008;**37**(12):1101-1109. DOI: 10.1007/s00256-008-0546-0. Epub 2008 Jul 23

[30] Takebayashi S, Takasawa H, Banzai Y, et al. Sonographic findings in muscle strain injury: Clinical and MR imaging correlation. Journal of Ultrasound in Medicine. 1995;**14**(12):899-905. DOI: 10.7863/jum.1995.14.12.899

[31] Petersen J, Thorborg K, Nielsen MB, et al. The diagnostic and prognostic value of ultrasonography in soccer players with acute hamstring injuries. The American Journal of Sports Medicine. 2014;**42**(2):399-404. DOI: 10.1177/0363546513512779. Epub 2013 Dec 11

[32] Brukner P. Hamstring injuries: Prevention and treatment—An update. British Journal of Sports Medicine. 2015;**49**(19):1241-1244. DOI: 10.1136/bjsports-2014-094427

[33] Drakonaki EE, Sudoł-Szopińska I, Sinopidis C. High resolution ultrasound for imaging complications of muscle injury: Is there an additional role for elastography? Journal of

Ultrasonography. 2019;**19**(77):137-144. DOI: 10.15557/JoU.2019.0020. Epub 2019 Jun 28

[34] Frankewycz B, Henssler L, Weber J, et al. Changes of material elastic properties during healing of ruptured achilles tendons measured with shear wave elastography: A pilot study. International Journal of Molecular Sciences. 2020;**21**(10):3427. DOI: 10.3390/ijms21103427

[35] Aubry S, Nueffer JP, Tanter M, et al. Viscoelasticity in Achilles tendonopathy: Quantitative assessment by using real-time shear-wave elastography. Radiology. 2015;**274**:821829. DOI: 10.1148/radiol.14140434. Epub 2014 Oct 17

[36] Dirrichs T, Quack V, Gatz M, et al. Shear wave elastography (SWE) for the evaluation of patients with tendinopathies. Academic Radiology. 2016;**23**:1204-1213. DOI: 10.1016/j.acra.2016.05.012. Epub 2016 Jun 16

[37] Kawai T, Takahashi M, Takamoto K, et al. Hamstring strains in professional rugby players result in increased fascial stiffness without muscle quality changes as assessed using shear wave elastography. Journal of Bodywork and Movement Therapies. 2021;**27**:34-41. DOI: 10.1016/j.jbmt.2021.03.009. Epub 2021 Mar 20

[38] Paluch L, Nawrocka-Laskus E, Wieczorek J, et al. Use of ultrasound elastography in the assessment of the musculoskeletal system. Polish Journal of Radiology. 2016;**81**:240-246. DOI: 10.12659/PJR.896099. eCollection 2016

[39] Kjaer M, Magnusson P, Krogsgaard M, et al. Extracellular matrix adaptation of tendon and skeletal muscle to exercise. Anatolia.

2006;**208**(4):445-450. DOI: 10.1111/j. 1469-7580.2006.00549.x

[40] Mc Auliffe S, Mc Creesh K, Purtill H, et al. A systematic review of the reliability of diagnostic ultrasound imaging in measuring tendon size: Is the error clinically acceptable? Physical Therapy in Sport. 2017;**26**:S14 6630207-S146630203. DOI: 10.1016/j. ptsp.2016.12.002. Epub 2016 Dec 8

[41] Gatz M, Ljudmila Bejder L, Quack V, et al. Shear wave elastography (SWE) for the evaluation of patients with plantar fasciitis. Academic Radiology. 2020;**27**(3):363-370. DOI: 10.1016/j. acra.2019.04.009. Epub 2019 May 30

[42] Frara N, Fisher PW, Zhao Y, et al. Substance P increases CCN2 dependent on TGF-beta yet collagen type I via TGF-beta1 dependent and independent pathways in tenocytes. Connective Tissue Research. Jan 2018;**59**(1):30-44. DOI: 10.1080/03008207.2017.1297809. Epub 2017 Apr 12

[43] Stecco A, Stecco C, Raghaven P. Peripheral mechanisms contributing to spasticity and implications for treatment. Current Physical Medicine and Rehabilitation Reports. 2014;**2**:121-127. DOI: 10.1007/s40141-014-0052-3

[44] Urban M, Chen S, Fatemi M. A review of shearwave dispersion ultrasound vibrometry (SDUV) and its applications. Current Medical Imaging. 2012;**8**:27-36. DOI: 10.2174/1573405 12799220625

[45] Andonian P, Viallon M, Le Goff C, et al. Shear-wave elastography assessments of quadriceps stiffness changes prior to, during and after prolonged exercise: A longitudinal study during an extreme mountain ultra-marathon. PLoS One. 2016;**11**:e0161855. DOI: 10.1371/journal. pone.0161855. eCollection 2016

[46] Davis LC, Baumer TG, Bey MJ, et al. Clinical utilization of shear wave elastography in the musculoskeletal system. Ultrasonography. 2019;**38**:2-12. DOI: 10.14366/usg.18039. Epub 2018 Aug 23

[47] Gao Y, Waas AM, Faulkner JA, et al. Micromechanical modeling of the epimysium of the skeletal muscles. Biomechanics. 2008;**41**:1-10. DOI: 10.1016/j.jbiomech.2007.08.008. Epub 2007 Sep 27

[48] Stecco C, Stern R, Porzionato A, et al. Hyaluronan within fascia in the etiology of myofascial pain. Surgical and Radiologic Anatomy. 2011;**33**:891-896. DOI: 10.1007/s00276-011-0876-9. Epub 2011 Oct 2

[49] Cowman MK, Schmidt TA, Raghavan P, et al. Viscoelastic properties of hyaluronan in physiological conditions. F1000Research. 2015;**4**:622. DOI: 10.12688/f1000research.6885.1. eCollection 2015

[50] Głowacki A, Olczyk K, Sonecki P, et al. Glycosaminoglycans of normal and scarred fascia. Acta Biochimica Polonica. 1994;**41**:166-169

[51] Turrina A, Martínez-González MA, Stecco C. The muscular force transmission system: Role of the intramuscular connective tissue. Journal of Bodywork and Movement Therapies. 2013;**17**:95-102. DOI: 10.1016/j. jbmt.2012.06.001

[52] Stecco C, Macchi V, Porzionato A, et al. The ankle retinacula: Morphological evidence of the proprioceptive role of

DOI: http://dx.doi.org/10.5772/intechopen.102024

the fascial system. Cells, Tissues, Organs.
2010;**192**:200-210. DOI: 10.1159/
000290225. Epub 2010 Feb 27

[53] Huijing PA, Baan GC. Myofascial
force transmission causes interaction
between adjacent muscles and connective
tissue: Effects of blunt dissection and
compartmental fasciotomy on length
force characteristics of rat extensor
digitorum longus muscle. Archives
of Physiology and Biochemistry.
2001;**109**:97-109. DOI: 10.1076/
apab.109.2.97.4269